Living Low Carb

Living
Low
Carb

◆

Controlled-Carbohydrate Eating
for Long-Term Weight Loss

◆

Jonny Bowden, PhD, CNS
Foreword by Barry Sears, PhD

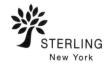

STERLING
New York

STERLING
New York

An Imprint of Sterling Publishing
387 Park Avenue South
New York, NY 10016

© 2013 by Jonny Bowden

First published by Sterling Publishing Co., Inc. © 2010 by Jonny Bowden

ISBN 978-1-4549-0351-2

Distributed in Canada by Sterling Publishing
c/o Canadian Manda Group, 165 Dufferin Street
Toronto, Ontario, Canada M6K 3H6
Distributed in the United Kingdom by GMC Distribution Services
Castle Place, 166 High Street, Lewes, East Sussex, England BN7 1XU
Distributed in Australia by Capricorn Link (Australia) Pty. Ltd.
P.O. Box 704, Windsor, NSW 2756, Australia

For information about custom editions, special sales, and premium and corporate purchases,
please contact Sterling Special Sales at 800-805-5489 or specialsales@sterlingpublishing.com.

Manufactured in the United States of America

6 8 10 9 7 5

www.sterlingpublishing.com

The low-fat–high-carbohydrate diet, promulgated vigorously by the National Cholesterol Education Program, National Institutes of Health, and American Heart Association since the Lipid Research Clinics-Primary Prevention Program in 1984, and earlier by the US Department of Agriculture food pyramid, may well have played an unintended role in the current epidemics of obesity, lipid abnormalities, type 2 diabetes, and metabolic syndromes.

This diet can no longer be defended by appeal to the authority of prestigious medical organizations or by rejecting clinical experience and a growing medical literature suggesting that the much-maligned low-carbohydrate–high-protein diet may have a salutary effect on the epidemics in question.

—"The Diet-Heart Hypothesis: A Critique"
S. L. Weinberg, *Journal of the American College of Cardiology* 43,
no. 5(March 3, 2004): 731–733.

"Never underestimate the convictions of the conventional, particularly in medicine."

—William Davis, MD

Contents

Foreword

There are three things in life that induce powerful visceral responses—religion, politics, and nutrition. Each is based on assumptions, and the adherents of each want to believe in their hearts that they are right; and of course they refuse to be confused by the facts. In the world of nutrition, nothing has generated as much heartburn as lower-carbohydrate diets. To the nutrition establishment, they are the equivalent of devil worship. To the medical establishment, they will cause massive increases in chronic disease and death. But to the millions of people who have used them, they seem to work. Obviously, there appears to be a disconnect between reality and fantasy. Are lower-carbohydrate diets actually safe? And what really is a lower-carbohydrate diet? Is a lower-carbohydrate diet the same as a high-fat or high-protein diet? Are there any magical supplements that can make you lose excess body fat? Into this quagmire of controversy steps Jonny Bowden.

I first met Jonny nearly 13 years ago. I had just written my first book, *The Zone*, and I was speaking about it in New York City. At the time, Jonny was a very well-recognized nutritionist working with a wide variety of clients ranging from those seeking weight loss to fitness enthusiasts. Like any typical New Yorker, he was skeptical of anything new, especially when it concerned diets. His skepticism was on especially high alert since my book not only recommended lower-carbohydrate diets for patients with diabetes and heart disease, but also for world-class athletes. After all, he had been training athletes for years using high-carbohydrate diets, and here was some pointy-head scientist telling him that all of his nutritional advice for athletes was wrong. Needless to say, he was ready to rake me over the coals. That is, until he heard my lecture. For the first time, he was introduced to the nuances of hormonal control theory using food as a drug. Although there was a lot of endocrinology (the science of hormones) being thrown around in the lecture, there were enough key points that Jonny had to take notice. After the lecture, he asked if we could talk. And for the next 2 hours, I went into more detail (probably more than he ever wanted to know) on the intricate dance of hormones that are controlled by the diet. Jonny then asked me, "If you are right about this, then everyone in nutrition is probably wrong." My reply was "Yes."

While Jonny was intrigued, he still remained skeptical. Jonny was also trained as an academic with a background in psychology and statistics, which guaranteed that any references I gave him on lower-carbohydrate diets (there wasn't much) as well as the science behind them (of which there was a lot) would be read and analyzed to the nth degree. As a result, he has not only become exceptionally knowledgeable about the nutritional science behind lower-carbohydrate diets, but he has also become my friend.

It's been many years since that first meeting with Jonny. The science dealing with the molecular biology of obesity has become more complex, but the basic concept remains: if you lower the carbohydrate content of the diet, you get better weight loss and better health. The trick is doing it for a lifetime.

I have always considered Jonny to be one of the better science writers I have ever met. That's why this book is so important for the general public. He lays out the history of lower-carbohydrate diets, explains in clear and concise language the underlying hormonal principles of such diets, and addresses the common misunderstandings of such diets, all in an entertaining and lively style.

As Jonny correctly points out, there is no one correct diet for everyone, since we are all genetically different. However, the hormonal principles are invariant for choosing an appropriate diet for your genetics. Once you understand the hormonal rules that govern lower-carbohydrate diets, you are in a position to become the master of your future. This book should be considered the starting point of that journey.

—Barry Sears, PhD
Author of *The Zone*
March 2009

Acknowledgments

Two sets of thanks here.

First . . . to my personal "brain trust" who gave so generously of their time.

Stacey J. Bell, PhD; Suzanne Bennett, DC; C. Leigh Broadhurst, PhD; Colette Heimowitz, MSc; Mary Enig, PhD; Joseph Evans, PhD; Oz Garcia, PhD; John Hernandez, MD; Malcolm Kendrick, MD; Ann Louise Gittleman, PhD, CNS; Mark Houston, MD, MS; Susan Lark, MD; David Leonardi, MD; Shari Lieberman, PhD, CNS; Linda Lizotte, RD; Lyle McDonald; Joe Mercola, DO; Liz Neporent, MS; Harry Preuss, MD; Uffe Ravnskov, MD, PhD; Donald S Robertson, MD, MSc; Ron Rosedale, MD; Alan Schwartz, MD; Diana Schwarzbein, MD; Barry Sears, PhD; Stephen Sinatra, MD; Allan Spreen, MD; Anton Steiner, MD; Jeff S Volek, PhD, RD. If this book is good, it's largely because of their stunning knowledge base.

And a really special "general principles" thanks to Robert Crayhon, MS and Jeffrey Bland, PhD, who have spent their professional lives making a difference by educating physicians, nutritionists, chiropractors and other health practitioners, challenging their boundaries and expanding their horizons. They certainly did mine.

The second part of this acknowledgments section is for the people who mean the most to me—the special people in my life without whom I might have still written books, but without whom I would not be who I am.

So to my family, chosen and otherwise: my brother Jeffrey, my sister-in-law Nancy, my nephew Pace, and my niece Cadence. And my LA family: Sky, Doug, Bootsie, Zack, Lukie, and Sage; my "person" and beloved friend Anja Christy; my brother from another mother Peter Breger; my lifelong friends Jeannette Lee Bessinger, Liz Neporent, Randy Graff, Janet Aldrich, Lauree Dash, Glen and Dawn Depke, Scott Ellis, Ketura Worthen, Diana Lederman, Kevin Hogan, Gina Lombardi, Kimberly Wright, Jerry White, Ann Knight, Amber Linder, Chad Ellingworth, Sue Wood, and Christopher Duncan.

And to Sky London again, just for good measure.

As always, to Howard, Robin, Fred, Gary, and Artie for putting a smile on my face for nearly 14 years.

To Werner Erhard—wherever you are, I love you and can never begin to repay you for what you've contributed to my life.

To the writers who taught me everything I know about writing, especially William Goldman (who could make the tax code interesting) and Robert Sapolsky, the greatest living science writer in America.

And a warm thanks to my first agent, Linda Konner, who put me on the map.

And to my current (and future) agent, Coleen O'Shea, who keeps me there.

And to the first editor of this book, Susan Lauzau, who had the patience to allow me to rant and rave about every comma change, most of which she was right about anyway.

And to the editor of the new expanded edition, Kate Zimmermann—ditto!

And especially to Michael Fragnito, who had the vision to imagine this book, the editorial skills to shape it, and an unfettered belief in me that allowed me to do my best work.

And to my mother, Vivienne Simon Bowden.

And to Michelle. Always, and forever.

Introduction

The Biggest Nutritional Experiment in History

The high-carbohydrate, low-fat diet has been the longest uncontrolled nutritional experiment in history.

The results have not been good.

Perhaps you've noticed.

Perhaps you have been one of its victims. You're unable to lose weight—or, if you have lost, it certainly hasn't been easy. You found yourself constantly fighting cravings, you were hungry a lot of the time, and you suffered with feelings of deprivation. You felt fatigued, like you were running on empty, and were still always battling the bulge, mostly unsuccessfully.

Maybe, like a lot of low-fat, high-carbohydrate dieters, you've noticed that your hair is dry, your nails brittle, your energy low, and your vitality sapped. And guess what? For all that, the weight *still* doesn't come off—or, if it does, it comes back on with a vengeance and you're right back where you started, except this time you feel even more discouraged.

Or maybe you're lucky enough to have never been on this delightful seesaw that I'm describing. Maybe you're just curious about all the fuss that's being made over low-carb diets and you want to learn more about how they work. Maybe you're thinking that you could stand to knock off a few pounds and are interested in low-carb dieting but don't know where to start. Or maybe you're already convinced that low-carb diets are for you but are concerned about some of the health implications that well-meaning people have warned you about.

Well, you've come to the right place.

Living Low Carb will help you understand three things:

1. What low-carb diets actually do to and for your body, and how they do it
2. Why some programs work for some people (and don't for others)
3. How you can adapt what you discover in this book to your own lifestyle

While I'd love to think that everyone who reads this book will devour it from cover to cover for its scintillating content and wealth of information, realistically I know that, with the possible exception of my girlfriend and my mother, few people will actually approach it that way. So I have designed *Living Low Carb* to be used like the I Ching: open it anywhere, and it will—hopefully—give you information you want.

I imagine that some of you will be interested in understanding more about the different popular diet plans, how they work, how they differ from one another, and what they offer. You guys should go straight for chapter 9, "Twenty-three Modern Low-Carb Diets and What They Can Do for You," find the plan or plans you are interested in, and read about them. You may find that reading further will spark some questions, which you're likely to get answered in chapter 10, "Frequently Asked Questions." Maybe, as you dig deeper into the book, you'll find yourself wanting to know more about the hormonal mechanisms in the body that drive weight gain and weight loss; you will find those issues addressed in chapter 3, "Why Low-Carb Diets Work," as well as the all-new chapter 4, "The Major Culprits in a High-Carb Diet: Wheat and Fructose."

Some of you may have already been on one of the plans discussed in chapter 9 but want more in-depth information about the questions, concerns, and controversies you have been hearing about—for example, cholesterol or ketosis or bone loss or kidney problems. You might head straight for chapter 6, "The Biggest Myths about Low-Carb Diets." When you get those concerns addressed, you may want to go back to chapters 3 and 4 to read more about the science behind low-carb eating and how it actually does its good work in the body.

The permutations are endless.

I also expect that there will be some dyed-in-the-wool low-carbers who have already experienced myriad health benefits, including weight loss, and simply want some tips for staying motivated, not getting bored, finding new things to eat, or breaking plateaus. All that information will be found in chapter 10, "Frequently Asked Questions," and chapter 11, "Tricks of the Trade: The Top 50+ Tips for Making Low-Carb Work for You."

Because I have designed this book to be extremely user-friendly and because I want you to be able to skip around as you like, some of the information and issues will be discussed in more than one place. For example, the subject of ketosis, which used to be so central to the Atkins diet and has been such a focus of criticism from the establishment (and which has caused such misunderstanding in the media), is discussed in three places. You will get a brief overview of ketosis in chapter 3, "Why Low Carb Diets Work"; but a much more in-depth discussion, which answers the criticisms leveled at ketogenic diets, appears in chapter 6, "The Biggest Myths about Low-Carb Diets." You will also find an abbreviated discussion of ketosis in chapter 10, "Frequently Asked Questions," since ketosis is definitely one of the topics about which I get the most questions when it comes to low-carb dieting.

Enjoy!

CHAPTER 1

Low-Carb Redux: The Updated Truth about Low-Carbohydrate Diets

"Low-carb diets are dangerous!" "All that meat can't possibly be good for you!"

"What about the China Study?" "You can't cut out an entire food group!"

"You need carbs for energy!" "I tried that Atkins diet once and it didn't work!"

"You lose weight on low-carb but then you gain it all back!" "Isn't low-carb bad for the heart?"

Sound familiar?

Low-carb eating continues to be one of the most misunderstood dietary strategies on the planet. Despite the fact that some form of low-carb dieting has been around since 1850, despite the enormous popularity of the Atkins diet, and despite mounting research implicating sugar and high-carb foods as instrumental catalysts to just about every major disease, the myths about low-carb diets simply behave like a Buddy Holly lyric and "won't fade away."

Maybe it's time to take a fresh look at low-carb diets and see if we can separate myth from reality.

Back in 2004, it seemed low-carb diets were at the top of the popularity charts. The Atkins diet—long a "fan favorite" but widely panned as "dangerous" by the medical establishment—had just been shown to produce more weight loss than either a low-fat diet or a Mediterranean diet in two studies published in the prestigious Annals of Internal Medicine.[1] Several other studies published around the same time confirmed these results and went even further, showing that the weight loss produced by low-carb dieting was not accompanied by any increase in the risk for heart disease. Quite the contrary—many of the studies showed improvements in triglycerides, no significant change in cholesterol, improved body composition, and significant improvements in risk factors for diabetes.

Low-carb was on a roll. Programs like *Protein Power, the Zone,* and *the South Beach Diet* were at the top of the diet book charts, Atkins was back in fashion, low-carb groceries were springing up, and even mainstream supermarkets began featuring low-carb sections (right along with their low-sodium and low-fat departments).

And then . . . it fizzled.

Or at least low-carb's status as a *media darling* fizzled. Low-carb continues to be used successfully as both a weight-loss strategy and as a dietary plan for overall health by millions of people. It's effective, safe, and has enormous health benefits that are obscured or played down by hopelessly out-of-date organizations like the American Dietetic Association. But make no mistake—low-carb is alive and well, and if you've been one of the folks who's dismissed it, it might be time to take a second look.

For years, low-carb suffered from bad publicity. Atkins—a superb nutritionist and very smart guy—couldn't shake the stigma of having "recommended" eating pork rinds (What he *actually* said was that pork rinds were probably better for you than sugar! And he was right.) People who didn't know any better also thought his diet forbade all carbohydrates, which it most certainly doesn't.

Then there was the ketosis confusion. Ketosis—a harmless metabolic state that the body goes into when carbohydrate intake is *very* low—became identified with low-carb diets largely because early editions of Atkins's books stressed ketosis as a desirable goal for the first stage of the Atkins diet (which limited carbs to 20 grams a day).

But very few—if any—low-carb diets put the body into ketosis.

The low-carb "movement" itself didn't help matters. Its supporters began to treat low-carb as something of a religion, becoming more focused on carb content than on the importance of good food. And many people forgot about the overarching, important message of controlled-carb eating—controlling blood sugar and eating whole foods—and instead replaced that message with a simple (and inaccurate) sound bite: *carbs are bad.*

This led to an explosion of junk-food products that engineered out the carbs but were still junk food (echoes of the low-fat movement of the '80s and early '90s—remember Snackwell cookies?). Junky low-carb processed foods now filled the shelves of the low-carb groceries and were also the reason those groceries are now out of business—they tasted terrible.

But that was then and this is now. A more twenty-first century controlled-carb approach requires more nuance.

First, we need some definitions. How exactly do we define low-carb, anyway?

What Exactly Is a Low-Carb Diet?

The American Dietetic Association designates "low-carbohydrate diets" as less than 130 grams a day (or 26% of calories from a 2,000-calorie diet). Though I hardly think this is "low," it seems to be a decent working definition, given that most Americans consume a whopping 300 grams of carbs a day! (Just for the record, carbohydrate consumption before the current obesity epidemic averaged 43% of daily calories, just about what is recommended by Dr. Sears in *The Zone.*)

According to Richard Feinman, PhD, professor of biochemistry at SUNY Downstate Medical Center and head of the Nutrition and Metabolism Society (of which I am a proud member), 26%–45% of calories from carbs is a good range for what we might call moderate- or controlled-carbohydrate eating, so let's use that as a working definition. According to Feinman, less than 30 grams a day should be referred to as a "very low-carbohydrate ketogenic diet" and reserved for the therapeutic approach to childhood epilepsy, for which it works quite well. I don't quite agree that a diet with 30 grams or less of carbohydrate should be reserved just for the treatment of childhood epilepsy, since many people do quite well on ketogenic diets, and some people may be so metabolically resistant that they need that level of carb restriction in order to lose weight.

Some low-carb diets for weight loss limit carbs to 20–30 grams a day, especially for the first couple of weeks, and then add them back gradually. But many health professionals and weight-loss experts believe that you can get most of the benefits of controlled-carb eating and still consume up to

100 grams a day (or even, in some cases, a bit more). And a copious amount of research—much of it in the last decade—supports the notion that even a *modest* reduction in carb intake is enough to stabilize blood sugar, reduce insulin, and, in the long run, facilitate weight loss.

Low-Carb Doesn't Have to Be Extreme to Work!

Low-carb diets don't have to be extreme to be effective, a concept that's been demonstrated many times. Take, for example, a study that was recently presented at the 91st Annual Meeting of the Endocrine Society in Washington, D.C.

The researchers gave one group of subjects a "standard" diet of about 55% carbohydrates, 18% protein, and 27% fat. A second group was given a diet of 43% carbs, 18% protein, and 39% fat. The number of calories consumed by both groups was identical, and the calorie level was set at just the amount needed to maintain weight.

The results showed that even when weight loss was not the goal, the group eating slightly *lower* amounts of carbs (Group Two) stayed full longer and reported being more satisfied. They also had healthier blood-sugar levels *and* lower levels of insulin, the fat-storage hormone.

Commenting on the study, lead researcher Barbara Gower, PhD, said, "Over the long run, a *sustained modest reduction in carbohydrate intake* may help to reduce [calorie consumption] and facilitate weight loss."[2]

Will Low-Carb Diets Harm Your Heart?

There isn't too much controversy anymore about the effectiveness of controlled-carbohydrate eating for weight loss, especially in the short term. The area of controversy concerns the question "At what cost?" Conventional wisdom—which is turning out to be far from wise on this subject—has held that only low-fat diets are effective for lowering the risk of heart disease, and even today, many conventional doctors recommend low-fat diets for diabetes, though emerging science suggests that this is precisely the wrong strategy.

Let's go to the videotape. An examination of data from the Nurses' Health Study involving over 85,000 women found that those consuming diets with the highest glycemic load (sugar, white rice, potatoes, low-fiber bread, and processed carbs) had a significantly higher risk of diabetes—

more than *twice* the risk of those consuming low-glycemic diets (fat, protein, vegetables, beans, fruits). Moreover, the women consuming diets rich in vegetable protein and fat had a modest *reduction* in the risk of diabetes.[3]

In a separate analysis, it was found that women in the study eating a low-carb diet with *higher* intake of animal fat and protein had a 6% *reduced* risk of cardiovascular disease! Considering that conventional wisdom would predict that the women eating the most animal fat and protein and the least carbs would have a vastly *higher* risk of heart disease, these results are pretty astonishing. When the researchers looked at women consuming a low-carb diet with higher rates of vegetable protein and fat, the reduction in risk went even higher, to a whopping 30%.[4]

Low-glycemic (low-carb) diets were also found to reduce the number of acne lesions.[5] They've been found to benefit women with polycystic ovary syndrome.[6] Low-carb diets were found to raise HDL ("good" cholesterol) by 10%.[7] And at least two different studies have shown that low-glycemic diets lower the risk for age-related macular degeneration.[8]

Add fiber to a low-carb diet, and your results are even better. In one study, researchers put 30 overweight or obese males on a carb-restricted diet. Half the subjects also got a soluble fiber supplement as well. The carb-restricted diet reduced body weight, percentage of body fat, systolic blood pressure, triglycerides, and waist circumference. Those consuming the fiber supplement along with their low-carb diet had a 14% reduction in LDL ("bad" cholesterol) *as well* as all the aforementioned benefits.[9]

The A–Z Diet Study: Atkins Wins, but the Good Part Was Left Out!

Back in March 2007, it seemed you couldn't swing a bat without seeing a headline proclaiming that the Atkins diet was finally vindicated. "Atkins beats Zone, Ornish, and U.S. diet advice," proclaimed CNN. "Atkins Diet Tops Others in Study," said the Washington Post.

Good news for low-carb diets, but as usual, the headlines did not tell the whole story.

First, some background. Researchers at Stanford University[10] took 311 premenopausal women, all of them overweight or obese, and assigned them to four diet groups: Atkins, Ornish, the Zone, and the LEARN plan, a conventional eating program based on US dietary guidelines. "We wanted a range of diets, from high-carbohydrate to low," explained lead researcher Christopher Gardner, PhD.[11] The Atkins diet is famously low in carbohydrates (and can be high in either fat, protein, or both), the Ornish diet is extremely low in fat (about 10% of intake), and the Zone is right in the middle (technically 40% of the diet comes from carbs and 30% each from protein and fat). The LEARN diet is based on conventional recommendations of about 55–65% carbs and less than 10% saturated fat.

The researchers were interested primarily in weight loss, though other measures were taken as well (more on that in a moment). "In the weight-loss department, there was a modest advantage for the Atkins group," Dr. Gardner told me. Those in the Atkins group lost the most amount of weight (10 pounds on average).

But there were some problems. For one thing, the women in the study were far from meticulous about following the dietary regimen to which they were assigned. While the women in the Atkins group were aiming for between 20–50 grams of carbohydrate a day, by the end of the study they were eating well over 125 grams. The Ornish group, aiming for 10% fat, was eating almost 30%. Zone dieters shooting for 30% protein wound up eating 20%, and even the women attempting to follow the conventional LEARN diet had reduced their carbs to just over 47%. Critics—including the designers of the diets that bore their names—complained loudly that the study results were not valid because the diet strategies under investigation had not been followed to the letter.

Actually, this is the good part.

In real life, people rarely follow diets exactly as they're laid out in the diet books. So it's hardly a surprise that the folks in the Atkins group didn't achieve the target of 20–50 grams of carbs a day. What's worth noting—and what the media largely missed—is that merely *attempting* to reduce carbs resulted in vast improvements in weight and overall health. The folks in the study may have been aiming for 20–50 grams, but the 125 grams they wound up consuming was still well within the definition of low-carb, represented a huge reduction from their baseline consumption, and wound up giving them terrific results.

"So what we're seeing here in terms of deviation from the exact principles of each diet is a very real-world scenario," said Dr. Gardner. "It's what happens when even motivated people follow diet books. We think that's extremely relevant."

He has a great point. While the women may not have followed the diets to the letter, they *did* make changes in some important areas according to the principles of the respective plans. For example, the Atkins women had started the program consuming about 215 grams of carbohydrate a day (about 45% of their diet). By the end of the 12 months, they were down to about 34%. That's a big deal. At the end of the day they were eating a higher percentage of carbs than they were aiming for, sure, but they had *still* managed to reduce their carb intake substantially compared to where they started out. They may not have achieved perfection, but they did achieve results, and those results shouldn't be overlooked simply because the women didn't follow the diets perfectly. After all, who can?

It's worth mentioning that the women in the Atkins group also improved some of their risk factors. The HDL ("good") cholesterol at 12 months was *significantly* higher for the Atkins group than for the group on the low-fat Ornish diet, and triglycerides for the Atkins group went down by 29%, more than twice the percentage of any other group. The decrease in average blood pressure for the Atkins group was significantly greater than any other. The effect on LDL ("bad") cholesterol, the type that many health professionals warned would worsen on the Atkins diet, was the same among all of the diet groups after 12 months. These are important findings, particularly in view of the negative press low-carbohydrate diets have gotten for their supposed bad effects on cardio-vascular health. In this study, at least in the short term, the opposite appeared to be the case.

So what's the takeaway? "I think one advantage that the Atkins diet had was the simplicity of the message," Dr. Gardner told me. "A lot of people say that the main Atkins message is to eat all the steak and brie that you want, but that's not it. The main message is this: you can't have any refined sugar. None. No soda, no white bread, no high-fructose corn syrup. It's simple and direct and easy to understand and I think it may turn out to be one of the most important messages of all."

Matching the Diet to the Person

Further analysis of the data from the A–Z diet study revealed something even more important. While the low-carb approach worked well for every-one, it worked spectacularly well for a subgroup in the population with a condition known as "insulin resistance." Briefly, these are folks who don't process carbs very well to begin with. When they do eat carbs—particularly grains, rice, cereal, bread, and sugar—their blood sugar goes up way more than it should; in response to that increased blood sugar, their pancreas secretes more insulin than is healthy, and they have a fiendishly difficult time losing weight. They are also at high risk for diabetes.

When Gardner analyzed the effects of the Atkins diet on this subgroup of people, he found the results were even more impressive than they were in the population as a whole (more weight loss and even better blood tests).

The idea that low-carb diets are even more effective for those with metabolic conditions like insulin resistance was given another boost by a study involving 73 obese young adults (18–35). Half of the subjects were given a low-glycemic diet similar to the Zone (in this case, 40% carbs, 35% fat, 25% protein) and half were given a standard low-fat diet (55% carbs, 20% fat). Among those subjects whose bodies released the "normal" amount of insulin in response to food, the diets had an equally beneficial effect, but in those who had high levels of insulin secretion to begin with (insulin resistance), the low-carb diet was the much better performer, resulting in greater weight loss and reduction in body-fat percentage.[12] The researchers speculate that many of these diet studies produce different results for one simple reason: *individual differences*. Those with "high" insulin secretion do much better on low-carb diets than on low-fat ones, a finding exactly in accordance with what Gardner found in the A–Z diet study.

What about Deprivation?

Low-carb diets are always trashed in the mainstream media for being "restrictive" and leading to feelings of "deprivation," but the research—not to mention the daily experience of countless people—indicates the exact opposite. In one study involving 28 premenopausal overweight women, sticking to a low-carb/high-protein diet not only reduced these folks' body weight more than a high-carb/low-fat diet; it also reduced hunger.[13] The self-ratings of hunger for those on the low-carb diet went down over the course of the study, whereas hunger self-ratings remained essentially unchanged among the women eating high-carb/low-fat. It's always easier to stay on an eating plan if you're not starving, so this is an important consideration!

A separate study found that men and women put on a low-carb diet wound up consuming about ⅓ fewer calories without any special instructions to do so. In fact, these folks were told to limit their carbohydrates to a very low 21 grams per day (about the amount in the rigorous first stage of the Atkins diet) but were allowed to eat as much protein and fat as they wanted—they were even allowed limited amounts of cheese and cream cheese. Their insulin sensitivity improved by an incredible 75%, they lost weight, and they weren't hungry. Now there's a dietary trifecta![14]

What about Vegans?

Up until recently, conventional wisdom held that it's next to impossible to do a low-carb diet if you're a vegetarian or vegan. Once again, conventional wisdom turns out to be wrong, at least according to a study in the prestigious Archives of Internal Medicine, which investigated a diet they affectionately named "Eco-Atkins."[15]

The researchers wanted to see if they could design a low-carbohydrate diet that retained the proven weight-loss benefits of standard low-carb plans like Atkins but at the same time helped people improve their cholesterol.

The researchers put one group of participants on a vegan diet which met their definition of low-carb and high-protein. The diet contained not a single animal product or by-product, including eggs.

Protein (31% of total calories) came mainly from gluten, soy, and nuts, with typical foods being soy burgers, veggie bacon, and breakfast links. Most of the fat (43% of total calories) came from nuts, vegetable oils, soy products, and avocado. The rest of the calories on this vegan low-carb diet were carbohydrates (26% of total calories), mostly from fruits and vegetables and some cereals—common starchy items like bread, rice, potatoes, and baked goods were eliminated.

The researchers tested the Eco-Atkins diet against a standard low-fat lacto-vegetarian diet, which contained 58% of calories from carbs, 16% from protein, and 25% from fat and was designed to have both low saturated fat and low cholesterol; most of the protein on the "standard" diet came from low-fat or skim milk dairy products and egg whites. Both diets were calorie reduced (60% of estimated caloric requirement, with allowance for exercise). All subjects in both groups were overweight at the start of the study, which lasted one month.

Both groups lost weight, not surprising given the reduction in calories on both diets. And there were no significant differences between the two groups in weight loss—both groups lost about 4 kg (8.8 pounds), roughly the same amount of weight as would be expected on a more traditional low-carbohydrate Atkins diet. But there were some important differences between the two groups when it came to cholesterol.

The Eco-Atkins group saw their LDL-cholesterol (the so-called "bad" cholesterol) drop *significantly* more than the group on the low-fat vegetarian diet. As an added benefit, ApoB—a component of LDL that is related to heart disease—fell significantly more for the low-carb dieters than it did for the high-carbers.

Now you might easily argue that the Eco-Atkins diet—with its 130 grams of carbs a day—is very far from what we traditionally think of as a low-carb diet. And you might also argue that lowering cholesterol might not be nearly as important as the conventional medical establishment thinks it is (a position taken by myself and many other experts). But, that said, this is a really valuable piece of research, and here's why:

It's been a long, uphill, and sometimes discouraging battle to get the conventional medical community to accept low-carb in any form. Fixated on cholesterol, they worry that conventional low-carb diets don't lower cholesterol (ignoring the fact that these same diets have been shown to not only produce weight loss, but also lower triglycerides and insulin resistance). And—not without some justification—many conventional docs continue to be worried about overconsumption of meat. So here's a legitimate study in one of the most prestigious and conservative journals that demonstrates that low-carb can be adapted to even the rigorous vegan eating pattern, producing not only the expected weight loss, lowered insulin resistance, and lowered triglycerides, but lowered cholesterol *as well*. This study convincingly showed that a low-carb diet performed *better* than the low-fat vegetarian diets so many of these docs seem to adore! The results went a long way toward reassuring conventional docs that low-carb is a viable alternative to standard recommendations of low-fat/high carb diets, and can even "outperform" such diets on a number of variables.

Summing Up

Remember: as hard as it is to believe, your body has no physiological requirement for carbohydrate—astonishing, but 100% true.[16] That's not to say you shouldn't eat carbs—you should!

But if you're looking to lose weight and improve your health, you should get the vast majority of them from vegetables and fruits and beans, not from pasta, rice, bread, baked goods, cereal, and sugar-laden desserts.

Carbs from fruits and vegetables are loaded with vitamins, minerals, phytochemicals, fiber, and other good stuff that your body thrives on. And you can eat more vegetables and berries than you can imagine and still stay in the range of 100–130 grams of carbs a day!

Add to that about 100–120 grams of protein and about 60 grams of fat, and you've got a blueprint for health and weight management that will work for just about anyone.

CHAPTER 2

The History and Origins of Low-Carb Diets

*T*he first bona fide low-carb diet book came out in 1864, and it happened only because William Banting thought he was going deaf.

Banting was a prosperous London undertaker of sixty-six who was so overweight that he couldn't tie his own shoelaces. At 5 feet 5 inches in his stocking feet, he weighed in at 202 pounds and was so fat that he had to walk downstairs backward. On top of that, his eyesight was failing and he was having problems with his hearing. In August 1862, Banting took himself to an ear, nose, and throat surgeon named Dr. William Harvey, who examined him and promptly decided that Banting's problem wasn't deafness; it was obesity. His fat was pressing on his inner ear.

Here's what Banting was eating: "bread and milk for breakfast, *or* a pint of tea, with plenty of milk and sugar, and buttered toast; meat, beer, and much bread and pastry for dinner; more bread and milk at tea time; and a fruit tart *or* bread and milk for dinner."

Harvey promptly put Banting on a diet, and by December 1862, Banting had lost 18 pounds. By August 1863, he was down to 156 pounds. In a little less than a year, he had dropped almost 50 pounds and 12½ inches from his waistline. Banting also reported feeling better than he had at any time in the previous 26 years. His sight and hearing were normal for his age, and his other bodily ailments had become "mere matters of history."

Here's what he ate on the new plan.

Breakfast (9 A.M.): 5 or 6 ounces of either beef, mutton, kidneys, broiled fish, bacon, or cold meat of any kind except pork or veal.

A small biscuit or an ounce of dry toast. Large cup of tea or coffee without milk or sugar.

Dinner (2 P.M.): 5 or 6 ounces of fish, poultry, game, or meat, and any vegetable except potatoes, parsnips, beets, turnips, or carrots. An ounce of dry toast. Fruit. Two or three glasses of good claret, sherry, or Madeira (no champagne, port, or beer).

Tea (6 P.M.): 2 or 3 ounces of fruit. Toast and tea with no milk or sugar.

Supper (9 P.M.): 3 or 4 ounces of meat or fish as for dinner. A glass or two of claret or sherry.

Nightcap (if required): a tumbler of gin, whisky, or brandy with water but no sugar, or a glass or two of claret or sherry.

The man did like to drink.

Here's what he did *not* eat: milk, sugar, beer, potatoes, or pastry. And what he ate *way* less of: bread (3 ounces total, about a slice).

The calorie as a measurement was unknown at that time, but we know now that Banting was eating about 2,800 calories a day—not exactly a low-calorie diet. Banting may not have known much about the science and chemistry of food and weight, but he knew enough to observe that the *amount* of food he was eating didn't seem to be the determining factor in his weight loss. In Banting's words, "I can now confidently say that *quantity* of diet may be safely left to the natural appetite; and that it is the *quality* only which is essential to abate and cure corpulence."

In other words: it's *what* you eat, not how much, an idea that even then flew in the face of conventional wisdom. (It's worth noting that Banting was not completely right—as it turns out, it's *both* what you eat *and* how much. But he opened the door to the discussion that *quality* mattered as much as quantity, and that was a significant change from conventional thinking. Still is.)

Banting became a man on a mission. Excited and inspired by his results on this high-calorie, low-carbohydrate diet—which was made up almost entirely of protein, fat, alcohol, and what was then called "roughage"—he published, at his own expense, the first commercial low-carb diet book, *Letter on Corpulence.*[1]

Banting identified sugar as the main cause of his own obesity, and his physician, Dr. Harvey, promptly put both flour and sugar on the forbidden list.

It worked.

The book eventually went into 4 editions, with the first 3 selling 63,000 copies in England alone, and it was translated into French and German and sold heavily in those countries, as well as in the United States. The fourth edition included letters of testimony from at least 1,800 readers who had written to Banting to support his assertions and praise the diet.

Once I did some reading, I realized that low-carb diets aren't brand new—they've been advocated by some forward-thinking scientists for more than a century.

—Gary S.

Banting, by the way, kept the weight off and lived comfortably until the age of 81.

With Banting's book, the nascent debate—is it *what* you eat or *how much* you eat that makes you fat?—was born, and it continues, alive and kicking, to this day. But the controversy didn't gather its full steam until Wilbur Atwater figured out how to measure calories.

It's the Calories, Stupid! The Dominating Hypothesis in Weight Loss Is Born

Sometime between 1890 and 1900, an agricultural chemist named Wilbur O. Atwater got the bright idea that if you stuck some food in a mini-oven called a calorimeter and burned the food to ash, you could *measure* the amount of heat it produced. He called the unit of measurement a calorie (technically, the amount of heat it takes to raise the temperature of 1 gram of water from 14.5 to 15.5 degrees centigrade). He went to town. He constructed vast tables of the caloric content of various foods. (It's important to remember that calories are not actually found *in* food; they're a measure of how much heat or energy can be *produced* by food.) The idea that the human body behaves exactly like the chamber used in Atwater's experiments—that we all "burn" calories exactly the same way and our bodies behave like calorimeters—has been the dominating hypothesis in weight loss to this day.

And man, is it wrong. (More coming—stay tuned.)

Later, some enterprising scientists extended the calorie theory even further. They began to measure how much heat was produced (read: how many calories were "burned") in the course of daily activities, from resting to vigorous exercise, from sleeping to digesting food to running marathons.

It was now possible to form an equation: calories in versus calories out. The guiding concept of weight management was officially born.

That theory is called the *energy balance theory*, and it goes something like this: if you take in more calories than you burn up, you'll gain weight. If you burn up more calories than you take in, you'll lose weight. It doesn't matter where those calories come from. It's as simple as balancing a checkbook: spend more than you make, and you're calorically in the red (and dipping into your fat stores to make up the difference); make more than you spend, and you're in the black (and buying bigger jeans).

It was the first law of thermodynamics in action. What goes in must either come out in some other form (like heat) or stay in (in the form of fat or muscle). What it *can't* do is simply disappear.

Yet Banting, unscientific though he was, had made an interesting observation, which was that *what* he ate made more of a difference to his fat cells than *how much* he ate. This notion was heresy to the calorie theorists who believed, to paraphrase Gertrude Stein, that a calorie is a calorie is a calorie. It wasn't until much later that the idea surfaced that calories from certain kinds of food (or combinations of food) might have a greater tendency to be stored in the body than others, or that people might vary widely in their metabolic ability to "burn" calories as opposed to "saving" them, or that the type of food eaten might actually trigger bodily responses that say "stay" or "go."

Meanwhile, calorie-counting had taken off with a vengeance. In 1917 (the same year, coincidentally, in which the ultraconservative American Dietetic Association was founded), an LA physician named Dr. Lulu Hunt Peters published what had to be the first calorie-counting book ever, *Diet and Health, with Key to the Calories*. She sold 2 million books, making it the first best-selling diet book in America. And here's the thing: by making calorie-counting equivalent to weight control, she also injected her own view of morality into the equation. People who couldn't control their calories (and therefore their weight) just lacked self-discipline. We can thank Dr. Peters for popularizing the concept that being overweight is a sign of moral weakness. And the idea that people are fat simply because they lack self-control is still very much alive and well today—witness, for example, the recent work of Dr. Phil McGraw.[2]

Calories in/calories out remains the dominant view of most mainstream weight-loss experts to this day, and it is even embraced to a degree by some of the gurus of the low-carb movement, albeit not nearly to the same extent as the mainstreamers, who have made it a virtual religion. All of the low-carb theorists have to be seen against the backdrop of this calorie-counting orthodoxy. But throughout the twentieth century and into the twenty-first, observations have indeed been made—and experiments performed—that have cast huge doubts on whether the calories in/calories out theory was the whole story or even the most important part of the story. No one claims it is not *part* of the story—the argument is whether or not it is the *whole* story. Answer: It's not.

Eat and Grow Thin: Low-Carbing Reappears on the Scene

In 1914, Vance Thompson, a nonscientist and the husband of a famous actress of the day, published a book called *Eat and Grow Thin*,[3] which touted the virtues of a low-carb diet. It suggested that corpulence was caused by eating the wrong *kinds* of food, not merely the wrong amounts, and singled out "starches, sugars, and oils" as particular culprits—pretty much what you'd expect from a guy whose most famous saying was "To the scientist there is nothing so tragic on earth as the sight of a fat man eating a potato." His list of forbidden foods included the fattiest meats (like bacon); bread, biscuits, crackers, macaroni, and anything else made from the flour of wheat, corn, rye, barley, or oats, which included all breakfast foods and cereals; rice; potatoes, corn, dried beans, and lentils; milk, cream, butter, and cheese; oils and grease of any kind; pies, cakes, puddings, pastries, custards, ice cream, sodas, candies, bonbons, and sweets; and wines, beers, ales, and spirits.

One can only imagine how many times he was asked the question we hear so often today: so, *what's left to eat?*

As it turns out, a lot. According to Thompson, the only things that had really been taken away were sugar, starch, oil, and alcohol. The rest of his book consisted of menus that included:

- All kinds of meat (except pig in any form)
- All kinds of game
- All kinds of seafood—fish, lobsters, oysters, etc.
- All kinds of fruit (except bananas and grapes)
- All kinds of salad
- Virtually all vegetables

The low-carb gurus of today would have loved this, except they would have added some good fat to the mix.

The book also contained this little caveat: "Never, under any circumstances—even when you have reduced to the desired weight and have, to some degree, discontinued the diet—*eat potatoes, rice, white bread, macaroni, or sweets.*"

Calories were never once mentioned in Thompson's book, which went through 113 printings by 1931 and was still in circulation when a little problem arose at the DuPont company.

The Problem at the DuPont Company: The Work of Alfred Pennington, MD

DuPont executives were getting fat.

Really fat. No kidding.

Shortly after World War I, the medical department of E.I. DuPont, a large American chemical firm, became concerned about the growing obesity problem among the staff. The company hired Dr. Alfred Pennington and entrusted him with the job of finding out why the traditional low-calorie diets of the time were bombing when it came to losing weight. Pennington applied his considerable brain power to an analysis of the scientific literature and came to the conclusion that our old friend—the formerly fat undertaker William Banting—was right all along: obesity was due not to overeating, but instead to the body's inability to use carbohydrates for anything other than making fat.

Pennington put the DuPont executives on a high-fat, high-protein, low-carbohydrate, *unrestricted-calorie* diet. He limited their carb intake to 60 grams a day, allowed them at least 24 ounces of meat and fat (more if they wanted it), and restricted them to one portion a day of any one of the following: potatoes, rice, grapefruit, grapes, melon, bananas, pears, raspberries, or blueberries.

Pennington published a number of articles in prestigious journals such as *The New England Journal of Medicine*,[4] but he summed up his results with the fat executives best in an interview he gave to *Holiday Magazine*. I've added the italics for emphasis.

Of the twenty men and women taking part in the test, all lost weight on a diet in which the total calorie intake was unrestricted. The basic diet totaled about 3,000 calories per day, *but meat and fat*

in any desired amount were allowed those who wanted to eat still more.
The dieters reported that they felt well, enjoyed their meals and
were never hungry between meals. Many said they felt more energetic
than usual; none complained of fatigue. Those who had high
blood pressure to begin with [no longer did]. The[se] twenty
obese individuals lost an average of twenty-two pounds each, in an
average time of three and a half months. The *range of weight loss
was from nine pounds to fifty-four pounds,* and the range of time was
from about one and a half months to six months.[5]

Chalk up another one for the low-carb approach to weight loss.

Then, in 1928, something really interesting happened at the dietetic
ward of Bellevue Hospital in New York City. But to understand why it happened, you have to understand the experiences of a rugged young explorer
named Vilhjalmur Stefansson.

Stefansson and the Eskimos: All Meat, All Fat, All the Time

Kicked out of school at age 23 for inciting a protest within the student body,
Vilhjalmur Stefansson picked up the pieces of his life and entered the world
of his true love, anthropology. By 1906, at the age of 27, he had managed to
get a master's degree at Harvard, where he became an assistant professor of
anthropology and got really interested in the diets of other people. Not
much for city life, Stefansson dumped Harvard and decided that it would
be more fun to join the Anglo-American Polar Expedition, which was kicking off that year, and travel to the Arctic.

A couple of years after his first foray, he persuaded the American
Museum of Natural History in New York to give him the money to do it
again, and he departed on his second expedition in 1908; this time, he
stayed 4 years. He discovered a previously isolated group of natives called
the Copper Inuit (so named because they used copper tools), and he lived
with them for his entire stay. His third and final expedition began in 1913
and lasted for 5 years.

Later, he wrote: "In 1906 I went to the Arctic with the food tastes and
beliefs of the average American. By 1918, after eleven years as an Eskimo
among Eskimos, I had learned things which caused me to shed most of
those beliefs."[6]

One of the beliefs Stefansson took to the Arctic was the prevailing notion that the less meat you ate, the better off you'd be. The view then—as now—was that if you ate a lot of meat, you would develop, among other things, hardening of the arteries, high blood pressure, and, very likely, a breakdown of the kidneys.

But this is what he found: the Eskimos he lived with ate a diet that consisted almost exclusively of meat (or fish) and fat. And they were as healthy and robust as a bunch of wild horses. High blood pressure, coronary infarctions, and strokes were virtually unknown. The women rarely suffered with breast-feeding problems, complications in pregnancy, or difficult births. And prior to their contact with mainstream civilization, Eskimos seldom suffered from cancer. (Today, about a century after their contact with "civilization" and the modern diet, they routinely suffer from all of the above.)

Ever the anthropologist, Stefansson lived with an Eskimo family for much of his time in the Arctic and adopted all their eating habits. Though he had hated fish all his life, he ate it night and day. He ate it raw, baked, and boiled. He ate the heads and the tails. He even came to like the Eskimo delicacy of rotten fish, which he likened to his first taste of Camembert. It was the beginning of an aggregate of 5 years on a diet that consisted almost exclusively of protein, fat, and water.

> I've always found it easier to stay on a low-carb diet than on any other kind of diet. I just never feel as hungry so I don't really feel like I'm dieting."
>
> —Doug M.

According to the prevailing dietary wisdom of the times, he should've been dead.

He wasn't. And, by the way, he never gained weight. He also never saw a fat Eskimo.

He wrote:

> Eskimos, when still on their home meats, are never corpulent—at least, I have seen none who were. Eskimos in their native garments do give the impression of fat, round faces on fat, round bodies, but the roundness of face is a racial peculiarity and the rest of the effect is produced by loose and puffy garments. See them stripped, and one does not find the abdominal protuberances and folds which are so in evidence on Coney Island beaches and so persuasive an argument against nudism.[7]

The guy did have a sense of humor.

By the way, lest anyone think that Eskimos were somehow genetically or racially immune to getting fat, Stefansson was quick to point out how quickly they fattened up when they ate mainstream American or European diets. In other words, they stay nice and slim on a high-fat diet, but as soon as they start eating starch and sugar, guess what happens?

Stefansson was genuinely curious to see if this strange diet had produced any ill effects that he perhaps hadn't noticed. And there were plenty of doctors who were just as curious as he. A committee was convened, and Stefansson was put through as rigorous an examination as a potential astronaut would get today. The findings were published in *The Journal of the American Medical Association* on July 3, 1926, in an article titled "The Effects of an Exclusive Long-Continued Meat Diet." The result? The committee had failed to find even *one trace of evidence* of all the supposed harmful effects of the diet.

This brings us to the dietetic ward of Bellevue Hospital in 1928. Stefansson and Dr. Karsten Anderson, a colleague who had been on one of the expeditions with Stefansson, agreed to act as human guinea pigs in a two-person experiment. Stefansson had not only survived but thrived on a diet that was supposed to have killed him, but this experience had never really been verified under scientific conditions. So Stefansson and Anderson agreed to live in the dietetic ward of Bellevue Hospital under the strictest of medical supervision, eating an exclusive diet of meat, for a solid year. The aim of the project was not to "prove" something, but merely to get at the facts and answer the prevailing questions of the time: Would the men get scurvy? Would they suffer from other deficiency diseases? What would be the effect on the circulatory system? On calcium levels? On the kidneys? On their weight?

Lest anyone think this was a quaint little "experiment" supervised by a couple of country quacks, let's look at the committee assembled to supervise this dietetic experiment: from Harvard University, Dr. Lawrence Henderson, Dr. Ernest Hooton, and Dr. Percy Howe; from Cornell University Medical College, Dr. Walter Niles; from the American Museum of Natural History, Dr. Clark Wissler; from Johns Hopkins University, Dr. William McCallum and Dr. Raymond Pearl; from the Russell Sage Institute of Pathology, Dr. Eugene DuBois and Dr. Graham Lusk; from the University of Chicago, Dr. Edwin O. Jordan; from the Institute of American Meat Packers, Dr. C. Robert Moulton; and a physician in private practice, Dr. Clarence W. Lieb.

Not exactly "The Gang That Couldn't Shoot Straight."

This is how the experiment went: For the first 3 weeks, Stefansson and Anderson were fed the standard diet of the time: fruits, cereals, bacon and eggs, and vegetables. (Notice that there were no fast foods, no snacks, and no vending-machine fare available then, so by today's standards, the "ordinary" diet was already light-years better than what we eat now.) During those first 3 weeks, the two guys were given preliminary checkups and were basically free to come and go as they pleased. After the first 3 weeks, they went on the all-meat diet and were more or less under house arrest. Neither of them was permitted at any time, day or night, to be out of sight of a supervising doctor or a nurse.

One interesting sidebar: Anderson was able to eat anything he liked as often as he wanted, provided that it came under the experimental definition of meat: steaks, chops, brains fried in bacon fat, boiled short ribs, chicken, fish, liver, and bacon. But because Stefansson had reported in one of his books, *My Life with the Eskimo*, that he had become very ill when he had to go 2 or 3 weeks on just *lean* meat ("caribou so skinny that there was no appreciable fat"), DuBois, who headed the experiment, suggested that for a while they try a *lean-meat-only* diet on Stefansson to contrast the results with those of Anderson, who was eating whatever mix of fat and meat he felt like. They continued to give Anderson as much fat as he liked, but Stefansson was limited to chopped fatless meat.

Stefansson wrote:

> The symptoms brought on at Bellevue by an incomplete meat diet (lean without fat) were exactly the same as in the Arctic, except that they came on faster—diarrhea and a feeling of general baffling discomfort. Up north the Eskimos and I had been cured immediately when we got some fat. DuBois now cured me the same way, by giving me fat sirloin steaks, brains fried in bacon fat, and things of that sort. In two or three days I was all right, but I had lost considerable weight. If yours is a meat diet then you simply must have fat with your lean; otherwise you would sicken and die.[8]

For the rest of the year, both men were kept on a diet of meat and fat in whatever proportion they liked, and the experiment went off without a hitch. Every few weeks, with DuBois supervising, they would run around the reservoir in Central Park, then run up to DuBois's house, going up the stairs two or three at a time, after which they would plop down on cots and have their breathing, pulse rate, and other measurements taken. These tests showed that their stamina increased the longer they stayed on the meat diet.

In 1930, DuBois and associates published the results of the study in the *American Journal of Biological Chemistry*. The title of the paper was "Prolonged Meat Diets with Study of Kidney Functions and Ketosis." Here's a summary of what they wrote: Stefansson, who was about 10 pounds overweight at the beginning, lost his excess weight in the first few weeks on the all-meat diet. His total caloric intake ranged from 2,000 to 3,100 calories per day. His metabolic rate rose—from 60.96 to 66.38 calories per hour during the period of the weight loss, indicating an increase of almost 9%. His blood cholesterol at the end of the year was 51 milligrams lower than it had been at the start. He wound up choosing a ratio of somewhere around 3:1 (in grams) of lean meat to fat. He con-tinued the diet a full year, with no apparent ill effects.

Stefansson wrote about his experiences in a fascinating and very long three-part piece called "Adventures in Diet" in *Harper's Monthly Magazine* between Novem-ber 1935 and January 1936. His conclusions were surprisingly mod-erate: "So you *could* live on meat if you wanted to; but there is no driv-

> *Everyone warned me that if I went on a high-protein diet my cholesterol and triglycerides would go through the roof. Meanwhile, the exact opposite happened.*
>
> —Pamela R.

ing reason why you *should*. Apparently you can eat healthy on meat without vegetables, on vegetables without meat, or on a mixed diet."

What he did not say, but undoubtedly would have had he been alive today, was this: you *cannot* eat "healthy" if most of your food comes from 7-Eleven.

The low-carbers of today would've loved him.

A postscript: it seems that in the twenty-or-so-year interim between his days in the Bellevue dietetic ward and his life in the 1950s as a scholarly (and relatively sedentary) academic, Stefansson suffered a mild cerebral thrombosis, put on a few pounds, and became quite a grump. According to Mrs. Stefansson, her husband had mostly recovered from the thrombosis but couldn't dump the extra weight. Her words: "By will power and near starvation, he had now and then lost a few [pounds] but [they] always came back when his will power broke down." Mrs. Stef also noted that he had become a real pain in the butt. As she delicately put it, "Stef had grown a bit unhappy, at times grouchy."[9]

Stef then asked Mrs. Stef if she wouldn't mind if he went on the "Stone-Age Eskimo sort of all-meat diet" he had thrived on during the most active part of his Arctic career. Mrs. Stef was not exactly a stay-at-home wife. She lectured, she wrote books about the Arctic, she was the director of a course called the Arctic Seminar, and she sang in madrigal groups. She had better things to do with her time than to prepare two different menus. But she bit her tongue and said, "Of course, dear. That will be fine."

So back it was to *all meat, all fat, all the time* in the Stefansson household. Mrs. Stef wrote:

> When you eat as a primitive Eskimo does, you live on lean and fat meats. A typical Stefansson dinner is a rare or medium sirloin steak and coffee. The coffee is freshly ground. If there is enough fat on the steak we take the coffee black, otherwise heavy cream is added. Sometimes we have a bottle of wine. We have no bread, no starchy vegetables, no desserts. Rather often we eat half a grapefruit. We eat eggs for breakfast, two for Stef, one for me, with lots of butter.
>
> Startling improvements in health came to Stef after several weeks on the new diet. He began to lose his overweight almost at once, and lost steadily, eating as much as he pleased and feeling satisfied the while. He lost seventeen pounds; then his weight remained stationary, although the amount he ate was the same. From being slightly irritable and depressed, he became once more his old ebullient, optimistic self.
>
> An unlooked-for and remarkable change was the disappearance of his arthritis, which had troubled him for years and which he thought of as a natural result of aging. One of his knees was so stiff he walked up and down stairs a step at a time, and he always sat on the aisle in a theatre so he could extend his stiff leg comfortably. Several times a night he would be awakened by pain in his hip and shoulder when he lay too long on one side; then he had to turn over and lie on the other side. Without noticing the change at first, Stef was one day startled to find himself walking up and down stairs, using both legs equally. He stopped in the middle of our stairs; then walked down again and up again. He could not remember which knee had been stiff!
>
> Conclusion: The Stone-Age all-meat diet is wholesome. It is an eat-all-you-want reducing diet that permits you to forget you are dieting—no hunger pains remind you. Best of all, it improves the temperament. It somehow makes one feel optimistic, mildly euphoric.[10]

A post-postscript: Stefansson remained married to the former Evelyn Schwartz Baird (Mrs. Stef) for 21 years; continued his research, writing, and public speaking at Dartmouth College; and died, by all accounts happy, on August 26, 1962, at the age of 83.

Meanwhile, back at the ranch . . .

In 1944, cases of obesity were being treated at New York City Hospital by a cardiologist named Blake Donaldson. After a year of unsuccessful results with traditional low-calorie diets, he decided to investigate alternative methods. He took himself to the American Museum of Natural History, where, using teeth as an indicator of both body condition in general and diet specifically, he hit the mother lode when he looked at skeletons dug from Inuit burial grounds. Looking further into Inuit diets, he consulted with Vilhjalmur Stefansson and became convinced that a meat-only diet was the answer for his obese patients. Donaldson allowed his patients to eat as much as they liked, but the *minimum* was one 8-ounce porterhouse steak *3 times a day*, with a cooked weight of 6 ounces lean meat and 2 ounces fat, the same 3:1 ratio of lean to fat that had worked so well in the Stefansson–Anderson experiment (and the same one that Pennington had used with his DuPont execs).

Foreshadowing many of the low-carb diets of the 1990s, Donaldson kept his patients on a strict version of the diet until they reached their target weight, at which point they could add back certain "prohibited" foods, unless they began to put on weight again. Donaldson treated some 15,000 patients and claimed a 70% success rate using this diet. He also claimed that the 30% who were unsuccessful failed to lose weight not because of any fault in the diet but because they couldn't stay on it. He wrote a book in 1960 called *Strong Medicine*,[11] so named because Donaldson knew that his diet was not for the faint of heart—it took a lot of willpower and dedication to stick with it, and he knew that not everybody would be up for the challenge.

Then came a seminal moment in the history of low-carb theory, one that served as an acknowledged inspiration to the main guru of the low-carb movement of the late twentieth century, Robert Atkins. It happened in the 1950s and 1960s, and it happened in London.

Inspiration for Atkins

Professor Alan Kekwick was director of the Institute of Clinical Research and Experimental Medicine at London's Middlesex Hospital, and Dr. Gaston L.S. Pawan was senior research biochemist of the hospital's medical unit. These two researchers joined forces in the middle of the twentieth century to perform some visionary experiments.[12] They wanted to test the theory that different proportions of carbs, fat, and protein might have different effects on weight loss _even if the calories were kept the same._

In one study, they put obese subjects on a 1,000-calorie diet but varied the percentages of protein, carbs, and fat. Some subjects were on a diet of 90% protein, some 90% fat, and some 90% carbs. The subjects on the 90% protein diet lost 0.6 pounds per day, the ones on the 90% fat diet lost 0.9 pounds per day, and the ones on 90% carbs actually gained a bit.

In another study, subjects didn't lose anything on a so-called "balanced" diet of 2,000 calories; but when these same subjects were put on a diet of primarily fat with very low carbohydrate, they were able to lose even when the calories went as high as 2,600 per day. The February 1957 issue of the American journal _Antibiotic Medicine and Clinical Therapy_ reported: "If . . . calorie intake was kept constant . . . at 1,000 per day, the most rapid weight loss was noted with _high-fat diets_ . . . But when the calorie intake was raised to 2,600 daily in these patients, _weight loss would still occur provided that this intake was given mainly in the form of fat and protein._" (Emphasis mine.)

Still, the criticism from the medical establishment was enormous—this work contradicted the mantra that a calorie is a calorie is a calorie. One of the criticisms leveled at the two researchers was that the weight their patients lost was "just water weight." So Kekwick and Pawan did water-balance studies that showed water loss to be only a small part of the total weight lost. Interestingly, as recently as 2002, a very well-designed study done at the University of Cincinnati and Children's Hospital Medical Center[13] compared weight loss on a very low-carbohydrate diet to weight loss on a calorie-restricted low-fat diet, and found again that the greater weight loss experienced by the low-carb dieters was _not_ due to water loss. The exact words: "We think it is very unlikely that differences in weight between the two groups . . . are a result of [water loss] in the very low-carb dieters." Yet to this day, the myth persists that the majority of weight lost on low-carbohydrate diets is mainly from water.

Eat Fat and Grow Slim and the Theory of Metabolic Disorder

The dietary establishment remained firmly convinced, as it does to this day, that the only thing that mattered when it came to weight reduction was calories; but there were pockets of dissent popping up throughout the 1950s, '60s, and '70s. One of the leaders of this dissent was Dr. Richard Mackarness, who ran Britain's first obesity and food allergy clinic and who in 1958 wrote *Eat Fat and Grow Slim* (which was revised and expanded in 1975).[14] He argued that it was *carbohydrates*, not calories, that were the culprit in weight gain. The following lines, from the foreword to the book, give the reader some idea of what's coming. They were written by Sir Heneage Ogilvie—a consultant surgeon at Guy's Hospital in London, the editor of *The Practitioner*, and a former vice president of the Royal College of Surgeons, England.

> There are three kinds of foods—fats, proteins, and carbohydrates. All of these provide calories. *But the carbohydrates provide calories and nothing else.* They have none of the essential elements to build up or to repair the tissues of the body. *A man given carbohydrates alone, however liberally, would starve to death on calories.* The body must have proteins and animal fats. *It has no need for carbohydrates,* and, given the two essential foodstuffs, it can get all the calories it needs from them.

You heard it here first, folks. And you'll be hearing it again throughout this book: *the body has no physiological need for carbohydrates.* You cannot live without protein. You cannot live without fat. But you can survive perfectly well without carbohydrates. No one is saying you *ought* to, or that you *have* to—just that you *can.* This is simple, basic human biochemistry. There is no "minimum daily requirement" for carbohydrates—which raises the question worth keeping in the back of your mind as you read through the rest of the book: why would the dietary establishment—including the American Dietetic Association—continue to insist that the only healthful diet consists of one in which the *majority* of the calories come from the *one macronutrient for which we have no physiological need?*

But I digress.

Sentiments similar to those of Ogilvie were echoed in the Mackarness book's introduction, written by Dr. Franklin Bicknell:

> The cure of obesity . . . can be, of course, achieved by simple starvation, but as Dr. Mackarness explains, this is both an illogical and an injurious treatment, while [a treatment] based on eating as much of everything one likes except starches and sugars and foods rich in these, is both logical and actively good for one's

health, quite apart from the effect on one's weight. *The sugars and
starches of our diet form the least valuable part and contribute nothing
which cannot better be gained from fat and protein foods like meat and
fish, eggs and cheese, supplemented by green vegetables and some fruit.*
Such a diet provides an abundance . . . of vitamins, trace
elements, and essential amino acids—an abundance of all those
subtle, yet essential, nutrients which are often lacking in diets
based largely on the fat-forming carbohydrates.

A little context: ever since 1829, when William Wadd, surgeon-extraordinary
to the prince regent, proclaimed that the cause of obesity was "an over-
indulgence at the table" (i.e., eating too darn much!), the conventional
wisdom was that fat people are fat because they eat too much food. Period.
This view, that only the quantity and not the quality of food that people eat
makes a difference, had a stranglehold on mainstream medicine—a stranglehold that continued through the twentieth century with the cooperation
of the sycophantic American Dietetic Association and is only now, in the
twenty-first century, beginning to loosen.

To give you a sense of the spirit of the era, the medical correspondent
of The London Times, on March 11, 1957, wrote at the time of Mackarness's book: "It is no use saying as so many women do: 'But I eat practically
nothing.' The only answer to this is: 'No matter how little *you imagine* you
eat, *if you wish to lose weight you must eat less.*'" (Emphasis mine.)

Mackarness comes out swinging, right in his author's introduction,
leaving no doubt what "side" of the quality-versus-quantity argument he's
on: "Starch and sugar are the causes of obesity. Particularly modern refined
and processed starches and sugars, the ever ready, highly publicized carbohydrate foods of twentieth-century urban man." He puts forth the interesting argument—foreshadowing much of what we hear today in the
discussions of metabolic type—that there are two kinds of people, whom he
characterizes as Mr. Constant-Weight and Mr. Fatten-Easily.

According to Mackarness, if you give both types the same exercise and
feed them the same food, one will stay the same weight while the other will
gain. When Mr. (or Ms.) Constant-Weight—people we hate who seem to be
able to eat anything and not gain an ounce—take in too much carbohydrate, the extra food simply causes a revving-up in their metabolism that
burns the extra calories consumed, and they stay the same weight. Nothing
is left over for laying down fat. "But," MacKarness writes, "when Mr. Fatten-
Easily eats too much bread, cake, and potatoes, the picture is entirely different: his metabolic rate does not increase. Why does he fail to burn up the

excess? The answer is the real reason for his obesity: Because he has a defective capacity for dealing with carbohydrates."

Mackarness was suggesting a metabolic disorder, and he was on to something. He was really the first diet-book author to postulate some sort of metabolic defect in the way some people process food (especially carbohydrates) that causes them to send much of what they eat to their fat stores. Dr. Alfred Pennington (of the DuPont-execs study) had come to the same conclusion. Summing up a 1953 paper called "Obesity: Over-nutrition or Disease of Metabolism?" published in the *American Journal of Digestive Diseases,* Pennington wrote: "Analysis of the results . . . appear[s] to necessitate an explanation of obesity on the basis of some intrinsic metabolic defect."

Writing for the general public, Mackarness had a simpler way of putting it. He came up with a great analogy: the steam engine.

> The orthodox view is that a fat man's engine is stoked by a robot fireman, who swings his shovel at the same pace whether fat, protein, or carbohydrate is in the tender. This is true for Mr. Constant-Weight, but as he does not get fat anyway, it is only of academic interest to us. It is certainly not true for Mr. Fatten-Easily, with whom we are concerned. Mr. Constant-Weight has a robot stoker in his engine. The more he eats—of whatever food—the harder his stoker works until any excess is consumed, so he never gets fat. Recent research has shown that Mr. Fatten-Easily's stoker is profoundly influenced by the kind of fuel he has to shovel. On fat fuel he shovels fast. On protein slightly less fast *but on carbohydrate he becomes tired, scarcely moving his shovel at all.* His fire then burns low and his engine gets fat from its inability to use the carbohydrate which is still being loaded into the tender. *Mr. Fatten-Easily's stoker suffers from an inability to deal with carbohydrate.*

At the back of his book, Mackarness lists foods that can be eaten without reservation, which are meat, poultry, game, fish and other seafood, dairy products, fats and oils, most vegetables, and some fruits; foods that can be eaten in moderation with some caution, including nuts and higher-carb vegetables and fruits; and foods that could be eaten once a day, such as beans, beets, corn, potatoes, and bananas. While some low-carb theorists of today might quibble with the inclusion of dairy, what's more interesting is the Mackarness list of "never eat" foods. Are you ready? Don't shoot the messenger.

- breakfast cereals
- bread and rolls
- biscuits and crackers
- macaroni products, noodles, spaghetti, and other pastas
- rice
- jellies, jams, and preserves
- ice cream, cakes, pies, and candy
- sauces and gravies thickened with flour or cornstarch
- beer
- sweet wines and liqueurs
- sodas (and all "sweetened fizzy drinks")
- sugar

The Mackarness diet suggests that carbs be kept as low as possible—no more than 60 grams a day for most people (and in some cases 50 grams or fewer a day). This figure is in the ballpark of the recommendations of many low-carb diet books of today (*Life Without Bread*[15] recommends a maximum of 72 grams a day, and the ongoing weight loss and maintenance programs of the Atkins diet and Protein Power are in the Mackarness range, as is the beginning program for overweight sedentary people adhering to the Schwarzbein Principle. It is also practically identical to the generic program for beginners that I recommend in chapter 12.)

We should not leave Mackarness without mentioning that he was one of the first to note the emotional and psychological component of overeating. Here's what he said, in words that will undoubtedly ring true for thousands of people today. (Emphasis mine.)

> So far, then, two big factors in the production of obesity have emerged.
>
> A *defect in dealing with carbohydrates* which makes a person fatten easily on an ordinary mixed diet;
>
> Overeating, especially of sugars and starches as a result of *loneliness, fear or emotional dissatisfaction.*
>
> When the two factors are present, weight is gained very rapidly.
>
> *So anyone who finds himself tempted to overeat for emotional reasons and who shows a tendency to get fat, should be careful to choose low-carbohydrate foods.*[16]

Overeaters Anonymous

Mackarness was not the only one to notice the emotional component of overeating. Interestingly, on the other side of the ocean, in 1959—less than a year after the publication of Mackarness's book and 24 years after the founding of Alcoholics Anonymous—two women in Los Angeles began the fellowship now known as Overeaters Anonymous. A spiritual program to address compulsive overeating, it was based on the same 12-step principles as its predecessor, but with one significant difference. While alcoholics and drug addicts could conceivably abstain from their drug of choice, compulsive overeaters could not. They had to eat to survive.

This presented an entirely different set of issues, since for overeaters, complete "abstinence" from their "drug" (food) was not possible. Many of the original participants in OA attended because they were terribly overweight, but most understood that there was a compulsive emotional component to their overeating that could not be addressed by simple diets or by the prescription drug of the day, *dextroamphetamine*, sold under the brand name *Dexedrine*. What's especially interesting for our purposes is a particular subgroup of OA that developed in Los Angeles in the early '60s. This group had noticed that, even though many people lost weight in Overeaters Anonymous, many were nibbling their way back to obesity and that certain foods seemed to feed the compulsion to eat more than others.

Can you guess what the culprits were?

Yup.

By 1963, there was a very vocal minority of OA members who were convinced that carbohydrates sabotaged any weight-loss plan because they produced cravings and addictive eating behavior. The OA contingent called them "binge foods." One of the founders of this faction—which later came to be known as the Grey Sheet Group—wrote "I wonder if we have an *allergy of the body* too. Are we going to help the Doctors understand obesity just as the alcoholic had to educate the medical profession?"[17]

From that time on—although it is little known—there has always been a faction of OA that believes strongly that "abstaining" from carbohydrates (with a very low-carbohydrate diet) is a necessary component of emotional sobriety when it comes to food, just as it is a necessary strategy for weight loss in carbohydrate-sensitive individuals. Could this be another case of the patient profoundly understanding the disease far in advance of the medical professionals?

Calories, Carbs, or Just Plain Fat?
The Roaring '60s

In the 1960s, two books came out in favor of the low-carb approach, both of which got a lot of attention. One of them deserved it; the other did not. The one that did was a thoughtful, if somewhat misguided, treatise called *Calories Don't Count* by a New York doctor named Herman Taller. Taller had been a fat man all his life, at one time almost 100 pounds over his ideal weight. He described himself as one of those who "only had to look at a platter of spaghetti to gain [weight]." He struggled with every version of the low-calorie diet available with virtually no results. A physician friend of his was sure that Taller had to be lying about how much he was eating, so Taller hatched a plan. Reading his experience will no doubt produce quite a number of nodding, sympathetic heads.

> I proposed an interesting vacation test [to the physician who was certain I was cheating]. We would go away together for ten days, stay in each other's company continually, eat and drink the same things, and check the results. He accepted, and we went off to a resort. I followed what was then the accepted method of weight control: a low-calorie diet. I concentrated on salads, which I now know was a mistake, ate fat sparingly, another mistake, and, since this was a vacation, drank a cocktail each night before dinner. My physician friend, who was slim, did the same. At the end of the vacation, he had lost a pound or two and I had gained nine pounds. "I don't understand it" he said as we drove back to New York. Neither did I.[18]

Taller didn't reject the calorie theory at all. On the contrary, he wrote: "No one, least of all myself, would dispute the concept that led to the calorie fad. Any person will lose weight when he burns up more energy than he eats. This is a simple chemical law. Why, then, didn't a low-calorie diet work? Why did people lose weight on high-calorie, high-fat diets?" Taller postulated that all calories are not the same and that carbohydrates present a different problem to the body, *at least for some people.* He rightly pointed out that low-fat diets were by nature high in carbohydrates, thus stimulating insulin and creating more fat, particularly in people who were sensitive to carbohydrates. (It is noteworthy that, almost four decades later, Eleftheria Maratos-Flier, director of obesity research at Harvard's prestigious Joslin Diabetes Center, said, "For a large percentage of the population, perhaps

30 to 40 percent, low-fat diets are counterproductive. They have the para-doxical effect of making people gain weight.") Taller completely agreed that the underlying reason people get fat is an imbalance between calories taken in and calories burned. But he suggested that for some people there is a disturbance in the metabolism, with three results, none of them good: (1) the body forms fat at a rate that is faster than normal; (2) the body stores fat at a rate that is faster than normal; and (3) the body disposes of stored fat at a rate that is slower than normal. Taller summed up: "The crux of the matter is not how many calories [we] take in, but what [our bodies do] with those calories."[19]

Taller did not recommend a diet devoid of carbohydrates—in fact, a typical day's menu contained up to three slices of "gluten bread," some-thing no low-carb advocate today, including myself, would recommend (there are far more healthful starchy carbs to choose from, including sprouted-grain or gluten-free breads). The rest of the day's food came from meat, poultry, seafood, and plenty of vegetables as well as some oils. There was no counting of calories.

Now here's where it gets interesting.

In the '50s and '60s, when Taller was writing, a scientist named Ancel Keys had begun studying heart disease and diet—research that culminated in what has come to be known as the diet-heart hypothesis. Keys concluded that cholesterol is a cause of heart disease, saturated fat causes a rise in cholesterol, and therefore saturated fat causes heart disease. Keys's seven-country study[20] became the basis for dietary policy for more than three decades, indirectly birthed the fat phobia of the '80s, and directly spawned an entire bureaucracy devoted to lowering cholesterol (the National Cho-lesterol Education Program) and also to producing some of the most profit-able pharmaceutical drugs in history. Note for now that there are serious problems with this theory, and it is finally being reexamined.[21]

Taller, a product of the time, accepted the demonization of cholesterol and believed that if you could reduce it in the diet, you could significantly lower heart-disease rates. He was very concerned about the saturated fat in the low-carb diets of the past, so he came up with what he thought was a perfect solution: his version of the diet would incorporate tons of polyun-saturated fats. Problem was, he lumped all unsaturated fats together. He was correct in pointing out how healthy marine fats are (the famous omega-3s from fish and flaxseed), but he was dead wrong in advocating excessive amounts of man-made refined vegetable oils like safflower, sunflower, and corn oils, which we now know are associated with a host of diseases, inflam-matory conditions, and cancers.[22]

Taller's book went through eighteen printings and ultimately had more than a million copies in circulation, but his career came to an unfortunate end when he was convicted of six counts of mail fraud for using the book to promote a particular brand of safflower capsules, which the court called "a worthless scheme foisted on a gullible public."[23] Too bad. By all reports, he was a good guy and very sincere in his efforts to bring healthy low-carb living to the masses.

The other low-carb book published in the '60s—also against a backdrop of the fledgling no-fat madness started by the flawed Keys research—was one that didn't deserve much attention, though that little detail didn't stop it from selling 5½ million copies. *The Doctor's Quick Weight Loss Diet*,[24] otherwise known as the Stillman diet, put forth a high-protein solution that attempted, at the same time, to satisfy the low-fat contingent. On the Stillman diet, you ate nothing—and I mean nothing—but protein with every drop of fat trimmed from it. You could eat all you wanted from the following selection: lean meats with all possible fat trimmed; chicken and turkey without skin; all nonfatty fish; eggs made in nonstick pans without butter, margarine, oil, or other fat; cottage cheese and other soft cheeses made only from skim milk; and at least eight glasses of water a day. We know from the Stefansson experiment that this diet, if followed for any length of time, would make you very sick precisely because of the *absence* of fat.

The Stillman diet was a dumb idea and should not be followed for any reason. Although the Stillman all-protein plan was in fact a low-carb diet, it's important to remember that not all low-carb diets are *high-protein* diets. Even the Atkins diet, which will be discussed at greater length in chapter 9, is not necessarily high-protein. In fact, the average protein content of all three major phases of the Atkins diet is only 31% (the average *fat* content is 56%); and during the Atkins maintenance phase, the average protein content is only 5% higher than Weight Watchers (25% versus 20%)![25] Some of the diets discussed in this book don't even approach high-protein: for example, Barry Sears's Zone diet (see chapter 9) has often been called a high-protein diet by magazine writers who have either not read his books or not understood them, and by members of the American Dietetic Association, who have frequently done neither. The point is that *low-carb does not necessarily equal high-protein,* and the Stillman diet is Exhibit A in making the case that all low-carb diets are not the same.

Atkins, Yudkin, and the Question of Sugar

By 1970, the Keys research had been published and was being picked up by the media; the low- or no-cholesterol brigade was gearing up for an assault on the consciousness of the American public. In 1972, Robert Atkins published the first edition of the *New Diet Revolution*, the Cadillac of low-carb diet plans, which became the de facto poster child for the low-carb movement two decades later.

Atkins was the first popular diet-book author to seriously focus on insulin as a determinant in weight gain. He preached the virtues of something he called "the metabolic advantage": benign dietary ketosis (a process that, because it is so central to the discussion of low-carb diets and so misunderstood, will receive much further attention in chapter 6). Because his high-fat, high-protein, low-carb diet went so dramatically against the conventional "wisdom" of the times, Atkins was attacked mercilessly in the press and vilified by the medical mainstream, who turned him into a pariah in the medical community. His voice was drowned out by the low-fat, no-cholesterol, calorie-counting establishment, and although he remained active, he didn't catch on big time until the early 1990s, when an updated edition of the *New Diet Revolution* was published.

The public, with their rapidly expanding waistlines, was growing weary of the low-fat dogma and beginning to realize that their low-fat diets were accomplishing very little in the way of weight loss; people were finally ready to look elsewhere for a solution.

In the same year in which Atkins published the first edition of his book, which firmly took the position that the problem in obesity was carbohydrates, not fat, a brilliant English doctor named John Yudkin was making waves by politely and reasonably suggesting to the medical establishment that perhaps their emperor, while indeed cholesterol-free and low-fat, was nonetheless naked as a jaybird. A professor of nutrition at Queen Elizabeth College, London University, and the surgeon-captain of the British Royal Navy, Yudkin was a highly respected scientist and nutritionist and the possessor of both an MD and a PhD, with dozens of published papers in such august peer-reviewed journals as *The Lancet, Cardiovascular Review, British Medical Journal, The Archives of Internal Medicine, The American Journal of Clinical Nutrition*, and *Nature* to his credit.

Yudkin was typically portrayed by his detractors as a wild-eyed fanatic who blamed sugar as the cause of heart disease, but in fact he was nothing of the sort. In his 1972 book, *Sweet and Dangerous*, he was the embodiment of reason when he called for a reexamination of the data—which he considered highly flawed—that led to the hypothesis that fat causes heart disease. (These data, as you will recall, came originally from a study of seven countries published by Ancel Keys, a study that conveniently omitted a substantial amount of data that did not fit his hypothesis.)[26]

Yudkin pointed out that statistics for heart disease and fat consumption existed for many more countries than those referred to by Keys, and that these other figures didn't fit into the "more fat, more heart disease" relationship that was evident when only the seven selected countries were considered. He pointed out that there was a better and truer relationship between *sugar consumption* and heart disease, and he said that "there is a sizable minority—of which I am one—that believes that coronary disease is *not* largely due to fat in the diet." (Three decades later, Dr. George Mann, an associate director of the Framingham Study, arrived at the same conclusion and assembled a distinguished group of scientists and doctors to study the evidence that fat and cholesterol cause heart disease, a concept he later called "the greatest health scam of the century."[27] Around the same time, the brilliant Danish scholar Uffe Ravnskov, MD, PhD, reanalyzed the original Keys data and came to the identical conclusion. His exemplary scholarship is supported by hundreds of referenced citations and studies from prestigious, peer-reviewed medical journals and can be found in book form[28] and at the website http://www.ravnskov.nu/cholesterol.htm.)

While Yudkin did not write a low-carb diet book per se, he was one of the most influential voices of the time to put forth the position that sugar was responsible for far more health problems than fat was. His book called attention to countries in which the correlation between heart disease and sugar intake was far more striking than the correlation between heart disease and *fat*. And he pointed to a number of studies—most dramatically of the Masai in Kenya and Tanzania—where people consumed copious amounts of milk and fat and yet had virtually no heart disease. Interestingly, these people also consumed almost no sugar.[29]

Yudkin patiently explained that sugar consumption is *one* of a *number* of indices of health. Heart disease is associated with many of these indices, including fat consumption, overweight, cigarette smoking, a sedentary lifestyle, and television viewing. It is *definitely* associated with a high intake of sugar. He never said that sugar *causes* the diseases of modern civilization, just that a case could easily be made that it deserved attention and study—certainly as much, if not more than, fat consumption. (Yudkin himself performed several interesting studies on sugar consumption and coronary heart disease. In one, he found that the median sugar intake of a group of coronary patients was 147 grams, twice as much as it was in two different groups of control subjects who didn't have coronary disease; these groups consumed only 67 and 74 grams, respectively).[30]

As Yudkin put it, "It may turn out that [many factors including sugar] ultimately have the same effect on metabolism and so produce coronary disease by the same mechanism." What is that mechanism? Fingers are beginning to point suspiciously to an *overload of insulin* as a common culprit at the root of at least some of these metabolic and negative health effects like heart disease; controlling insulin was the main purpose of the original Atkins diet and has become the raison d'être of the low-carb approach to living. (In the next chapter, we will explore some of the connections between high levels of insulin and heart disease, hypertension, obesity, and diabetes.)

Cholesterol Madness

Yudkin's warnings against sugar and Atkins's early low-carb approach to weight loss were mere whispers lost in the roar of antifat mania. By the mid-1980s, fat had been utterly and completely demonized, and fat phobia was in full bloom, with hundreds of no-cholesterol foods being foisted on a gullible public (despite the findings that dietary cholesterol had little or no effect on serum cholesterol, a fact acknowledged even by Ancel Keys himself, who, in 1991, said that dietary cholesterol only mattered if you happened to be a rabbit!).[31] In November 1985, the National Heart, Lung, and Blood Institute launched the National Cholesterol Education Program with the stated goal of "reducing illness and death from coronary heart disease in the United States by *reducing the percent of Americans with high blood cholesterol.*"[32] (Emphasis mine.)

Though high cholesterol *doesn't* cause heart disease and, in fact, has turned out to be a relatively poor predictor of it, the juggernaut was already in full swing, and the cry of "hold the butter" was heard all over America. Fat-free foods were everywhere. Snackwells replaced Oreos as the best-selling cookie in America. In 1976, Nathan Pritikin opened his Pritikin Longevity Center in Santa Barbara, California, and for the next decade he preached the super-low-fat dogma to all who would listen, which included most of the country. Jane Fonda ushered in a new generation of aerobicized exercise fanatics whose motto was "no pain, no gain" and who looked upon fat of any kind as a Tootsie Roll in the punch bowl. (Later, Apex, a supplement company based in California, got a strong foothold in health clubs as nutrition "experts" largely by being the hand-maiden of the American Dietetic Association, and Apex's people taught gullible trainers and their clients the dogma of high-carbohydrate diets for weight loss while they railed against the "dangers" of high protein and ketosis.)[33] It became a point of pride to exorcise any hint of fat from the diet: egg-white omelets became de rigueur on every urban menu, and waiters across America became accustomed to orders without butter, oil, or fat of any kind.

Pritikin died in 1985, but his mantle was quickly taken up by Dr. Dean Ornish. Ornish's reputation—and much of the public's faith in the low-fat diet approach—was fueled by his famous 5-year intervention study (the Lifestyle Heart Trial), which demonstrated that intensive lifestyle changes may lead to regression of coronary heart disease.[34] Ornish took 48 middle-aged white men with moderate to severe coronary heart disease and assigned them to two groups. One group received "usual care," and the other group received a special, intensive 5-part lifestyle intervention con-sisting of (1) aerobic exercise, (2) stress management training, (3) smoking cessation, (4) group psychological support, and (5) a strict vegetarian, high-fiber diet with 10% of the calories coming from fat.

When Ornish's study showed some reversal of atherosclerosis and fewer cardiac events in the 20 men who completed the 5-year study, the public perception—reinforced by Ornish himself—was that the results were largely due to the low-fat diet. This is an incredible leap that is in no way supported by his research. The fact is that *there's no way to know* whether the results were due to the low-fat diet portion of the experiment (highly unlikely in the view of many), the high fiber, the whole foods, the lack of sugar, or some combination of the interventions. It is entirely possible that Ornish would have gotten the same or better results with a program of exercise, stress management, smoking cessation, and group therapy plus a whole foods diet of high protein, good fats, high fiber, and low sugar. (Interestingly, critics of low-carb diets frequently proclaim with great righ-teousness that the only reason a low-carb diet works is because it is a low-calorie diet in disguise. They never level that criticism at Ornish, whose diet, in a recent analysis, turned out to be *lower* in calories [1,273 calories] than the Atkins ongoing weight-loss phase [1,627 calories], the Atkins maintenance phase [1,990 calories], the Carbohydrate Addict's Diet [1,476 calories], Sugar Busters! [1,521 calories], the Zone [approximately 1,500 calories], and even Weight Watchers [1,462 calories].)[35]

The Tide Turns: A Reexamination of the Low-Carb Solution

By the 1990s, it was pretty obvious that low-fat dieting wasn't getting results. The country was fatter than ever, diabetes was becoming epidemic, and people were getting more and more frustrated and confused. The time was right for another look at the low-carb wisdom that had been around in one form or another since Banting's day in the 1800s. To the chagrin of the medical establishment and the American Dietetic Association, Atkins resurfaced with a vengeance with his newly updated *New Diet Revolution* in 1992, followed by perhaps the most influential nutrition book of the 1990s, Barry Sears's *The Zone*, in 1995, a year that also saw the publication of the brilliant *Protein Power* by Drs. Michael and Mary Dan Eades.

After massive resistance by the establishment, serious research was finally comparing low-carb diets to traditional diets, and the results were impressive. While it would be incorrect to say that low-carb diets always produced greater weight loss than the traditional kind, they *often* did; they frequently produced it faster (a huge motivating force for many people); and they almost always produced better health outcomes such as blood-lipid profiles, precisely the measures that the anti-low-carb forces had predicted would be disastrous on these regimens (see chapter 3). In what will probably turn out to be a signal event in the death of the high-carb dictatorship, Dr. Walter Willett—chairman of the Department of Nutrition at Harvard University's School of Public Health and one of the most respected mainstream researchers in the country—recently came out publicly against the 1992 USDA Food Guide Pyramid, which for a decade had promoted 6 to 11 servings a day of grains, breads, and pastas.[36]

Internecine battles among advocates of different diets were hardly something new. What was different this time was that the arguments were finally taken public. On February 24, 2000, the US Department of Agriculture hosted a major symposium, "The Great Nutrition Debate," which featured, among others, Dr. Robert Atkins (the Atkins diet), Dr. Barry Sears (the Zone diet), low-fat advocates Dr. Dean Ornish and Dr. John McDougall, and various representatives of the dietary establishment.[37]

Then, on July 7, 2002, *the New York Times* published a cover story in its Sunday magazine section titled "What If It's All Been a Big Fat Lie?" in which Gary Taubes, a brilliant science journalist and three-time winner of the National Association of Science Writers' Science in Society Award, brought to the table massive evidence that the low-fat diet had been the dumbest experiment in dietary history. The article created a predictable uproar, with defenders of the faith rallying to discredit Taubes—not an easy task, I might add—and the low-carbers beaming ear to ear with I-told-you-so grins.

An interesting side note: on the Dietitian Central website (a dietitian Internet community), the following post was found on July 14, a week after the Taubes article appeared: "Please, dietitians, download from the NY Times Magazine section from last Sunday, July 7, the article 'What If It's All Been a Big Fat Lie?' by Gary Taubes. *It is full of information that could rock our world.* As dietitians, we need to be prepared and informed re: changes that may be completely different from what we have learned and have been educating people about." (Taubes has since published a superb full-length book based on that article called Good Calories, Bad Calories—highly recommended.)

Low-carbing had come back, but this time with a clarity and a scientific validation that had simply not been present in previous decades. It's time now for a reassessment of the twin sacred cows of dietary commandments—*high carbohydrates* and *low fat*—and for a clearer look at just what could be gained in terms of health and weight loss by following a diet more like the one that sustained the human genus for 2.4 million years and sustained modern man for at least 50,000 years.

It's time to revisit the low-carb wisdom of the past, evaluate the wisdom of the present, and see what they have to teach us about living healthy in the twenty-first century.

CHAPTER 3

Why Low-Carb Diets Work

In other fields, when bridges do not stand, when aircraft do not fly, when machines do not work, when treatments do not cure, despite all the conscientious efforts on the part of many persons to make them do so, one begins to question the basic assumptions, principles, theories, and hypotheses that guide one's efforts.

—Arthur R. Jensen, PhD Professor of psychology at the University of California at Berkeley, in Harvard Educational Review, winter 1969

On November 1, 1999, Woody Merrell—the Muhammad Ali of doctors, loved, respected, and admired across the entire political spectrum of medicine and nutrition—wrote an article in *Time* magazine about weight loss. This is how it started:

"In my 25 years of medical training and practice in Manhattan, I've seen a wide range of diets come and go. *Virtually none of them work.*"

A few paragraphs later, Merrell wrote: "For most of my professional career, I adhered to the generally recognized dictum of weight management. *I advised my patients to count their calories and follow a low-fat diet.*"

He then talks about his experience with a few patients who weren't getting anywhere, no matter what they tried. Skeptically, he put them on a low-carb diet.

Finally he wrote: "I have become a convert. Carbohydrates . . . are often prime saboteurs of our weight. [O]f all the diets I've seen over the past few decades, the moderate-fat, lower-carbohydrate ones are the most success-ful. *They stress not how much food you eat but what kinds. Calorie counting is not as important as carbo counting.* " (All emphases mine.)

The article is titled "How I Became a Low-Carb Believer."[1]

What convinced Merrell—and what is convincing more and more of his colleagues—is the fact that lower-carbohydrate diets *really work* for many, many people. The evidence of the senses is hard to argue with. People lose weight, feel better, and, equally important, have major improvements in their health. Chronic complaints and ailments have been known to disappear. Some of these people had tried every possible diet, had adhered to every conventional cholesterol-lowering, fat-reducing program, and wound up in exactly the same place as when they started—and sometimes were even worse. Yet on lower-carb diets, they do great.

GENIUS AND ANTIAGING GURU CHOOSES LOW-CARB DIET!

Ray Kurzweil is a scientist, inventor, and recipient of the National Medal of Technology. Largely considered a genius (the *Wall Street Journal* called him "the restless genius," and Forbes called him "the ultimate thinking machine"), his fans range from Bill Gates to Bill Clayton.

Recently Kurzweil teamed up with Terry Grossman, MD, the founder and medical director of the Frontier Medical Institute in Denver and the author of *The Baby Boomers' Guide to Living Forever*. The two turned their not-inconsiderable brain power and experience to studying the science of life extension.

In their seminal book, *Fantastic Voyage: The Science Behind Radical Life Extension*, they discuss genes, diet, exercise, stress, genomics, and cutting-edge research on gene manipulation.

They also discuss their personal dietary programs, arrived at after consuming and digesting hundreds—if not thousands—of research papers related to even the most obscure areas of health and longevity.

These guys are serious about health and life extension.

Would you like to know what they personally eat?

Low-carb diets. Both men consume no more than 80 grams a day of carbs, or ⅙ (about 16%) of their total calories from carbohydrates on a daily basis.

Food for thought.

How can something that is so counterintuitive work? (And it *is* counterintuitive for most of us—after all, even Gary Taubes, in his seminal article "What If It's All Been a Big Fat Lie?"[2] said he couldn't quite get over the feeling that the bacon and eggs on his plate were going to somehow jump up and kill him.) We need to remember that low-carb eating is counterintuitive precisely *because*

> *My doctor kept telling me not to try a low-carb diet because he thought it was so dangerous. Then his wife lost 50 pounds on Protein Power and now he's really done a 180.*
>
> *—Adele P.*

we have all been taught a number of "truths" that we have internalized as nutritional gospel but which may in fact be nutritional hogwash.

We "know" low-carb diets can't work because they are often high in fat or cholesterol (which we "know" causes heart disease), are often high in protein (which we "know" causes heart disease, bone loss, and possibly cancer), and may be higher in calories (which we "know" causes weight gain). Yet people eating the low-carb way are losing weight and lowering their risk for heart disease, hypertension, diabetes, and obesity. There is even some indication that they may be lowering their risk for some cancers.[3] How do we explain this? It is as though all three of Christopher Columbus's ships returned home with great bounty from the New World, but the people back in Spain shook their heads in disbelief, saying, "How can this be? It must be a trick. The ships had to have fallen off the earth because we *know* the earth is flat!"

I've got news for you: low-fat is the flat-earth theory of human nutrition.

See, all theories of weight loss fit into one of two major categories of thought—*all of them*. There is no exception to this rule. If you understand the two categories, you're immediately better informed than half the population on the subject of dieting and weight loss.

Let's call category one the Checkbook Theory. This is the idea that when it comes to calories and weight loss, the human body is like a checking account. You eat a certain number of calories, and you burn up a certain number of calories. If you eat *more* than what you need, you *gain* weight. If you eat *less* than what you need, you *lose* weight. Much like a checking account, if I deposit (take in) more money than I write checks for, I have some extra cash (i.e., I gain weight). If I spend (put out) more than I take in, I have to dip into that cash (i.e., I lose weight). If what I *deposit* exactly equals what I *spend*, I have a zero balance (i.e., my weight stays the same).

Let's call category two the Telephone Theory of weight loss, based on the game of Telephone you may have played as a child. You line ten people up, and then whisper something in the ear of the first person. That person whispers it to the second person, and so on down the line, until the words are repeated to the last person, who then says them out loud. What usually happens is that you start out with something like "A rose is a rose is a rose" and you wind up with "Gardenias don't grow on the planet Mars." Applied to weight loss, the theory goes something like this: the stuff that goes on *in between* the calories coming in and the calories going out is *much* more important than the actual number of calories involved. There are so many enzymes, cofactors, energy cycles, hormones, neurotransmitters, eicosanoids, genes, and other variables in the human body that determine the fate of the food coming in, that it is impossible to predict what's going to happen to someone's weight just by knowing the number of calories that go in. It would be like predicting the outcome of Telephone simply by knowing the phrase that was originally said. Sure, if everything goes perfectly, "A rose is a rose is a rose" comes out as "A rose is a rose is a rose." More often, though, it comes out as "Adam Sandler's latest movie stinks."

The checking-account model, known as the *energy-balance theory*, has been the dominant theory of weight loss for years. The entire low-fat movement has been built on it: take in fewer calories and burn more, and you will lose weight. You have probably been hearing this advice for years. While this view is not entirely without merit, it's so far from the whole picture as to almost constitute dietary malpractice.

The thinking behind low-carbing belongs to the second category of theories about weight loss, the Telephone Theory. This view asks a critical question: what goes on inside the body once those calories are taken in? Why do some people store everything as fat and others don't? What determines whether what you eat goes on your hips or is burned up as energy and disappears as heat into the atmosphere?

The answer is one word: hormones.

Hormones control just about every metabolic event that goes on in your body, and you control hormones via your lifestyle. Food—along with several key lifestyle factors such as stress—is the drug that stimulates hormones, and those hormones direct the body to store or burn fat, just as they direct the body to perform a gazillion other metabolic operations. (Dr. Barry Sears has said that "food may be the most powerful drug you will ever encounter because it causes dramatic changes in your hormones that are hundreds of times more powerful than any pharmaceutical.") Hormones are the air-traffic controllers determining the fate of whatever flies in. *If*

*your food is stimulating the wrong hormones or creating a hormonally unbalanced
state, you will find it extremely difficult, if not impossible, to lose weight and keep
it off.*

In this chapter, you will learn why it is so vitally important to balance
your hormones if you want to lose weight. It is probably as important as—or
more important than—counting calories, and it is *certainly* more important
than reducing dietary fat. But managing our hormones has even bigger
consequences. Insulin—the hormone most targeted by the low-carb diet
plans discussed in this book—is at the hub of a significant number of diseases of civilization. When you control insulin, you hugely increase the
odds that you will be able to control your weight. But, as you will see, you
also reduce the risks for heart disease, hypertension, diabetes, polycystic
ovary syndrome, inflammatory diseases, and even, possibly, cancer.

So let's get to know the players in our hormonal dance. If I've done my
job, at the end of this chapter you'll have a much better understanding of
what has now come to be popularly known as "Endocrinology 101": how the
body *makes* fat, *stores* fat, and, finally, *says good-bye* to fat. You'll also understand why the same eating plan that helps you lose weight *also* has the positive "side effect" of preventing you from becoming a medical statistic.

THE STAR OF THE SHOW:
EXPERTS WEIGH IN ON INSULIN

"Insulin is the key to the vast majority of chronic illness."
—Joe Mercola, DO

"There is an epidemic of insulin resistance in the world at large."
—Gerald Reaven, MD

*"When you have excess levels of insulin, it's like a loose cannon on
the deck of a hormonal ship."*
—Barry Sears, PhD

*"Insulin sensitivity is going to determine, for the most part, how long
you are going to live and how healthy you are going to be. It
determines the rate of aging more so than anything else we know
right now."*
—Ron Rosedale, MD

The Good, the Bad, and the Ugly: Insulin and Its Discontents

Insulin, a hormone first discovered in 1921, is the star actor in our little hormonal play. It is an anabolic hormone, which means it is responsible for building things up—putting compounds (like glucose and amino acids) inside storage units (like cells). Its sister hormone, glucagon, is responsible for breaking things down—opening those storage units and releasing their contents as needed. Insulin is responsible for *saving*, glucagon is responsible for *spending*. Together, their main job is to maintain blood sugar within the tightly regulated range it needs to be in, to keep your metabolic machinery running smoothly.

And to keep you from dying. Without insulin, blood sugar would sky-rocket and the result would be metabolic acidosis, coma, and death, the fate of virtually every type 1 diabetic in the early part of the twentieth century prior to the discovery of insulin. On the other hand, without glucagon, blood sugar would plummet and the result would be brain dysfunction, coma, and death. So the body knows what it's doing. This little dance between the forces that keep blood sugar from soaring too high and those that prevent it from going too low is essential for survival. It's interesting to note that while insulin is the only hormone responsible for preventing blood sugar from rising too high, there are several other hormones besides glucagon—cortisol, adrenaline, noradrenaline, and human growth hormone—that prevent it from going too low. Insulin is such a powerful hormone that five other hormones counterbalance its effects.

How a High-Carbohydrate Diet Raises Both Cholesterol and Triglycerides

Let's follow the nutrients you eat on their journey through the body. When you eat food—any food—it mixes with acids and enzymes from the stomach, pancreas, and liver that break it down into smaller molecules. The nutrients are then absorbed through the intestinal walls, while the indigestible parts of the food pass through the digestive system as waste. Proteins break down into amino acids, carbohydrates into glucose, and fats into fatty acids. These pass through the intestinal walls into the portal vein, which is like their private passageway into the liver, the central processing plant of the body. After the liver works its magic, often repackaging these compounds into different forms, the new forms are released into the general circulation of the bloodstream, where they are transported to cells and tissues to be either used or saved for a rainy day.

As these smaller units pass through the portal vein en route to the liver, the pancreas immediately takes notice of the parade and responds by secreting our star player, insulin. It secretes *some* insulin in response to protein; but when it sees carbohydrates in the passageway, its eyes light up, and it brings out the big guns and goes to town. (Fat doesn't even rate a "hello" from the pancreas and has no impact on insulin.)

Under the influence of this incoming insulin, the liver does a number of things. First, it decides how much of the sugar coming in is excess. It makes that decision based largely on how much insulin the pancreas has decided to send along to accompany the payload. If there's a lot of insulin, the liver says, "*Woo-hoo, we've got a truckload of sugar on our hands; let's get busy.*" Some of the incoming sugar will pass right through (as glucose) to the bloodstream to be transported to muscle cells—which can use a hit of sugar now and then for energy—and to the brain, which needs sugar (or ketones, which we'll discuss in detail later) to think and do all the other good things that brains like to do. Part of the excess sugar will be converted to the storage form of glucose, called glycogen, much of which will stay right there in the liver. (Glycogen is also stored in the muscles, but muscle glycogen is like a private bank account that can be used only by the muscle in which it is stored.) The liver doesn't hold a lot of glycogen, so if there is still excess sugar, which there almost always is after a high-carbohydrate meal, it is packaged into triglycerides (fats found in the blood and in the tissues). The high level of insulin accompanying the high-carbohydrate meal stimulates the cholesterol-making machinery: the body starts churning out more cholesterol, which it then packages (together with triglycerides) into little containers called VLDLs (very low-density lipoproteins), most of which eventually become LDLs (low-density lipoproteins), or "bad" cholesterol. This is how a high-carbohydrate diet raises both triglycerides and cholesterol.

Which Is Worse, Sugar or Fat? No Contest!

Why, you may ask, does the liver feel this compelling need to get rid of the excess sugar, anyway? Why doesn't it just give it a pass and let it go into the bloodstream as is? Why create all this work for itself? Why bother to turn it into triglycerides in the first place?

That's a very good question, and the answer is central to understanding the health effects of a lower-carbohydrate diet: *sugar is far more damaging to the body than fat.* In a very real sense, what the liver is doing is *detoxifying* sugar into triglycerides.

As you just read, eating high-carb foods usually makes your cholesterol go up. Here's why: insulin turbocharges the activity of a particular enzyme—with the unwieldy name of HMG-coenzyme A reductase, or HMG-CoA reductase—that runs the cholesterol-making machinery in the body. (Glucagon inhibits the HMG-CoA reductase enzyme, so your body makes less cholesterol.) So high levels of insulin basically signal the liver to ramp up the production lines on cholesterol, and high levels of sugar signal it to ramp up the production of triglycerides. (Interestingly enough, if you ate a diet of almost 90% fat, your cholesterol numbers would probably drop, because there would not be enough insulin around to power the cholesterol-making machinery.) However, the American diet—high-fat *and* high-carbohydrate—virtually guarantees both high cholesterol and high triglycerides. Your Honor, the body had *motive, means,* and *opportunity.* Motive—to get rid of the excess sugar. Means—fat and sugar. Opportunity—tons of insulin to drive the works. Case closed: when there's plenty of excess sugar and insulin around, triglycerides skyrocket and so does cholesterol.

At this point, it may start to occur to you that since sugar is made into triglycerides, then maybe one of the reasons that blood levels of triglycerides are lowered on a low-carb diet is because there's less excess sugar coming in to require packaging into triglycerides in the first place. And you'd be absolutely, 100% right. (Cholesterol sometimes comes down as well, but as you'll see later, that doesn't matter nearly as much.) This lowering of triglycerides is one of the major health benefits of a low-carb diet—high triglycerides are far more of a danger sign for heart disease than high cholesterol ever was.

You may also be thinking that the higher levels of fat that are frequently (though not always) part of low-carb diet plans may not be so bad after all, if they're not accompanied by the high insulin levels that go with high-carb diets. You'd be right on that count as well.

Insulin Prevents Fat Loss

An important thing to remember just from a weight-loss point of view is that insulin isn't only responsible for getting sugar into the cells and out of the bloodstream: it's also responsible for getting *fat* into the fat cells *and keeping it there.* Insulin actually prevents fat burning. That's why a low-carb diet usually produces more weight loss than a high-carb, low-fat diet with the same calorie count. By lowering insulin, you open the doors of the fat cells and allow the body to release fat.

One of the ways insulin interferes with fat burning is by inhibiting carnitine, an amino acid–like compound in the body that is responsible for escorting fatty acids into the little central processing units of the muscle cells, where those fats can be burned for energy. By inhibiting carnitine, insulin inhibits fat-burning. That's one reason you shouldn't eat a big meal before going to bed—the resulting high levels of insulin virtually ensure that your body will not be breaking down fat as you sleep but instead will be busy storing whatever is around in the bloodstream. (A side note: many years ago, an American health magazine decided to do a weight-loss story on sumo wrestlers. The writers reasoned that the wrestlers knew everything there was to know about putting on weight, so if we could just learn what it was they did, we'd know what *not* to do if we wanted to slim down. One of the major rituals of the sumo wrestlers was eating a huge meal and then going right to bed.)

So on a high-carbohydrate diet, you've got all this sugar coming into your system—because all carbs eventually break down into sugar—and your liver can basically do one of three things with it:

1. Pass it right through and send it into the bloodstream
2. Transform it into glycogen and store it (in the liver or the muscles)
3. Use it to make triglycerides

Remember, as far as your body is concerned, the most important thing is to prevent blood sugar from getting too high. Your insulin may very well be able to keep your blood sugar in the normal range, but the high level of insulin needed to do the job—plus the high levels of triglycerides and VLDLs being created at the same time—are silently laying the foundation for future damage: you are slowly on your way to becoming overweight and/or insulin-resistant.

Insulin Resistance: The Worst Enemy of a Lean Body

Insulin resistance makes losing weight incredibly difficult and is a risk factor for heart disease and diabetes. It is not something you want, and you *can* do something about it. Here's how insulin resistance develops: the muscle cells don't want to accept any more sugar (this is especially true if you have been living a sedentary life). They say, "Sorry, pal, we're full, we don't need any more, we gave at the office, see ya." Muscle cells become *resistant* to the effects of insulin. But the fat cells are still listening to insulin's song. They hear it knocking on their doors and they say, "Come on in; the water's fine!" The fat cells fill up and you begin to put on weight.

Meanwhile, back in the bloodstream, those little packages called VLDLs that we talked about earlier are carrying triglycerides around trying to dump them. After the VLDL molecules drop off their triglyceride passengers to the tissues and the ever-expanding fat cells, most of them turn into LDL ("bad") cholesterol.

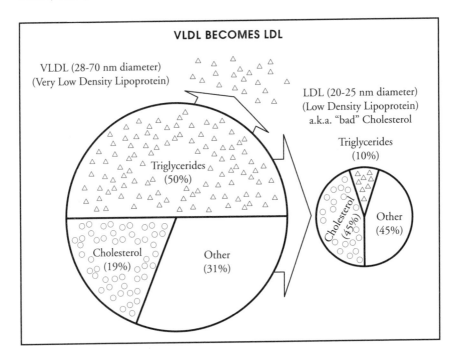

VLDL BECOMES LDL

VLDL (28-70 nm diameter)
(Very Low Density Lipoprotein)

LDL (20-25 nm diameter)
(Low Density Lipoprotein)
a.k.a. "bad" Cholesterol

Triglycerides
(50%)

Cholesterol
(19%)

Other
(31%)

Triglycerides
(10%)

Cholesterol
(45%)

Other
(45%)

Now you're overweight, with high triglycerides, high LDL cholesterol, and *definitely* high levels of insulin, which the pancreas keeps valiantly pumping out in order to get that sugar out of the bloodstream. From here, two scenarios are possible, neither of them good.

In one scenario, your hardworking pancreas will somehow be able to keep up with the workload and keep your blood sugar from getting high enough for you to be classified as diabetic. But you will be paying the price for that with high levels of insulin and the increased risk factors for heart disease that go with them. In the other scenario, your poor pancreas will eventually become exhausted—even its most valiant efforts to shoot enough insulin into the system won't be adequate for the job. The sugar will run out of places to go, so it will stay in the blood and your blood-sugar levels will rise. Now you'll have elevated insulin *and* elevated blood sugar, plus, of course, high triglycerides and abdominal obesity. If your blood sugar continues to rise even more, beyond the capacity of your insulin to reduce it, you'll eventually have full-blown type 2 diabetes.

Welcome to fast-food nation.

What's So Bad about a Little Sugar?

Obviously, the body knows how important it is to protect the tissues, the brain, and the bloodstream from excess sugar. So what exactly does sugar do that's so damaging to the body that the body is willing to risk the effects of large amounts of insulin and dangerously high levels of triglycerides just to prevent it?

Well, for one thing, excess sugar is sticky (think cotton candy and maple syrup). Proteins, on the other hand, are smooth and slippery (think oysters, which are pure protein). The slippery nature of proteins lets them slide around easily in the cells and do their jobs effectively. But when excess sugar keeps bumping into proteins, the sugar eventually gums up the works and gets stuck to the protein molecules. Such proteins are now said to have become *glycated.* The glycated proteins are too big and sticky to get through small blood vessels and capillaries, including the small vessels in the kidneys, eyes, and feet, which is why so many diabetics are at risk for kidney disease, vision problems, and amputations of toes, feet, and even legs. The sugar-coated proteins become toxic, make the cell machinery run less efficiently, damage the body, and exhaust the immune system.[4] Scientists gave these sticky proteins the acronym AGEs—which stands for advanced glycolated end-products—partially because these proteins are so involved in aging the body.

For another thing, high blood sugar is also a risk factor for cancer—cancer cells consume more glucose than normal cells do.[5] Researchers at Harvard Medical School suggested in the early 1990s that high levels of a sugar called *galactose*, which is released by the digestion of lactose in milk, might damage the ovaries and even lead to ovarian cancer. While further study is necessary to definitively establish this link, Walter Willett, MD, DrPH,—chairman of the Department of Nutrition at the Harvard School of

Public Health and one of the most respected researchers in the world—says, "I believe that a positive link between galactose and ovarian cancer shows up too many times to ignore the possibility that it may be harmful."[6]

Sugar depresses the immune system. It makes the blood acidic, and certain white blood cells (lymphocytes) that are part of our immune system don't work as well in an acidic environment.[7] A blood-sugar level of 120 reduces the phagocytic index—a measure of how well immune-system cells gobble up bacteria—by 75%.[8] Since refined sugar comes with no nutrients of its own, it uses up certain mineral reserves of the body that are needed to metabolize it, which, in turn, throws off mineral balances and results in nutrient depletions.[9] (One of the minerals that refined sugar depletes is chromium, which is needed for insulin to do its job effectively!) Since minerals are needed for dozens of metabolic operations, these mineral deficiencies can wind up slowing down your metabolism and creating havoc with your energy level. Finally, sugar reduces HDL, the helpful, "good" cholesterol, adding yet another risk factor for heart disease to its résumé.[10]

Is it any wonder people drastically improve their health when they switch to a diet lower in sugar?

Why Should We Care about High Levels of Insulin?

Now you understand the problems caused by high levels of sugar in the blood. But what problems are associated with high levels of *insulin?* See, insulin doesn't just bring blood sugar down, call it a day, and go home. It affects many other systems as well. Bringing in a huge amount of insulin to fix the sugar problem is like importing twenty thousand workers to fix a broken power plant in a city. The city can't run efficiently without electricity— hospitals are in danger, computers shut down, there's no public transportation, and you can't cook. So the prime order of business is to fix the emergency. At first, city officials aren't thinking about the effect of that influx of workers on the *rest* of the city's business; they just want to get the immediate problem fixed. Yet all those workers are going to have a major impact: the roads will be overcrowded, pollution will increase, crime may go up, and there will be additional demands for housing and food. But the city is faced with a life-and-death situation, so it imports however many people are needed to fix the problem. The same thing happens when the body produces high levels of insulin to cope with high blood sugar: damn the torpedoes, full steam ahead—the body will worry about the consequences later.

Insulin and Heart Disease

One of insulin's many effects on the body is to make the walls of the arteries thicker. It does this by encouraging growth and proliferation of the muscle cells that line those artery walls. Insulin also makes the walls stiffer, reducing the "flow space" inside and increasing blood pressure. Smaller arteries are also more prone to plaque.

As we've seen, insulin also increases LDL cholesterol (the so-called "bad" cholesterol) in the blood. But despite what you may have heard, we don't really care about that until that LDL becomes damaged (oxidized) and then gets deposited on the lining of the artery walls. *Now* we have something to worry about. Damaged LDL attracts cells called macrophages, little Pac-Man–like creatures that come out to feast on the LDL like sharks on a bleeding carcass. When LDL is not damaged, the macrophages leave it alone, but as soon as damage occurs, the macrophages zoom in and feed, gorging themselves until they're full, at which point they're called "foam cells." These foam cells group together and make a fatty streak, the first step in the formation of plaque.

How does the LDL get damaged in the first place? By two processes— *oxidation*, the interaction with oxygen that produces the same kind of "rusting" damage you see when you leave a cut apple out in the air; and *glycation*, bumping into sticky sugar. We just discussed how glycosylated proteins cause all sorts of damage in the body. This same process of glycation damages LDL, and damaged LDL attracts macrophages like red flags attract bulls.

So insulin increases the amount of LDL in the system, and excess sugar damages the LDL, leading ultimately to plaque. If this were not enough to increase your risk for heart disease, you're also going to have lowered levels of magnesium, a mineral that is absolutely essential for the health of the heart. Why is your magnesium level lowered? Because insulin, in addition to storing sugar and fat in the cells, is also responsible for storing magnesium, so when your cells become resistant to insulin, you lose the ability to store some of that magnesium. Magnesium relaxes muscles, including those in the arterial walls. When you can't store magnesium, you lose it and your blood vessels constrict, causing a further increase in blood pressure. The loss of magnesium can also lead to heart arrhythmia and other cardiac problems.[11] And because magnesium is required for virtually all energy production that takes place in the cells, you may also find yourself with lower energy to boot.

How Does a Low-Carb Diet Lower Your Risk of Heart Disease?

There are numerous ways in which a low-carb diet can significantly lower your risk for heart disease. Lowering your insulin levels is certainly one of the most important. Raising your HDL ("good" cholesterol) is another. A third—the importance of which it is difficult to overstate—is by lowering triglycerides. Researchers from the cardiovascular divisions of Brigham and Women's Hospital and Harvard Medical School, in a study led by J. Michael Gaziano, looked at various predictors for heart disease and found that the ratio of triglycerides to HDL was a better predictor for heart disease than anything else, *including* cholesterol levels. They divided the subjects into four groups according to their ratio of triglycerides to HDL and found that those with the highest ratio (i.e., high triglycerides to low HDL) had *a sixteen times greater risk of heart attack* than those with the lowest ratio (low triglycerides to high HDL).[12]

There's more. Most of us are familiar with "good" cholesterol (HDL) and "bad" cholesterol (LDL), but what is not as well known is that both types of cholesterol have subparts that behave very differently from one another. What *kind* of LDL you have turns out to be much more important than just the *amount* of LDL you have (several LDL-"particle tests" are now widely available to tell you what kind of LDL you have). For example, LDL cholesterol comes in two basic flavors: it can be a big, fluffy, cotton ball–like molecule (LDL-A type), or it can be more like a dense, tight, BB-gun pellet (LDL-B type). The big, fluffy LDL-As are pretty harmless. They are far less likely to become oxidized or damaged and cause problems. But the little LDL-Bs are a different story. Those are the ones that cause problems, and those are the ones you should be concerned about. The Gaziano study found that high triglycerides correlate strongly with high levels of the dangerous LDL-B particles, and low levels of triglycerides correlate with higher levels of the harmless LDL-As. In other words, the higher your triglycerides, the greater the chance that your LDL cholesterol is made up of the B-particles (the kind that is way more likely to lead to heart disease). The take-home point: reduce your triglycerides (and raise your HDL), and you reduce your risk of heart disease.

Insulin and Hypertension

As you saw in the previous paragraphs on heart disease, high levels of insulin can narrow the arterial walls which, in turn, will raise blood pressure, since a more forceful pumping action is required to get the blood through the narrower passageways. But there's an even more insidious way in which insulin raises blood pressure.

It talks to the kidneys.

Insulin's message to the kidneys is this: *hold on to salt*. Insulin makes the kidneys do this even if the kidneys would much prefer not to. Since sodium, like sugar, is controlled by the body within a very tight range, the kidneys figure, "Listen, if we have to hold on to all this salt, we'd better bring on more water to dilute it so that it stays in the safe range." And that's exactly what they do. Increased sodium retention results in increased water retention. More fluid means more blood volume, and more blood volume means higher blood pressure. Fully 50% of people with hypertension have insulin resistance.[13]

Insulin will also ultimately raise adrenaline, and adrenaline will raise both blood pressure and heart rate. We'll discuss the insulin–adrenaline axis a little more under the topic of obesity in the next section.

How Does a Low-Carb Diet Lower Your Risk of Hypertension?

Lowering insulin levels will intercept the message to the kidneys to hold on to salt. You will almost immediately lose water weight, and bloat and blood pressure will go down. Lowering insulin is actually such an effective strategy for lowering blood pressure that it sometimes works too well too fast. In rare cases, your blood pressure might dip too low, and you may experience lightheadedness or dizziness upon standing up. This is why some clinicians recommend increasing salty foods or adding a teaspoon of salt to your food on a daily basis if you find this happening to you.[14]

When the kidneys dump excess sodium, potassium sometimes gets caught in the crossfire and you wind up dumping potassium as well. This is even truer if you exercise and sweat a lot. You don't want to lose too much potassium, because that can cause muscle cramps, fatigue, and breathlessness. This is why I always recommend potassium supplements, especially during the first week of a low-carb diet, and particularly when you are on one of the very restricted carbohydrate plans such as the induction phase of Atkins or the first 2 weeks of Protein Power. Potassium supplements come in 99-milligram tablets, and you can get them at any drugstore or health-food store. Take one or two at each meal. Foods rich in potassium, such as liver, broccoli, and avocados, are also a good idea, as is using over-the-counter salt substitutes like Morton's Lite Salt or No Salt, which are both potassium salts.

Insulin and Obesity

The connection between a high-sugar diet, high levels of insulin, and becoming overweight or obese should be painfully obvious by now. The more sugar—i.e., carbohydrates—you take in, the more sugar you need to store and the more your insulin levels rise. The more your insulin levels rise, the less fat you burn and the more sugar you store in fat cells, along with those extra triglycerides that the liver made from excess sugar. The more you store, the fatter you get. The fatter you get, the more insulin-resistant you become.

When there are consistently high levels of insulin floating around, the body will put out more cortisol and adrenaline (the "breakdown" hormones) to counteract the "building-up" effects of insulin and attempt to bring the body back into balance. Cortisol in part breaks down muscle, further reducing your metabolic rate. Too much adrenaline can eventually lead to even *more* insulin, as insulin will eventually be secreted to combat the effects of too much adrenaline! The interaction of insulin and cortisol/adrenaline is the particular aspect of low-carbohydrate dieting central to the metabolic healing work of Diana Schwarzbein, who feels that this kind of constant imbalance—often brought on by yo-yo dieting, high levels of stress, and a diet high in sugar—ultimately damages the metabolism. If getting off this particular seesaw sounds interesting to you, be sure to read about the *Schwarzbein Principle* in chapter 9.

Even if you don't remember the basic biochemistry discussed here, tattoo the following on the inside of your eyelids: *insulin is the fat-storage hormone.* It is also the hunger hormone. When it finally does its job of lowering blood sugar, it causes blood sugar to go really low, setting you up for a cycle of craving (and eating) more high-carb foods. Result: higher blood sugar, more insulin, and more fat storage as the cycle continues.

How Does a Low-Carb Diet Help You Lose Weight?

When you eat a lower-carb diet, you stimulate less insulin but you also stimulate more glucagon, its sister hormone, which responds more to protein (remember that neither hormone is stimulated by fat). Glucagon liberates the fat from storage sites and gets it ready to burn for energy. Meanwhile, since you no longer have elevated levels of insulin, you are not suppressing carnitine, which, you may remember, is the compound in the body responsible for escorting fat into the central furnaces of the cells, where it can be burned for fuel.

Along with insulin and glucagon, a pair of enzymes plays a major role in the whole fat-storage/fat-release equation: *lipoprotein lipase* and *hormone-sensitive lipase*. Lipoprotein lipase is responsible for storing fats: it breaks down triglycerides in the bloodstream and shoves the fatty-acid parts into fat cells. People who are trying to lose weight are not fond of this enzyme. It's very persistent; in fact, when people lose weight, the activity of lipoprotein lipase is ramped up, almost as if the body is fighting to hold on to fat. This is one of the reasons it's so difficult to keep weight off. (Lipoprotein lipase is also suppressed when you smoke and increases when you stop smoking, one of the reasons people usually put on a few pounds when they first give up cigarettes.)

Hormone-sensitive lipase, on the other hand, reaches into fat cells and releases fatty acids into the bloodstream when they are needed—for example, if you're doing a long aerobic exercise session and your legs need some fuel. Its ability to liberate fat is really intense. Consider this: there's a protein called *perilipin* that shields fat from the fat-burning effects of hormone-sensitive lipase. Mice that don't have any perilipin to protect their fat from hormone-sensitive lipase don't get fat no matter what they eat![15] The fat-burning effect of hormone-sensitive lipase is that intense.

Insulin and glucagon have profound effects on both lipoprotein lipase and hormone-sensitive lipase. Can you guess what effects they have? By now it should come as no surprise: insulin *stimulates* lipoprotein lipase (the fat-storing enzyme) and *inhibits* hormone-sensitive lipase (the fat-releasing enzyme). If you want your fat cells to let go of fat, you want all the hormone-sensitive lipase activity you can scrounge up—you certainly don't need high levels of insulin turning down the volume. Glucagon, on the other hand, has exactly the opposite effect on these enzymes. It *inhibits* the fat-storing enzyme and *stimulates* the fat-releasing one. This is just one more way that restoring a healthy balance between insulin and glucagon helps you to lose weight.

Fat Cells Know How to Protect Their Existence!

When you do lose weight, you stack the hormonal deck in your favor even more. We used to believe that fat cells were these inert little sacks of blubber that basically didn't do anything metabolically—they just took up space and held on to a gazillion calories' worth of energy that never got burned up fast enough. We now know that fat cells are anything *but* inactive. They are actually endocrine glands that releases a host of hormones—including estrogen—and other substances that can have a profound effect on our weight.

Many of the hormones that are released by the fat cells have one major purpose—to keep those fat cells in business! In this way, you might say that fat actually perpetuates its own existence by releasing hormones that make it harder for the body to get rid of it.

One of the hormones released by fat cells is *resistin*. The more fat cells you have, the more resistin gets released into your body. Mice given extra dosages of resistin develop insulin resistance in 2 days;[16] and, as we've just seen, insulin resistance is a major obstacle to fat loss. Another substance released by the fat cells is TNF-alpha 1, also known as tumor necrosis factor. This is a good guy, at least some of the time: it's part of the immune system's arsenal, and as you can tell by the name, it's involved in destroying tumors. But TNF-alpha 1 is also found in fat tissue, and in the circulatory system it appears to act like a hormone. In low amounts, it *inhibits* the ability of insulin to lower blood sugar, essentially making insulin's job harder to accomplish and thereby forcing the pancreas to put out even more insulin to get the job done.[17] Once again, a hormone-like compound released by the fat cells raises insulin and makes fat loss difficult. As you can see, the fat cells *themselves* contribute to the difficulty in losing weight by releasing substances that offer "fat-protection insurance"—chemicals that, in essence, help your fat cells stay in business. By lowering your fat stores with a low-carbohydrate diet, you will also lower the amounts of these fat-protecting substances in the bloodstream.

A Low-Carb Diet Helps Reduce Insulin Resistance

When you are insulin-resistant, your cells stop making insulin receptors to import sugar and fat into the cells. This process is called down-regulation. Receptors are like job recruiters. When the market is flooded with unemployed workers, companies don't have to go hunting for job applicants because there are so many knocking at the door. When you're insulin-resistant, you've got a hell of a lot of insulin—applicants—knocking at the cell door. The cells figure there's enough insulin hanging around, beating on the doors, so they stop sending out "recruiters" to the surface of the cells. When you bring your insulin down with a low-carb diet, suddenly there's not so much insulin banging at the doors of the cells. Now you begin to lose weight. Eventually, the cells start to send up more receptors to bring in the fuel, a process called up-regulation. The cells are now gradually becoming more insulin-*sensitive*—a condition you most decidedly want. Insulin sensitivity always improves when you lose weight.

There are other ways in which a low-carb lifestyle will help you lose weight. One way has to do specifically with protein itself, which is usually more plentiful on lower-carb diets. Protein has less of an effect on insulin, has a greater effect on glucagon, and increases metabolic rate considerably more than carbohydrates do. Specific amino acids found in protein may also play a role in weight loss. Several papers by D.K. Layman demonstrated greater body-fat loss on a high-protein diet than on a high-carb diet,[18] and in one paper he argued that *leucine*—an amino acid—may be one of the reasons.[19] Other studies have also suggested the possible role of specific amino acids in weight loss. In one animal study, a diet deficient in the amino acid lysine resulted in the accumulation of larger amounts of fat both in the bodies of the animals and in their livers.[20] Increasing the proportion of protein to carbohydrates appears to be more *satiating* during weight loss—it makes you feel fuller.[21] And metabolic rate, technically called thermogenesis— the heat production in our bodies from burning calories—is turned up after eating protein. In one study, thermogenesis was 100% higher with high-protein meals—even 2½ hours after eating—in young, healthy women.[22]

You may have heard that it is easier to stay on a low-carb diet than it is to stay on a traditional high-carb, low-fat diet. Let me say one word about that: *appetite.* A low-carb diet contains built-in appetite controls—it's like having your own little diet pill built into the meals. Here's how it works. One of the major hormones involved in telling the brain that you are full is *cholecystokinin* (CCK), which is secreted in the intestines in response to a meal. (You may have also heard, correctly, that it takes about 20 minutes for this hormone to reach your brain and tell you you've had enough—another reason to listen to your grandmother and eat slowly if you want to lose weight!) But here's the thing: CCK, being part of our ancient digestive system, recognizes protein and fat very well because they've been the mainstay of our diet for as long as the human genus has been on the planet. But CCK does *not* respond very well to carbohydrates. It barely recognizes them! That's why it is so easy to overeat carbs—you really have no idea when you've had enough.

Insulin Resistance and Diabetes

Insulin resistance is a huge risk factor for the development of both heart disease and diabetes.[23] Eighty percent of the 16 to 17 million Americans who have diabetes are insulin-resistant.[24] Dr. David Leonardi, founder of the Leonardi Medical Institute for Vitality and Longevity in Denver, insists that insulin resistance is reversible and that many type 2 diabetics can be cured. He says: "Diabetics die from *diabetes complications, all of which are a direct or indirect result of high blood sugar.* Normalizing the blood sugar prevents disease, normalizes life expectancy, and profoundly enhances quality of life. Cured or not, they're winners either way."

In case you hadn't noticed by now, low-carb diets are all about normalizing blood sugar. Insulin resistance *is* reversible. And it's hardly a rare phenomenon. The prevalence of insulin resistance has skyrocketed 61% in the last decade alone, according to Daniel Einhorn, MD, cochair of the AACE Insulin Resistance Syndrome Task Force and medical director of the Scripps Whittier Institute for Diabetes.[25] In fact, the prevalence of insulin resistance has probably been underestimated from the beginning. Gerald Reaven of Stanford University did the original work on insulin resistance in the 1980s. Here's how he approximated the number of people who were insulin-resistant: He divided his test population—nondiabetic, healthy adults—into quartiles and tested their ability to metabolize sugar and carbohydrates. He found that while the top 25% of the population could handle sugar just fine, the bottom 25% could not—they had insulin resistance (or, in the parlance of researchers, impaired glucose metabolism). So for a long time, it was thought that the number of people with insulin resistance was one in four.

DIABETES AND COMPLICATIONS

- *80 percent of diabetics are insulin-resistant.*

- *2,200 people are newly diagnosed each day.*

- *Diabetes is the seventh leading cause of death in the United States.*

- *60–70 percent of diabetics have mild to severe forms of nerve damage.*

- *Diabetes is the leading cause of lower-extremity amputations in the United States.*

- *86,000 amputations a year are related to complications from diabetes.*

- *The five-year mortality rate after amputation is 39–68 percent.*

- *Diabetics are two to four times more likely to have heart disease.*

- *Heart disease is present in 75 percent of diabetes-related deaths.*

- *Diabetes is the leading cause of new cases of kidney disease.*

- *Diabetes is the leading cause of new cases of blindness in adults.*

But there's a problem.

What happened to the 50% of the people *between* those two extremes? It turns out they had neither the terrific glucose metabolism of the top 25% nor the full-blown insulin resistance of the bottom 25%; instead, they fell somewhere in between. One could easily argue that since only 25% of the population had flawless glucose metabolism, the rest of us—up to 75% of the population—have *some* degree of insulin resistance! Remember, too, that Reaven used young, healthy adults as subjects, and their numbers are definitely not representative of the population as a whole—the fact is, insulin sensitivity actually decreases as you get older. The take-home point: insulin resistance isn't just something that happens to other people. Recently, the American Association of Clinical Endocrinologists estimated that one in three Americans is insulin-resistant.[26]

As of 2011, there are approximately 26 million diabetics in the United

States, of which 7 million are not yet diagnosed.[27] Approximately 80% of them are insulin-resistant. Even if you are insulin-resistant and somehow manage to dodge the diabetes bullet, you are still at serious risk for heart disease. Being overweight (having a body mass index of greater than 25 or a waistline of greater than 40 inches for men and 35 inches for women) is a risk factor for insulin resistance—a big one. So are hypertension (high blood pressure), elevated triglycerides, and low-HDL cholesterol.[28] It's estimated that 47 million Americans have some combination of these risk factors.[29] As you have seen in this chapter, all of them are related to insulin, and virtually *all of them improve substantially on a low-carbohydrate diet.*

How a Low-Carb Diet May Help Prevent—or Even Reverse—Diabetes

Dietary treatment for diabetes is currently one of the hottest topics of debate in the diabetes community.[30] Some factions are passionately holding on to the old recommendations of a high-carb diet, while other clinicians are making strenuous arguments for lower-carb, higher-fat, higher-protein diets.[31] The precise dietary treatment for full-blown type 2 diabetes is beyond the scope of this book, though it is a fascinating subject and in my opinion has great relevance for nondiabetics as well. What can we say for sure? A number of studies have shown that people on low-carbohydrate diets experience increased glucose control, reduced insulin resistance, weight reduction, lowered triglycerides, and improved cholesterol.

Excess Insulin and PCOS

One in ten women has polycystic ovary syndrome (PCOS), the most common reproductive abnormality in premenopausal women, which puts them at high risk for both cardiovascular disease and diabetes.[32] One of the major biochemical features of PCOS is the combination of insulin resistance and hyperinsulinemia (elevated insulin levels). The ability of obese women with PCOS to use glucose is significantly impaired, and they have a marked reduction in insulin sensitivity.[33]

When we talk about insulin resistance, we often forget that not all tissues and cells become resistant at the same time, and some do not become resistant at all. For example, overweight people may—at least in the beginning—have very nonresistant fat cells. Their muscle cells refuse to take any more sugar, but the fat cells still have open arms. These cells are said to be insulin-sensitive. The ovaries also tend to remain insulin-sensitive.

LOW-GLYCEMIC DIET AND DIABETES

Low-glycemic foods—beans, peas, lentils, pasta, rice boiled briefly, and breads like pumpernickel and flaxseed—do a better job of managing glycemic control for type 2 diabetes and risk factors for coronary heart disease than diets based around the "traditional" high-fiber foods such as whole-grain breads, crackers, and breakfast cereals.

That's the finding of a 2008 study published in the *Journal of the American Medical Assocation.*[*]

Although the American Dietetic Association continues to mindlessly parrot the "conventional" wisdom about whole-grain breads and cereals, the truth is that most of these whole-grain products are fiber lightweights. (Read the label—whole grains typically offer 1–2 grams of fiber at best, compared to 11–17 in a cup of beans.) And if you check the glycemic index/glycemic load tables, you find that the difference between a processed grain like white rice and its whole-grain counterpart (brown rice) is—from a *blood-sugar* point of view—almost negligible.

Obviously, whole grains are better than white junk, but only because they contain slightly more vitamins and other nutrients. From a blood-sugar—and from a food-sensitivity or allergy—standpoint, they're not that much of an improvement. If you've got a gluten sensitivity—which is way more common than you might think—whole grains will be just as much a problem for you as the processed kind.

In the JAMA study, researchers found that hemoglobin A1c—a very important marker for diabetes—decreased *significantly* more in subjects on the low-glycemic diet than it did for people eating the "traditional high-fiber" choices with cereal fiber. The low-glycemic group also saw a significant *increase* in HDL (the so-called "good" cholesterol) as well as a significant *reduction* in LDL (the so-called "bad" cholesterol).

The low-glycemic diet group did eat some breads—like pumpernickel, rye pita, and quinoa bread with flaxseed—and some cereals—like real oatmeal—but they were all low-glycemic.

Bottom line: just because a cereal or bread product says "made with whole grains" *doesn't* mean it's the best food for you. Many of these products raise your blood sugar to a level that is way too high, and manufacturers are notorious at trading on the "whole grain" buzz to

*David J. Jenkins, Cyril W. Kendall, Gail McKeown-Eyssen, et al., "Effect of a low-glycemic index or a high-cereal fiber diet on type 2 diabetes." *Journal of the American Medical Association* 300 (2008): 2742–2753.

LOW-GLYCEMIC DIET AND DIABETES (CONTINUED)

create ridiculous products like "whole grain Cocoa Captain Sugar Krispies" (I made that one up, but you get the point).

Glycemic impact is very important and should be paid attention to by anyone interested in his or her health. And you don't have to walk around with a bunch of scientific formulas to figure out whether a food has high or low glycemic impact: just look for foods that have minimal processing, maximum color (the exception is oatmeal and cauliflower), and as much fiber as possible.

If there's a genetic predisposition for these glands to overproduce andro-gen hormones—as there is with women who have PCOS—the excess insulin that's sent into the bloodstream to deal with the excess sugar bathes these nonresistant tissues in an ocean of insulin that is way too much for their needs. One of the responses to all that insulin hitting the ovaries is that they produce even more testosterone and androstene, which leads to hair loss, acne, obesity, infertility, and other symptoms of PCOS.

Interestingly, those affected with PCOS often have relatives with adult onset diabetes, obesity, elevated triglycerides, and high blood pressure.[34] Sound familiar? This is why a low-carb diet is the dietary treatment of choice for PCOS. It's a common enough problem that many of the community bulletin boards on the low-carb sites listed in the Resources section have specific areas for PCOS.

Excess Insulin and Inflammation

Essential fatty acids, notably members of the omega-6 and omega-3 family, are the parent molecules for an entirely different group of fascinating hormones called *eicosanoids*. Eicosanoids, also known as *prostaglandins*, live in the body for only seconds and act on the cells that are in their immediate vicinity—they don't travel in the bloodstream. They are very, very powerful modulators of human health. Like many other systems in the body, they need to be in balance. Sometimes, as a shorthand, we'll talk about "good" eicosanoids (the prostaglandin 1 series, or PG1), which inhibit clotting, promote vasodilation (the relaxing of the blood vessels), stimulate the immune response, and are anti-inflammatory, versus the "bad" eicosanoids (the prostaglandin 2 series, or PG2), which have the opposite effects, pro-moting clotting, constriction, and inflammation. But this shorthand is not completely accurate, as you need a *balance* of the two. For example, if you clot too much and too easily, you can have a stroke, but if you didn't clot at all, you'd bleed to death from a hemorrhage!

Here, too, insulin leaves its mighty footprint. Insulin inhibits a critical enzyme called *delta-6-desaturase*, which is responsible for directing traffic into the production line for the "good," anti-inflammatory eicosanoids. Inflammation has been implicated in a host of conditions, from heart disease to Alzheimer's to arthritis to food allergies. In fact, the modulation of insulin for the purpose of controlling eicosanoid production and reducing the risk of heart disease was the major reason for the development of the Zone diet by Barry Sears. If you're interested in learning more about this diet, be sure to read about it in chapter 9.

Excess Insulin and Aging

"If there is a single marker for life span," asserts Dr. Ron Rosedale, author of The Rosedale Diet (see chapter 9), "it's insulin sensitivity."[35] He's right. In 1992, researchers collected data on people who were both mentally and physically fit and were at least 100 years old. The researchers looked carefully to find the factors these folks might have in common, the ones that could be predictors for a long and healthy life. They came up with three. The first was low triglycerides. The second was high-HDL cholesterol. Can you guess the third? A low level of fasting insulin![36] You've learned in this chapter how a lower-carbohydrate diet almost always improves all three of these variables. Since this kind of diet is what our ancestors ate for eons, it makes sense that we would live the longest and stay the healthiest by adhering to it.

By the way, the only dietary strategy shown to actually *increase* life span in laboratory animals has been calorie restriction. When we humans try calorie restriction on a standard high-carb, low-fat diet, we generally hate it—we're hungry all the time. With a diet higher in protein, higher in fat, and lower in carbohydrates—and high in fiber—we're more satiated and our appetite is much more under control. Insulin—the hunger hormone— is no longer out of control, blood sugar is manageable, and weight becomes stabilized. We can actually wind up eating fewer calories and feeling more satisfied in the bargain. That's a recipe for an antiaging, health-producing diet *without* creating cravings or hunger pangs.

Senior Moment? Maybe It's Your Blood Sugar!

Is the phrase "I'm having one of those senior moments" becoming an increasingly common utterance?

Research suggests that it might be related to your sugar levels.

The research, published in the December 2008 Annals of Neurology,* focused on a particular section of the hippocampus—an area of the brain associated with memory and learning. This section—the *dentate gyrus*—is typically affected by changes seen with aging.

"In this study, we were able to show the specific area of the brain that is impacted by rising blood sugar," said Scott Small, MD, the lead researcher on the study, which was partly funded by the National Institute on Aging. Using special high-resolution brain imaging, Small and his team found that rising blood sugar was directly associated with decreased activity in the dentate gyrus.

The result: you forget where you put your keys!

The important point here is that the research strongly suggests that keeping blood sugar under control could be the key to preventing "senior moments" and lapses in memory, even in healthy individuals with no hint of diabetes!

"Our findings suggest that maintaining blood sugar levels, even in the absence of diabetes, could help maintain aspects of cognitive health," said Small.

Two of the most effective measures to manage blood sugar are exercise and a controlled-carb diet!

*S. A. Small, *Annals of Neurology*, December 2008; online edition.

Switching to a Fat-Burning Metabolism: The Meaning of Ketosis

When you go on a low-carbohydrate diet, you restrict the amount of sugar coming into your system. That's a good thing. But what happens when there's a severely reduced amount of sugar coming down the pike? What does the body use for fuel?

The body does have basic glucose (sugar) requirements. The brain, for example, needs about 150 to 200 grams of glucose daily. If you're eating only about 20 grams of carbs a day—probably the lowest amount you would consume on the first phase of the strictest diets—where does the other 130 to 180 grams of glucose come from? Equally important, where does the body get the rest of the fuel it needs for its many other metabolic activities, such as exercise and breathing?

Well, the body gets sugar from a process called *gluconeogenesis*, a word that literally means "the creation of new sugar." Gluconeogenesis is a metabolic process by which sugar is created from *noncarbohydrate* sources. For example, the body will make sugar by using the glycerol molecule in triglycerides (making sugar from fat). It will also make some sugar from protein (e.g., from certain amino acids). And here's the really good news for the overweight person: if carbohydrates in the diet are sufficiently limited, the majority of the fuel the body needs for its day-to-day operations will come from fat, specifically from a breakdown product of fat called *ketones.*

The body loves ketones. The heart works fine on them, and so does the brain. Here's how they work. Fats are oxidized, or broken down, by a process called beta-oxidation, in which the long chain of carbons that constitutes a fatty acid is split into pairs of two carbon molecules each, called acetyl fragments. These acetyl fragments join with a compound called CoA (coenzyme A) to form the appropriately named acetyl CoA. Incidentally, acetyl CoA is also the end product of the breakdown of carbohydrates, so both carbohydrates and fats eventually wind up as acetyl CoA.

When there are enough carbs in the pipeline, the acetyl CoA do-si-dos into something called the Krebs cycle, in which the acetyl CoA is burned for energy. But if there's not enough sugar, acetyl CoA doesn't get its all-access pass into the Krebs cycle. Instead, it accumulates at the door and eventually turns into three ketone bodies (first acetoacetic acid, then beta-hydroxybutyric acid and acetone, for the science-minded among you). Most of these ketone bodies are sent to the tissues—including the heart and brain—to be used for energy, and some are excreted in the urine and breath. This is what the low-carb diets that stress ketosis are talking about when they speak of changing from a sugar-burning metabolism to a fat-burning metabolism. Ketones are the by-product of fat breakdown.

Ketosis—which happens when there are enough of these ketones to be detectable in the urine—is a topic of such misunderstanding, controversy, and criticism that it will get a much fuller discussion later on. For now, let's just say that this process is a part of normal metabolism and is not—I repeat, *not*—dangerous.

Ketosis is *not necessary* for weight loss. You could be in ketosis and not lose weight, just as you could lose weight without being in ketosis. You won't burn your stored fat (and the ketone bodies made from it) if you have a surplus of fuel coming into the pipeline from the food you're eating. If you're eating 10,000 calories of fat and no carbs, you'll definitely be producing a ton of ketones but you won't lose a pound. However, if you are eating a moderate number of calories *and* you are in ketosis, it is a good sign that you are burning fat and not sugar as your primary energy source.

If you switch to a higher-fat, higher-protein, lower-carb (and higher-fiber!) diet, you won't have enough sugar coming in to burn as fuel, and your body will have to make its own, mostly from fat and certain amino acids, and/or happily use ketones as fuel. If calories are at reasonable levels at this point—which they probably will be because you'll be a lot less hungry and have a lot fewer cravings—you will lose weight. You will also improve your blood-lipid profiles (lower triglycerides, higher HDL) *and* your insulin sensitivity. Not only will you get slimmer, but your risk for heart disease, diabetes, and hypertension will plummet.

Not a bad deal, right?

How a Low-Carb Diet Keeps You Healthy and Slim

We've talked about what sugar does to the body and why eliminating it is such a good idea. Obviously, a low-carb diet removes a great deal, if not all, of the refined sugar you've probably been eating. The health benefits of this reduction are enormous. But a low-carb diet can also remove three other substances that are a huge problem, albeit for very different reasons. One is trans-fats. The other two are wheat and fructose. (The latter two are discussed at length in chapter 4).

The subject of trans-fatty acids is one of the hottest topics in nutrition today and has been the center of a great deal of debate in the area of public policy regarding food and food labeling. It has been discussed extensively elsewhere, particularly in the writings of Dr. Mary Enig, a lipid biochemist widely considered to be the leading authority on trans-fats in the country, if not the world. For now, let's just say that in the opinion of many experts, saturated fats have gotten a raw deal and have in fact been blamed for damage done, for the most part, by trans-fats. We know that trans-fats raise LDL cholesterol, probably way more than saturated fats do, and that these damaged trans-fats actually *increase* the risk for type 2 diabetes.[37] They also lower HDL cholesterol and raise the risk for heart disease. A prediction was made in the prestigious medical journal *Lancet* as far back as 1994 that trans-fats would turn out to be a major factor in insulin resistance;[38] that was the same year that the Center for Science in the Public Interest petitioned the FDA to require that Nutrition Facts labels disclose amounts of trans-fat. On July 10, 2002, the National Academy of Science's Institute of Medicine issued a report that concluded that "the only safe intake of trans-fats is

> *After learning of the dangers of trans-fats, I began avoiding fast-food lunches—it's better for me and my kids.*
>
> *—Gina D.*

zero." After much hemming, hawing, and stalling, the FDA finally mandated that trans-fat content be listed on food nutrition labels, a ruling that went into effect in 2006.

The intelligent low-carb diet is almost *always* naturally low in trans-fats, which may be one of the many reasons it can impart such health benefits. Consider this: the top sources of trans-fats are baked goods, muffins, cakes, cookies, doughnuts, granolas, crackers, pies, fast food, french fries, anything deep-fried, partially hydrogenated vegetable oils, and most margarines. The intelligent low-carb diet naturally contains almost none of these foods, or if it does, they are present in extraordinarily low amounts. The health benefits of this restriction alone are incalculable.

The other ingredient that is either missing in action or has an extremely low profile on the low-carb diet is wheat. Now, most people are probably under the impression that wheat and grains are "good" for you. Maybe; maybe not. Certainly, foods made with whole grains—which are far harder to find than you might think and most certainly do *not* include most commercially available "wheat breads"—are better than foods made with the refined grains that constitute the vast majority of grains we eat. But grains, particularly wheat, have a high propensity for turning into sugar quickly, and wheat is also one of the foods most likely to be implicated in food sensitivities.[39] At one point, it was believed that celiac disease—an intolerance of gluten, which is found in most grains—was fairly rare, affecting only 1 in 1,700 people. Estimates are now running closer to 1 in 133; for those who have a parent, sibling, or child with celiac, the estimates are 1 in 22![40] And this doesn't include the hard-to-estimate number of people who have delayed food sensitivities, very often to grains in general or, at the very least, to wheat. A 2002 book by clinician James Braly, MD, suggests that gluten insensitivity may affect tens of millions of Americans.[41]

Dr. Joseph Mercola, medical director of the Optimal Wellness Center in Illinois, contends that grains—along with starches and sweets—trigger a "hormonal cycle of grain and sugar addiction, weight gain, and diabetes."[42]

And numerous studies link carbohydrates that have a high glycemic load—the tendency to turn into sugar quickly—with increased risk of coronary heart disease[43] and with risk of type 2 diabetes.[44] Most high-glycemic processed grains fall into this category, but these grains are virtually eliminated on low-carbohydrate diets.

Insulin: The Smoking Gun

Controlling insulin is the number one priority of all low-carb diets. The dietary approaches discussed in chapter 5 differ only in how they go about accomplishing it—what degree of carbohydrate restriction they believe is necessary to successfully control insulin, whether they emphasize protein or fat (or both) in the diet, what kinds of fat they recommend, other aspects of metabolism they stress, and whether they include a component on emotional eating and holistic self-care.

Once you understand what runaway insulin levels and unregulated sugar metabolism in general can do to your health, it's easy to understand why correcting those imbalances brings about not only weight loss but a myriad of wonderful health benefits.

In chapter 9, we'll explore exactly how a number of popular diet plans approach the issue of insulin control, and you'll be able to determine which one is best for you. But first, let's talk a little more about wheat and fructose. Then we'll dispel a few myths about fat, cholesterol and health.

HORMONES AND WEIGHT: A SHORT GUIDE TO THE PLAYERS

Insulin: *lowers blood sugar*
Also known as "the fat-storage hormone," insulin is secreted by the pancreas in response to elevated blood sugar. Its job is to escort the excess sugar into the muscles, where it can be burned for fuel. High levels of insulin effectively "lock" the doors to the fat cells by blocking glucagon (described next), whose job it is to open the fat cells and allow fatty acids to enter the bloodstream.

Glucagon: *raises blood sugar*
Like insulin, glucagon is secreted by the pancreas. But, unlike insulin, it's

secreted in response to low blood sugar, and it has an opposite effect—it raises blood sugar instead of lowering it. Sensing that blood sugar is low, glucagon prompts the release of sugar (glucose) from the liver as well as the release of free fatty acids from fat stores. Glucagon is stimulated by decreased blood sugar (hunger); it's inhibited by high levels of insulin.

Leptin: *tells the brain you're full*
Leptin is a hormone produced by the fat cells in the body. When things are working as they should, leptin travels to the brain while you are finishing up your meal, where it sends a message that the body is full and it's time to stop eating. In this way, it's essential to appetite regulation and plays a major part in minimizing the desire for food. Scientists originally believed that obese people simply didn't produce enough leptin, but research in the '90s showed that this wasn't the case at all. Obese people make plenty of leptin, but their brains aren't getting the message to stop eating. The leptin is there, but the brain cells are simply not "listening."In a very real sense, they have become leptin-resistant. High-carb diets, fructose, high triglycerides, and inflammation all contribute to leptin resistance.

Cortisol: *puts fat around the middle*
Cortisol is the main "stress" hormone produced by the body. It's a crucial hormone and necessary for survival. But high levels of cortisol—produced by chronic stress, intense physical activity, and sleep deprivation—prompt the body to store fat around the middle, even in relatively lean people. Cortisol also breaks down muscle, raises blood sugar, and increases insulin-resistance.

Resistin: *makes you more insulin-resistant*
Resistin is a hormone produced by the fat cells. It gets its name from the fact that it helps cause the condition known as "insulin resistance," which is a key player in obesity and diabetes. Insulin resistance is the name for the condition in which the cells have stopped "listening" to insulin, resulting in higher levels of blood sugar and insulin (both very bad news if you're trying to lose weight). Resistin is one of the ways fat cells protect their own existence. The more fat cells you have, the more resistin is produced, the more insulin-resistant you become, and the harder it is to lose weight.

Adiponectin: *makes you less insulin-resistant*
Adiponectin makes the cells more sensitive to insulin (i.e., it reduces insulin resistance). It's secreted by the fat cells. Low levels of it are found in

people who are obese; high levels are associated with a reduced risk of heart attack and type 2 diabetes.

Ghrelin: *makes you hungry*

Ghrelin, also known as "the hunger hormone," is an appetite stimulant. When we're hungry, ghrelin levels go up. They also go up when we're stressed or sleep-deprived. This is one reason why sleep disturbance often leads to overeating and why you'll eat anything in sight after pulling an all-nighter.

Neuropeptide Y (NPY): *makes you hungry*

Neuropeptide Y stimulates appetite, especially for carbohydrates, and is elevated by chronic stress, low protein intake, and high-carb diets.

Peptide YY (PYY): *makes you stop eating*

This hormone sends a message to the brain that says "stop eating." Protein stimulates a lot of PYY; carbs release very little. (This is why your bagel breakfast leaves you starving at 11 A.M.) PYY also improves sensitivity to leptin.

Glucagon-like peptide-1 (GLP-1): *makes you stop eating*

This hormone's message is similar to that of leptin (see previous entry). It sends a message to the brain that says "stop eating." It is released by the small intestine after you eat. GLP-1 levels are inversely correlated with body mass, meaning higher levels are associated with less body fat. Meals with a lower glycemic index (fewer carbs, more fat, and protein) seem to increase GLP-1.

Cholecystokinin (CCK): *makes you stop eating*

A gut hormone that tells the brain you're full. Levels go much higher after a high-fat meal than after a low-fat, high-carb meal, one reason why it's so easy to eat six bowls of cereal and not so easy to eat six marbled steaks.

CHAPTER 4

The Major Culprits in a High-Carb Diet: Wheat and Fructose

I f you're like most people, you've come to investigate low-carb diets because of a noticeable and visible concern: your body. You've read—or seen for yourself—that low-carb diets are effective for weight loss. That's probably the reason you picked up this book in the first place: to find a solution to a problem that's causing you pain. It's a problem you'd understandably like to solve.

When I first got involved in low-carb—certainly when I wrote the original edition of this book—that was really all I was concerned about as well. My mission was to debunk the myths about low-carbing and to show people how low-carb could be an effective and safe weight-loss strategy.

Which it is.

But over the years, the evidence has mounted that low-carb diets offer a heck of a lot more than that.

Lucky to Be Fat?

So many people are attracted to a low-carb approach because of a concern with their weight. Or they have some visible, noticeable health issue that they'd like to address immediately. If this sounds like you, you've come to the right place. I'd like to suggest that if you're reading this book to solve an immediate, pressing problem like being overweight, you are "lucky," and here's why.

You're lucky in the sense that your problem has caused you to seek out a solution, and that *very solution* may actually help you avoid an awful lot of problems down the road that may have flown under the radar for you. These problems—like high blood pressure, high triglycerides, and insulin resistance—might very well have *remained* under the radar right up until the point at which they began to cause serious (and perhaps even fatal) damage.

See, unlike being overweight, most of the conditions mentioned above don't have any real noticeable symptoms. High blood pressure certainly doesn't. Nor, really, does diabetes, at least not at first. High triglycerides is another condition that produces exactly zero symptoms or discomfort, even though it puts you at serious risk for heart disease. (Triglycerides drop like a rock on a low-carb diet.) You can walk around with full-blown heart disease without a single clue. Sadly, for many people, the first symptom of heart disease is sudden death. (Many risk markers for heart disease improve dramatically on a low-carb diet.)

You can't, however, be unaware of your own fat.

It's pretty easy to ignore some very important indicators of health, especially when they don't hurt and they're not "in our face" all the time. We're not constantly reminded of our triglycerides or blood pressure every time we look in the mirror. After trying to put on a pair of too-tight pants, we don't often find ourselves saying, "Note to self: today I *really* need to start doing something about my HDL cholesterol levels."

But we *do* look in the mirror and say, "I've *got* to do something about my weight."

Which is why I made the statement that being overweight makes you— in a very real sense—lucky.

You're lucky in the same way that a person who has a fire in her basement is lucky she has a smoke detector. Without the smoke alarm, the fire would burn unattended and, left alone, might actually inciner- ate the house. The alarm is a loud, annoying, pressing reminder that something is wrong and that someone better do something about it. The smoke alarm won't put out the fire, but it *will* call your attention to it in time for you to prevent your whole house from turning into a pile of smoldering ash.

Your fat is your smoke detector. It got you to pay attention. Which got you to this book. Congratulations on your new life!

Everything Is Related

Even a cursory glance at the copious amount of research on obesity shows that a number of diseases of civilization, including heart disease and diabetes, all overlap, so much so that it is almost difficult to talk about them as discrete entities. Hundreds of research papers that discuss obesity *also* touch on risk factors like high blood pressure, high triglycerides, abdominal fat, and uncontrolled blood sugar—all factors that are usually shared with heart disease and diabetes. Some of these risk factors cluster together so often that they have their own name: *metabolic syndrome*, also known as prediabetes.

Being overweight or obese puts you at much higher risk for metabolic syndrome, which is one of the fastest growing obesity-related health concerns in the United States.[1] According to the National Heart, Lung, and Blood Institute, a person who has metabolic syndrome is twice as likely to develop heart disease and a whopping five times more likely to develop diabetes than someone who doesn't have metabolic syndrome.[2] Having metabolic syndrome increases the risk of *dying* from heart disease by an incredible 74%![3]

Then there's diabetes. Almost 80% of diabetics are also overweight or obese,[4] and while being overweight or obese doesn't *always* lead to diabetes, it certainly puts you much more at risk. And diabetes and heart disease themselves are hardly strangers. Diabetics are twice as likely as nondiabetics to have heart disease or strokes,[5] and, as of September 2011, almost 26 million people in the United States alone have it, with about 2 million new cases a year being added to the list.[6] Hypertension (high blood pressure) is twice as common in adults who are obese,[7] and hypertension is a major risk for heart disease[8] as well as one of the hallmarks of metabolic syndrome.

Then there's the connection between weight and heart disease. A 2007 study in the Archives of Internal Medicine found that—completely independent of other risk factors like high blood pressure—being overweight increases the risk for cardiovascular disease by 17%, while being obese increases the risk by a whopping 40%![9]

Beginning to get the picture? These "diseases of civilization"—obesity, diabetes, hypertension, metabolic syndrome—are so intimately connected it's almost hard to talk about one without referencing the others. Living low-carb may be the solution to your extra padding, but it may *also* turn out to be the solution to heart disease and diabetes. The foods you wind up eliminating from your diet when you go low-carb are turning out to be powerful promoters of these diseases of civilization in ways that are only now beginning to be discovered.

We'll take a closer look at two of those foods in particular—wheat and fructose—in just a moment. But first let's talk a little more about the connection between carbs, appetite, fat cells, and health.

Your Fat Cells Don't Just Sit There

One of the biggest discoveries in recent years, at least in the area of fat metabolism, is that fat cells don't just sit there on your hips annoying the heck out of you. We all thought fat cells were just these little inert sponges of greasy stuff accumulating in all the places you didn't want them to accumulate, staying fat and jolly and sedentary until you somehow figured out how to get rid of them.

Nope.

Fat cells are busy little beavers.

We now know that fat cells behave more like endocrine glands. They secrete hormones—lots of them. They have names like *leptin, resistin, adiponectin,* and *ghrelin.* Some of those hormones protect fat cells themselves from extinction (like resistin, for example). Some are involved in appetite (leptin, ghrelin). The fat cells also secrete inflammatory chemicals called *cytokines,* which include *interleukin-6* and *tumor necrosis factor-alpha,* both of which contribute to the inflammation increasingly seen in obesity, diabetes, heart disease, Alzheimer's disease, and virtually every degenerative disease known to humankind.[10]

So your fat—your "smoke detector," if you will—may have brought you to this book, and you may be reading it with one specific goal: to lose weight and keep it off. But the fact is that by addressing that pressing, obvious problem—the one that painfully calls attention to itself every time you glance in the mirror—you will *also* be decreasing your risk for heart disease, diabetes, metabolic syndrome, and hypertension. Not least of all, you'll be reducing inflammation, which is turning out to be a much greater contributor to disease than anyone ever suspected, and which is turbocharged by the very fat cells you're trying to get rid of.

For you, the most important part of low-carb may be that it gives you the best chance of looking decent in a bathing suit. But in fact, that lower-carb diet will provide you with a range of health benefits you probably didn't even think about, including a dramatic decrease in your risk of developing cancer and heart disease.

See, all carbs are not created equal. "Carbohydrate" is what they call in politics a "big tent"—a category that encompasses a huge range of foods (and food "products") ranging from cauliflower to Twinkies. Unless all your carbs are coming from vegetables (which, for the average American, would be pretty uncommon), the majority of your carbs are coming from foods like cereals, breads, pasta, potatoes, rice, and an assortment of highly sweetened processed foods. These foods are almost always "high-glycemic," meaning they raise blood sugar very quickly, a fact which has all sorts of metabolic consequences, none of them good.

Emerging research continues to implicate high-glycemic diets in a host of conditions, including cancer[11] (cancer cells, after all, feed on sugar). Consuming carbohydrates with a high-glycemic index (meaning those that raise blood sugar quickly) is associated with an increased risk for coronary heart disease,[12] while *low*-glycemic diets have been reported to reduce measures of inflammation, aid in weight control, and lower the risk of diabetes and cardiovascular disease.[13] And by definition, lower-carb diets are almost always low-glycemic diets, since most of the carbs in a low-carb diet will be coming from vegetables, fruits, and the occasional healthy grain (like oatmeal), all of which have very low glycemic indexes.

Betcha Can't Eat Just One

One thing you probably know from experience is the effect high-glycemic foods have on your appetite. Remember one of the most successful ad campaigns in recent decades, the "Betcha Can't Eat Just One" ad? They weren't kidding. There's a reason it's so easy to go through three bowls of Cap'n Crunch while watching reruns of *Friends*. High-glycemic carbs make you hungry. Low-carb diets don't.

And that may be one reason why people do so much better on lower-carb diets. A 2005 study from Temple University School of Medicine found that the reason pounds melt off so quickly on low-carb diets is not at all related to water, metabolism, or boredom.[14] Nope. It's related to appetite.

"When carbohydrates were restricted," lead researcher Guenther Boden, MD, told *Science Daily*, "study subjects spontaneously reduced their caloric intake to a level appropriate for their height, did not compensate by eating more protein or fat, and lost weight." Boden added: "We concluded that excessive overeating had been fueled by carbohydrates."[15]

The path from eating a high-carbohydrate diet to being overweight is a pretty clear one: It has to do primarily with the ability of carbohydrates to raise blood sugar, which, in turn, raises a fat-storing hormone called *insulin*. When insulin is constantly elevated, it's darn near impossible to burn fat. (See chapter 3 for a full explanation.) But there are a few other "side effects" of lower-carb diets that may also have a lot to do with why lower-carb diets make it so much easier to lose weight and get healthy.

One of those "side effects" has to do with wheat. Another has to do with fructose.

Let me explain.

The Wheat Connection

Since virtually all low-carb diets recommend that you keep carb intake to somewhere under 100 grams a day (as low as 20 grams on the first stage of Atkins), one of the first things that gets eliminated—at least in the beginning—is wheat.

You can eat a ton of vegetables and still manage to keep your carbs under 100 grams a day; you can even eat some fruit. But once you start including bread, bagels, pasta, rice, and all the rest of the starches and grains, your carb allowance is quickly used up. (A single slice of bread has between 20 and 25 grams of carbs.) Not only that: all wheat products are high-glycemic, meaning they raise blood sugar quickly and keep it up there for a while, stimulating a ton of insulin, which essentially locks the doors to your fat cells.

I first experimented with eliminating bread from a client's diet back in 1990. I was a personal trainer, working at Equinox, and my nutrition knowledge was still pretty limited. Like most personal trainers, I received all my education in nutrition from American Dietetic Association–approved programs and instructors, so I totally bought into the low-fat, high-carb, lots-of-grains paradigm. But some of the other trainers had been experimenting with lower-starch diets for their clients, so I decided to try that approach with Lucy, a woman who came to me for the express purpose of losing some stubborn pounds she just couldn't seem to get rid of.

In a few short weeks, she dropped about 8 pounds.

But that's not the interesting part.

The interesting part was that Lucy had suffered from inexplicable headaches for most of her life. Not migraines, mind you, nor cluster headaches, but just regular, annoying, day-ruining garden-variety headaches that no doctor, naturopath, chiropractor, or nutritionist had ever been able to explain. When she came back to see me, she had some interesting news: "My headaches went away!" she exclaimed.

This was well before I knew much about gluten sensitivity, celiac disease, or delayed food reactions. I had taken bread out of her diet because I thought it would help her lose weight (which it did). I had no idea there would be a side effect like the elimination of a lifelong problem no one else had been able to fix.

As the years went by and my nutrition education continued, I did indeed learn all about celiac disease and gluten sensitivity. Gluten is a protein found in grains, particularly wheat, that triggers symptoms in a huge number of people; when your body responds to gluten with a full-blown autoimmune reaction, the condition is called *celiac disease*. But celiac disease, like many things, exists on a continuum. You don't have to have celiac disease to have a profound sensitivity to gluten, which is clearly what Lucy had. (Gluten sensitivity can lead to a host of symptoms like headache, bloating, weight gain, water retention, aches and pains, and digestive issues.) But, like most nutritionists at the time, I still thought the only problem with wheat was that it raised blood sugar—and insulin by extension—thus making it a good thing to avoid if you wanted to lose weight.

Most people still think the problem with wheat is limited to gluten, and gluten-free foods have taken off as a "niche" market that's growing like weeds. But the problems with wheat go a lot deeper than gluten. As you'll soon see, substances in wheat—particularly a type of starch called *amylopectin A*—can cause all sorts of problems in susceptible people. The most obvious problem is weight gain, but it's hardly limited to that.

Some Call It Fat, Some Call It "Wheat Belly"

In 2010, a brilliant cardiologist named William Davis, MD, published a book called *Wheat Belly*, which instantly (and deservedly) went to the top of the *New York Times* Best Seller list. Davis explains that the wheat we're consuming today is a genetically modified kind of wheat that had never been seen on earth before about 50 years ago. This wheat—called *dwarf wheat*—has replaced most of the other strains of wheat in the United States (and in much of the world). "Modern wheat, despite all the genetic alterations to modify hundreds, if not thousands, of its genetically determined characteristics, made its way to the worldwide human food supply with nary a question surrounding its suitability for human consumption," writes Davis.

In 2011, journalist/educator Tom Naughton interviewed Davis on the subject of wheat. (The interview is available on Naughton's website, www. fathead-movie.com.) One exchange was particularly telling:

> Naughton: *You're a cardiologist by profession, yet you just wrote an in-depth book about the negative health effects of consuming wheat. How did wheat end up on your radar? What first made you suspect wheat might be behind many of our modern health problems?*
>
> Davis: *If foods made from wheat raise blood sugar higher than nearly all other foods (due to its high-glycemic index), including table sugar, then removing wheat should reduce blood sugar. I was concerned about high blood sugar since around 80% of the people coming to my office had diabetes, pre-diabetes, or what I call "pre-pre-diabetes." In short, the vast majority of people showed abnormal metabolic markers.*
>
> *I provided patients with a simple two-page handout on how to do this, i.e., how to eliminate wheat and replace the lost calories with healthy foods like more vegetables, raw nuts, meats, eggs, avocados, olives, olive oil, etc. They'd come back three months later with lower fasting blood sugars, lower hemoglobin A1c (a reflection of the previous 60 days' blood sugar); some diabetics became non-diabetics, pre-diabetics became non-pre-diabetic. They'd also be around 30 pounds lighter.*
>
> *Then they began to tell me about other experiences: Relief from arthritis and joint pains, chronic rashes disappearing, asthma improved sufficiently to stop inhalers, chronic sinus infections gone, leg swelling gone, migraine headaches gone for the first time in decades, acid reflux and irritable bowel symptoms relieved. At first, I told patients it was just an odd coincidence. But it happened so many times to so many people that it became clear this was no coincidence: this was a real and reproducible phenomenon.*
>
> *That's when I began to systematically remove wheat from everyone's diet and continued to witness similar turnarounds in health across dozens of conditions. There has been no turning back since.*

Removing wheat—or grains in general—from the diet is a hard sell. For decades we've been sold a bill of goods on how healthful grains are and how "necessary" they are in our diet. We've heard the phrase "fruits, vegetables, and healthy whole grains" so many times it sounds like a vaudeville act, and the pairing of "healthy whole grains" with two things that actually *are* good for us has convinced most of us that grains—especially whole grains— are as wholesome and nutritious as vegetables.

Actually, that's not the whole truth.

THE STRANGE CASE OF MY TENNIS-PLAYING BUDDY

Every Wednesday morning, I play a couple of sets of tennis with a guy I'll call Marty. He's in his late '60s and in great shape. Recently he told me that he had atrial fibrillation, the most common kind of irregular heartbeat, a condition that has symptoms like heart palpitations and shortness of breath.

Two years ago, Marty told me, he had a "procedure" that effectively stopped the problem. Except that now, all of a sudden, it was coming back.

In the course of discussing his health, Marty also mentioned that he had constant bloating, gas, and other digestive problems.

Going for the low-hanging fruit (the digestive problems), I asked him if he'd considered a gluten-free diet. "Worth a shot," I said.

About a week later, I met him on the court and was greeted with good news. "This gluten-free thing seems to be really working. My gas and bloating is gone and I'm not having any stomach pains!"

I asked him how the atrial fibrillation was and if he had seen his doctor about it yet.

"Oh," he said, almost as an afterthought. "It seems to be gone! I haven't had any problems with it in a week."

As Davis points out in his book, the species einkorn was the great-granddaddy of wheat, and has the simplest genetic code. But einkorn and other wild and cultivated strands of wheat are no longer what we're eating. They've been preempted by literally thousands of man-made offspring of *Triticum aestivum*, which are genetically quite different from the original einkorn wheat. Today's wheat has been bred for greater yield and hardiness. It even looks different. Those "amber waves of grain" we sang about as children hardly exist anymore. They've been replaced by wheat varieties that barely stand two feet tall. The name for that stuff is dwarf or semi-dwarf wheat, and unless you've got access to a time machine, that's exactly what you're eating when you eat today's cereals, pastas, and breads.

Why does that matter?

Pull up a chair.

Wheat: The Real Story

Wheat—like all starches—is made up of two fractions: amylose and *amylopectin.* They have somewhat different effects on the body, something that's been known since at least 1989 when researchers fed men a diet containing 34% of calories as either 70% amylose starch or 70% amylopectin starch and measured the results. What's interesting is that there were no major differences—for the first 4 weeks. But when the meals were given after 5 weeks on each starch, some significant differences showed up. Blood-sugar and insulin responses were significantly lower when the amylose meal was compared to the amylopectin meal. Fasting triglyceride levels were also lower during the period when amylose was consumed.[16]

The complex carbohydrate in wheat is actually 75% amylopectin and 25% amylose. But the problem isn't just the amylopectin—it's the *type* of amylopectin. Amylopectin actually comes in several "flavors."Amylopectin C is found in beans and legumes and is the least digestible of the three; amylopectin B is found in potatoes and bananas, and it's a little more digestible than amylopectin C. But when it comes to digestibility, amylopectin A—the kind found in wheat—is the clear winner. It breaks down quicker than you can say "blood sugar hell."

That's why it's no surprise that whole wheat bread increases your blood sugar more than even pure sucrose (table sugar).[17] And—as you'll learn throughout this book—high blood sugar is quickly followed by a surge of the fat-storing hormone, insulin. This is exactly what you do *not* want if you're trying to control your weight. The higher your blood sugar, the higher your insulin, and the easier it is to store fat. Not only that: amylopectin A has a curious ability to keep that blood sugar/insulin surge going for about 2 hours.[18] That surge means there's going to be a big drop, and those drops in blood sugar—the aforementioned "blood sugar hell"—are largely responsible for cravings and hunger. That's why it's a breeze to binge on sugar-coated wheat cereal. Steak and broccoli? Not so much.

"Wheat is the Haight-Ashbury of foods, unparalleled for its potential to generate entirely different effects on the brain and nervous system," says Davis. Indeed. As anyone who recognized herself in the reference to the compulsive eating of cereal knows, wheat can stimulate addictive behavior. And there's a very good reason for that.

This Is Your Brain on Gluten

Gluten, you see, is broken down in the body to chains of amino acids called *polypeptides*. These polypeptides have a unique ability to get past the sentry who stands guard at the door of the brain, a structure called the *blood-brain barrier*. The blood-brain barrier functions like a bouncer at an exclusive night-club. The brain can't let just any riffraff get in, or it would be severely damaged by some of the crap floating around in our bloodstream. The blood-brain barrier protects it from this riffraff by being very selective about what it opens the door for. But the polypeptides that result from the breaking down of gluten somehow get a free pass. And when they get in, guess what they do?

They bind to the brain's morphine receptors.

One researcher—Christine Zioudrou at the National Institutes of Health—termed these sneaky polypeptides exorphins, a contraction of exogenous morphine–like compounds. The dominant one is called *gluteo-morphin*. And if you doubt that it can exert a drug-like effect on your brain, consider the following. (Faint-hearted readers beware: you may never feel the same way about that "wholesome" wheat bread of yours again.)

Naloxone is a drug given to reverse the effects of narcotic drugs. It's frequently given to addicts, and if you're stoned it will make you immediately *un*-stoned. Fine, you say, and what could that possibly have to do with me? Or, come to think of it, with wheat *or* with low-carb diets?

Well, in one ingenious study conducted at the University of South Carolina, two groups of healthy participants were let loose in the cafeteria, but one of them was first given a dose of naloxone. Those given the naloxone consumed ⅓ fewer calories at lunch and just under ¼ fewer calories at dinner, averaging about 400 fewer calories for the day.[19] In another study at the University of Michigan, researchers put binge eaters in a room loaded with all kinds of food and left them there for an hour. Those given the naloxone beforehand consumed a whopping 28% fewer wheat crackers, pretzels, and bread sticks.[20]

As Davis puts it, "block the euphoric reward of wheat, and calorie intake goes down, since wheat *no longer generates the favorable feelings that encourage repetitive consumption*." (Emphasis mine.)

Or, put another way: wheat is addictive. It's an appetite stimulant. Not only does it raise blood sugar more than any other carbohydrate—which alone would make it a disaster from a weight-control standpoint—but it also affects your brain in a way that makes overeating far more likely. "Just as the tobacco industry created and sustained its market with the addictive property of cigarettes, so does wheat in the diet make for a helpless, hungry consumer," says Davis. "From the perspective of the seller of food products, wheat is a perfect processed food ingredient: The more you eat, the more you want."

The Side Effects of a Wheat-Free Diet

Like Lucy, who stopped eating bread in order to lose weight but wound up losing her headaches, you may find that some other health conditions you've been worried about improve substantially if you cut out wheat. Bone density problems, for example. And here's why.

Wheat is one of the most acidic foods in our diet, and a diet that's highly acidic can cause problems with bone mineralization. Animal protein is acid-forming, and vegetables and fruits are alkaline, but if meat consumption is balanced with alkaline foods (such as vegetables), everything should be fine. (In fact, a number of studies have shown that animal protein does *not* affect the skeleton adversely[21] and that bone mineral loss is *greater* in people consuming low-protein diets.)[22]

But throw grains into the picture, and it's a whole different story.

Grains like wheat actually account for 38% of the acid load in the average American's diet. Researchers writing in the *American Journal of Clinical Nutrition* estimated the net amount of acid production in typical preagricultural Paleolothic diets (grain-free diets) and compared them to the average contemporary human diet. Even in a Paleolithic diet where a whopping 35% of calories came from animal foods, the overall effect of the diet was alkaline. But once grains came into the picture—the average contemporary diet—the picture changes drastically. Adding wheat shifted the diet from positive alkaline to positive acid. So while animal protein has been blamed for creating an acid state in the body (and for subsequent bone loss), it's actually grains that are doing the damage.[23] The researchers concluded that the shift from the alkaline diet of Paleolithic times to the acidosis induced by the modern diet is driven *primarily* by cereal grains and junk foods. "Wheat shifts a diet that had hopes of being net alkaline to net acid, causing a constant draw of calcium out of bone," writes Davis.

So there's a perfect example of the "side effects" of low-carb diets. You remove a food everyone has told you is healthy and necessary (wheat) because of its demonstrated connection to high blood sugar and fat storage, and you end up not only losing weight but improving health in literally dozens of ways across dozens of conditions.

Are you beginning to see why, in the beginning, I said you are "lucky"?

Fructose Makes You Fat—And It's Metabolic Poison

The other "food" that should get the pink slip on your low-carb diet is fructose. More specifically, (1) *high-fructose corn syrup*, which consists of 55% fructose and 45% glucose, and its kissing cousin,(2) *sucrose*, which is ordinary table sugar, composed of 50% fructose and 50% glucose.

Because high-fructose corn syrup (HFCS) has gotten so much heat in the press, some food manufacturers now proudly advertise that their products contain none of it, and are instead sweetened with "natural" sugar (meaning ordinary sucrose). Meanwhile, the National Corn Growers Association, essentially a lobbying arm of the sugar industry dedicated to whitewashing HFCS, has claimed that high-fructose corn syrup is being unjustly targeted and is no worse than "regular" sugar.

Sadly, they're right. But that's a little like saying Montezuma's revenge is "better" than diarrhea.

Fructose is the damaging part of sugar, and whether you get that fructose from regular sugar or from HFCS doesn't make a whit of difference. That doesn't absolve HFCS; it just means that "regular" sugar is *just as bad* as HFCS. It's the fructose in each of them that's causing the damage, and here's why.

Fructose and glucose are metabolized in the body in completely different ways. As "sugars," they are *not* identical. Glucose goes right into the bloodstream and then into the cells. It raises your blood sugar, causing a surge of insulin—the "fat-storage hormone"—leading to weight gain as well as the many other problems discussed in this book. Fructose *doesn't* raise blood sugar, but it damages the body nonetheless, albeit via different mechanisms. The end result is it still makes you fat, and it does some other significant damage as well.

Fructose is metabolized by the body like fat, and it turns into fat (triglycerides) almost immediately. "When you consume fructose, you're not consuming carbs," says Robert Lustig, MD, professor of pediatrics at University of California, San Francisco. "You're consuming fat." Once fructose enters the body, it goes right to the liver. A substantial amount of research has now implicated fructose in non-alcoholic fatty liver disease.[24] "Fructose is 'alcohol without the buzz,'" says Lustig. "[It's] a dose-dependent chronic hepatotoxin."[25] Research has shown that fructose is many times more likely than glucose to form artery-damaging, free radical-generating factories called AGEs (advanced glycation end-products). AGEs are dangerous compounds which play a major role in heart disease.[26] Research by Kimber

Stanhope at the University of California Davis has shown that when people consume 25% of their calories from fructose or high-fructose corn syrup, several factors associated with an increased risk for heart disease—including triglycerides and a nasty little substance called apolipoprotein B—go up significantly.[27]

The perfect example of how sugar is related to fat *and* to heart disease is *insulin resistance*. Insulin resistance is discussed throughout this book and is included in many of the diets we will review later, but here's the short definition so you don't have to go look it up: Insulin resistance is the condition in which the cells stop "listening" to insulin. That means insulin is *less* effective at getting sugar out of your bloodstream, even though the pancreas continues to pump out more and more of it in a futile attempt to make blood sugar go down. Eventually you have both high blood sugar *and* high insulin and you're basically—excuse my French—screwed. High blood sugar and high insulin are two of the features of metabolic syndrome, and when you have it, you're well on the road to diabetes, heart disease, or both. And you'll almost definitely find it impossible to lose weight.

The way in which sugar—especially fructose—damages the heart can be directly traced to insulin resistance. Varman Samuel of the Yale School of Medicine, a top researcher in the field of insulin resistance, told the *New York Times* that the correlation between fat in the liver (fatty liver) and insulin resistance is remarkably strong. "When you deposit fat in the liver, that's when you become insulin resistant," he says.[28]

And all together now, class: What causes fat to accumulate in the liver? Fructose.

If you want to watch a bunch of lab animals become insulin-resistant, all you have to do is feed them fructose. Feed them enough fructose and sure enough, the liver converts it to fat that then accumulates in the liver—with insulin resistance right behind it. This can take place in as little as a week if the animals are fed enough fructose, whereas it might take a few months at the levels we humans normally consume. In studies done by Luc Tappy in Switzerland, feeding human subjects a daily dose of fructose equal to the amount found in 8 to 10 cans of soda produced insulin resistance and elevated triglycerides within a few days.[29]

Fructose found in whole foods like fruits, however, is a different story. There's not all that much fructose in, for example, an apple, and the apple comes with a hefty dose of fiber, which slows the rate of carbohydrate absorption and reduces insulin response. But fructose extracted from fruit, concentrated into a syrup, and then inserted into practically every food we buy at the supermarket, from bread to hamburger buns to pretzels to cereals—well, that's a whole different animal.

High-fructose corn syrup was first invented in Japan in the 1960s and made it into the American food supply around the mid-1970s. It had two advantages over regular sugar, from the point of view of food manufacturers. Number one: because it's sweeter, theoretically you could use less of it. (Theoretically.) Number two: it is significantly cheaper than sugar. Manufacturers found that low-fat products could be made "palatable" through the addition of HFCS, so before long they were adding the stuff to everything. (Doubt this? Take a field trip to your local supermarket and start reading labels. See if you can find any processed foods that don't contain it.)

The result is that our fructose consumption has skyrocketed. Twenty-five percent of adolescents today consume 15% of their calories from fructose alone! As professor Robert Lustig, MD, points out in his brilliant lecture "Sugar: The Bitter Truth" (available on YouTube), the percentage of calories from fat in the American diet has gone down at the same time that fructose consumption has skyrocketed, along with heart disease, diabetes, obesity, and hypertension. Coincidence? Lustig doesn't think so, and neither do I.

Remember metabolic syndrome? It's that collection of symptoms—high triglycerides, abdominal fat, hypertension, and insulin resistance—all of which seriously increase the risk for heart disease. Well, rodents consuming large amounts of fructose rapidly develop it.[30] In humans, a high-fructose diet raises triglycerides almost instantly; the rest of the symptoms of metabolic syndrome take a little longer to develop in humans than they do in the rat experiments, but develop they do.[31] Fructose also raises uric acid levels in the bloodstream. Excess uric acid is well known as the defining feature of gout, but it also predicts future obesity and high blood pressure.

AGAVE NECTAR SYRUP: HOPE OR HYPE?

Agave nectar is an amber-colored liquid that pours more easily than honey and is considerably sweeter than sugar. The health food crowd loves it because it is gluten-free and suitable for vegan diets—*and*, most especially, because it's low-glycemic (we'll get to that in a moment). Largely because of its very low glycemic impact, agave nectar is marketed as "diabetic friendly." What's not to like?

As it turns out, quite a lot.

Agave nectar has a low-glycemic index for one reason only: it's largely made of *fructose*, which, although it has a low-glycemic index, is now known to be a very damaging form of sugar when used as a sweetener. *Agave nectar has the highest fructose content of any commercial sweetener (with the exception of pure liquid fructose).*

All sugar—from table sugar to HFCS (high-fructose corn syrup) to honey—contains *some* mixture of fructose and glucose. The proportion in table sugar is 50/50; HFCS is 55/45. Agave nectar is anywhere from 57% to a whopping 90% fructose, almost—but not quite—twice as high as HFCS.

In the agave *plant*, most of the sweetness comes from a particular kind of fructose called *inulin* that actually has some health benefits: it's considered a fiber. But there's not much inulin left in the actual syrup. In the manufacturing process, enzymes are added to the inulin to break it down into digestible sugar (fructose), resulting in a syrup that has a fructose content that is *at best* 57% and—much more commonly—as high as 90%.

"It's almost all fructose, highly processed sugar with great marketing," said Dr. Ingrid Kohlstadt, a fellow of the American College of Nutrition and an associate faculty member at Johns Hopkins School of Public Health. "Fructose interferes with healthy metabolism when (consumed) at higher doses," she told me. "Many people have fructose intolerance like lactose intolerance. They get acne or worse diabetes symptoms even though their blood (sugar) is OK."

Agave nectar syrup is a triumph of marketing over science. True, it has a low-glycemic index, but so does gasoline—that doesn't mean it's good for you.

Fructose and glucose behave very differently in the brain as well, as research from Johns Hopkins has suggested. Glucose decreases food intake while fructose increases it. If your appetite increases, you eat more, thus priming you for obesity, and likely an increased risk for heart disease. "Take a kid to McDonald's and give him a Coke," says Professor Lustig. "Does he eat less? Or does he eat more?"

M. Daniel Lane, PhD, of the Johns Hopkins University School of Medicine says, "We feel that [the findings on fructose and appetite] may have particular relevance to the massive increase in the use of high-fructose sweeteners (both high-fructose corn syrup and table sugar) in virtually all sweetened foods, most notably soft drinks. The per capita consumption of these sweeteners in the USA is about 145 lbs/year and is probably much higher in teenagers/youth that have a high level of consumption of soft drinks."[32]

If you've read my book *The Great Cholesterol Myth*, you already know that I think cholesterol is a very minor player in heart disease, and it doesn't predict heart disease very well at all. But hypertension, high triglycerides, and a high ratio of triglycerides to HDL cholesterol all *do*. Sugar, or more specifically *fructose*, raises *every single one* of those measures.

On top of that, high levels of sugar and insulin *damage* cholesterol particles, making them far more likely to start the process of inflammation. And even if you *don't* accept the theory that inflammation is at the "heart" of heart disease, it's worth pointing out that the metabolic effects of sugar are highly inflammatory to your artery walls.

And, by the way, to the brain. Elevated levels of glucose (sugar) in the brain actually impair the ability of nerve cells to repair themselves and regenerate, something greatly needed for cognitive health. It may be no coincidence that diabetics have almost twice the risk for Alzheimer's and cognitive impairment.[33]

The fact is that sugar is far more damaging to the heart—and to the brain—than either fat *or* cholesterol has never stopped the diet establishment from continuing to stick to their story that fat and cholesterol are what we ought to be worried about.

THE CASE AGAINST SODA

One clever study by Kimber Stanhope and her colleagues at Stanford investigated the effects of "moderate" soda drinking on health.

They took 29 healthy, normal-weight male subjects and ran each one of them through six different three-week experiments. In the first condition, the men drank what was called a "medium fructose" beverage; in the second condition they drank a "high fructose" beverage. In the third and fourth conditions they drank a "medium glucose" beverage and a "high glucose" beverage, and in the final two conditions they drank "medium sucrose" and "high sucrose" beverages.

So, again, we had two conditions where they drank beverages sweetened with plain sugar (sucrose), two conditions where they drank beverages sweetened just with glucose, and two conditions where they drank beverages sweetened with just fructose.

The results were not good news for soda drinkers.

First of all, in all conditions, fasting blood sugar and high-sensitivity C-reactive protein increased significantly. (C-reactive protein, by the way, is a measure of inflammation, so this study clearly shows that sugar in all forms is very inflammatory.) Second, particle size of their LDL—the so-called "bad cholesterol"—was reduced in both the high-fructose group and in the high-sucrose group. This is a really bad thing because we now know that not all LDL cholesterol is bad—only the small pellet-sized LDL molecules are the ones that cause damage, so shrinking the particle size of LDLs is a really bad outcome!

In addition, all the interventions containing fructose resulted in a significantly higher waist-to-hip ratio and there was a significantly higher percentage of body fat in the high-fructose intervention.

In another study, overweight and obese adults were instructed to eat their usual diet along with sugar-sweetened beverages. One group was asked to consume 25% of the day's calorie requirement as a specially made beverage sweetened with glucose. The other group was given an identical beverage sweetened with fructose. Both groups were allowed to eat as little or as much of their usual diet as they wanted, but were required to drink the sugar beverages.

"The subjects did not eat 25% fewer calories from their usual foods to make room for the sugar beverage calories. Instead, most of them ate more than their calorie requirement," Kimber Stanhope told me. Not surprisingly, all subjects gained weight. "But what was interesting and novel—and is a finding that needs to be confirmed—is that the fructose subjects gained intra-abdominal fat, whereas the glucose subjects did not," Ms. Stanhope said.

Why does this matter? Because intra-abdominal fat—the kind that makes you more of an apple than a pear—is the most dangerous kind of fat to carry around. It puts you at greater risk for diabetes, heart disease, and the constellation of symptoms called metabolic syndrome, an almost certain path to either heart disease or diabetes. "There was a definite increase in fasting insulin and in fasting glucose with the fructose consuming subjects," Stanhope explained. Elevated levels of fasting insulin and glucose (blood sugar) are both associated with a greater risk of metabolic syndrome and diabetes.

Triglycerides—a kind of fat found throughout the body and measured in a standard blood test—have long been recognized as an independent risk factor for heart disease. In many of the previous human studies on fructose, researchers have measured *fasting* triglycerides, and fructose didn't always have much effect on fasting levels. But in this study, researchers measured triglycerides after eating—what's called a postprandial measurement. "Fructose had a pronounced effect on postprandial triglycerides, while glucose did not," Ms. Stanhope said. "In the fructose group, postprandial triglycerides more than doubled."

While the research is preliminary and needs to be borne out by future studies, high-fructose consumption could well be setting consumers up for atherosclerosis. "The overweight men and women assigned to drink the fructose-sweetened beverages developed a more athrogenic lipid profile in just two weeks," said Stanhope. "In 2006, five different publications came out showing that adolescents, college students and adults under 50 were consuming as much as 15–20 percent of calories just from sugar-sweetened beverages—and that doesn't include the sugar calories from cakes and desserts."[*]

[*] Stanhope, et al., "Consumption of Fructose and High Fructose Corn Syrup Increase Postprandial Triglycerides, LDL-Cholesterol, and Apoliporotein-B in Young Men and Women" *The Journal of Clinical Endocrinology & Metabolism* 96, no. 10 (October 2011): E1596–1605.

So there you have it—the "side effects" of a low-carb diet. Lowered acid load (resulting in stronger bones), less likelihood of fatty liver disease, and a lower risk for heart disease, metabolic syndrome, and diabetes.

Not exactly a shabby list of accomplishments, and a heck of a lot better than the side effects of medicines.

CHAPTER 5

The Cholesterol Connection: Have We All Been Misled?

I t's been about 7 years since the first edition of *Living Low Carb* (then called *Living the Low-Carb Life*) was published. During that time I've witnessed a much greater appreciation for the value of low-carbohydrate eating, and a greater acceptance of the principles of low-carb among many (but not all) segments of the health professions.

But the conversation I listened to in between doubles sets on the tennis court the other day tells a much different story.

"My doctor says I have high cholesterol, so he put me on a statin drug," said one guy. "I can't understand why. I eat really healthy! No red meat, hardly any fat, lots of whole grains. Makes no sense!"

"My doctor just told me to eat low-fat foods and cut out meat. My cholesterol is OK, so I guess I don't have to worry," chimed in a second guy.

"I lost a ton of weight on that Atkins diet," said a third, "but my doctor told me it's really unhealthy. He says I might have lost weight, but I was putting myself at risk for heart disease from eating all that fat and osteoporosis from eating all that protein."

OK everyone, calm down and take a deep breath. We've got a lot of work to do.

The innocent conversation that took place on the tennis court in southern California—a conversation, mind you, among four reasonably smart, educated middle-aged men all of whom are health conscious enough to engage in regular exercise and affluent enough to afford good medical care—is a perfect object lesson in everything that's wrong with our collective thinking on diet and health.

Let me explain.

Low-Carb and Heart Disease: The Big Lie

"The big lie" was an expression coined—sorry to say—by Adolf Hitler, who used it in a completely different context. It's shorthand for the idea that if enough people repeat an untruth often enough, it becomes "accepted knowledge." Hitler meant it to refer to propaganda techniques. Though he was delusional about *who* was lying and what they were lying *about*, he was entirely correct about the propaganda part. Get enough people—and enough respected, mainstream organizations that dispense advice—to say that the world is flat, and before you know it, anyone who says differently is either crazy or subversive. After a while, everyone "knows" the world is flat, and anyone who says otherwise must be nuts.

Which brings us to low-carb diets and heart disease.

Those men who were worried about their cholesterol all bought into the "big lie" that cholesterol causes heart disease. (To disassemble this "big lie" would take a whole book. Cardiologist Stephen Sinatra, MD, and I wrote one: it's called *The Great Cholesterol Myth*. I hope you read it.)

What's important for our purposes here is the stuff that logically follows from that "big lie." The "big lie" that cholesterol causes heart disease—and the secondary fib that saturated fat always raises cholesterol—was the impetus for several decades worth of dietary advice that has led us down a path of ever-expanding waistlines and a virtual epidemic of obesity and diabetes. The dietary guidelines that flowed quite logically from the "big lie" about heart disease were nonsense when they were first issued in the late '70s and '80s, and they continue to be nonsense today.

If you think about it for a moment, every single time you've been warned off saturated fat it's for one reason only: it raises cholesterol. But really, it's not cholesterol you care about—it's heart disease. And they are *not* the same thing, though if you read the mainstream media, you'd never know it. The mainstream media and many mainstream medical organizations have got you convinced that cholesterol and heart disease *are* the same thing. By conflating cholesterol and heart disease they convinced us to avoid eating fat (especially saturated fat) since it *may* increase cholesterol. Since "everybody knows" that high cholesterol spells heart disease, anything that increases cholesterol *must* be bad, and that's precisely why your doctor tells you to avoid low-carb diets.

But if cholesterol isn't the demon mainstream medicine thinks it is, then the admonition to eschew saturated fat collapses like a house of cards. If the only "bad" thing saturated fat does is raise blood levels of an innocuous molecule that is turning out to have very little to do with heart disease anyway, then why are we avoiding saturated fat?

Fat and the Big Lie

Fat is the Rodney Dangerfield of the modern diet: "it don't get no respect."

For years we tried to eliminate it from what we eat, even though it's been a basic (and necessary) part of our diet since at least the first recorded Homo sapiens in Africa about 200,000 years ago, and likely from the beginning of the genus Homo roughly 2.4 million years ago. More recently, experts have begun—almost grudgingly, it seems—to admit that some fat is good, but a good number of them still continue to recommend that you reduce it as much as possible. (And—with the exception of the universally appreciated omega-3 fats—many experts are still for the most part woefully uninformed about which fats are actually "good" and why.) It's common for health-conscious people to collapse the terms "healthful" and "low-fat" as if they were synonyms (trust me, they're not). And the majority of fitness books continue to repeat low-fat nonsense that should have gone out of style a decade ago.

So it's probably safe to say that fat is the single most misunderstood component of the modern diet. And our thinking about fat deeply colors the way we think about low-carb diets

Here's why: Suppose, for the moment, that you're eating a typical American diet of 2,500 calories (or more), of which about half (or more!) comes from carbohydrates. If you remove a big chunk of the carbohydrates from your diet (the definition of a low-carb program, right?), one of two things *has* to happen: One, you simply cut out the carbs but keep everything *else* the same, effectively eating half as much food as before (this never happens). The second much more common and realistic option is that you replace all or some of those carbohydrate calories with something else.

Since there are only three other calorie-containing substances on the planet that you can replace those carbs with (protein, fat, or alcohol) and since most people don't replace their carbohydrates with a fifth of vodka, chances are your controlled-carb diet is now higher in either protein or fat (or both) than it was before and some registered dietitian will soon be screaming bloody murder about how dangerous your diet is because of "all that fat" and how you will quickly die of heart disease.

So, as you can see, it's all but impossible to speak about low-carb diets and evaluate them properly without treading on a lot of preconceived ideas about fat.

In case you've just joined us from another planet and haven't heard the argument that's been repeated ad infinitum for the last few decades, here it is in a nutshell: low-carb diets are bad *because* they have too much fat, and too much fat (especially saturated fat) is bad *because* fat raises cholesterol, and high cholesterol is bad *because* it increases the risk for heart disease.

Now, if your first thought on reading the above argument was "*Well, sure, that makes sense,*" it's only because you've heard this argument so many times that you no longer question whether any of it is true. The association of fat and heart disease has become what philosophers call a "meme"—a generally accepted cultural notion that is deeply embedded in the national consciousness. To question it almost puts you in the category of the crowd with the tinfoil hats.

Hence this chapter. Because we've been taught so much gibberish about fat, and because the *fear* of fat is intimately entwined with *both* the fear of cholesterol *and* the general prejudice against low-carb diets, arming yourself with some basic info on fat may help you understand why a higher fat diet is nothing to fear. Sure, the "conventional wisdom" says otherwise, but in this case the conventional wisdom is only conventional. It is anything *but* wise.

Bear with me if you know this stuff—and even if you think you do, it's probably worth reviewing. I'm going to question some widely held beliefs now, including some choice tidbits of information you may be sure are true, but remember—sacred cows make the best burgers!

And one more thing: I promise to make this short and sweet, and my mission is to write it in such a way that your eyes don't glaze over.

Interested? Read on.

Everything You Ever Wanted to Know about Fat (But Were Afraid to Ask)

"Fat" is actually the general, colloquial term for a collection of smaller units technically (and properly) called fatty acids. Each of these fatty acids has a team identity—it belongs to a *group* (saturated, unsaturated). When we call something like butter or olive oil a "fat," what we actually mean is that it's a *collection of individual fatty acids.* (When a food is "high in fat" that just means it's got a lot of fatty acids in it).

Almost all fats in food are some combination of the three main types of fatty acids—saturated, monounsaturated, and polyunsaturated—although we tend to identify a fat in food by the type of fatty acid that's *predominant* in the mix. For example, many foods that we call "saturated-fats foods" (like butter or steak) actually contain many "unsaturated" fatty acids, and most foods that we call "unsaturated fats" (like olive oil) contain some "saturated" fatty acids as well. And sometimes the mixture is actually quite different than you might think. (Would it surprise you to know, for example, that a typical sirloin steak has more *monounsaturated* fat than it does *saturated?* Or that fish oil—the ultimate unsaturated fat, and an omega-3 to boot—is about 25% saturated fatty acids? Both are true.)

In addition to belonging to one of the three major "groups" of saturated, monounsaturated, or polyunsaturated fats, each individual fatty acid *also* comes with a molecular description (don't ask) and a name (e.g., stearic acid, lauric acid). This is important because some individual fatty acids have important health benefits and have distinct effects on the body. Lauric acid, for example, is a saturated fatty acid found in coconut that has immune-system–boosting properties—it's both antimicrobal and antiviral. Stearic acid, another saturated fatty acid, has virtually no effect on cholesterol.

Every single fatty acid on the planet—regardless of whether it's saturated, monounsaturated, or polyunsaturated—is basically a *chain of carbon atoms* linked together by chemical bonds. Think of a little row of circles (carbon atoms), holding hands. You can also imagine these chains of carbon atoms as a bunch of little school kids on a day outing, joined together with one of those ropes that kindergarten teachers use when they take their kids on a field trip.

Now just as each of those kids in the kindergarten class has two arms that can "hold" something (like a book bag), each carbon atom has two "places" to which something can attach. In the case of the carbon atom, the only "thing" that can attach to those places are hydrogen atoms.

When all the "places" to which hydrogen atoms can attach are "filled" (i.e., "no seats left on the train"), the fatty acid is said to be "saturated." It's literally *saturated* with hydrogen. There's no more room at the table, so to speak. The places on the individual carbon atoms in the fatty acid are basically all occupied, so the fatty acid can't hold any more hydrogen passengers. (Trans-fats are a kind of "hybrid" saturated fat that's basically created in a lab by taking an "unsaturated" vegetable oil and blasting it with hydrogen atoms from the chemical equivalent of a turkey baster, forcing some hydrogen into the empty seats and producing "partially hydrogenized vegetable oil,"—or, as I like to call it, poison.)

Are you with me so far?

Good. Now, when there is one seat or more that's "unoccupied" on that chain link of carbons, the fatty acid is called *un*saturated—there are still places that could be occupied by hydrogen atoms. In other words, it's not yet a "full house." (If there's only *one* spot "open," it's called a *mono*unsaturated fatty acid; and if there's *more* than one spot "open," it's called a *poly*unsaturated fatty acid. More on that in a moment.)

So what happens when there's still "seating" on the carbon chain? Well, instead of holding on to two hydrogen atoms, that carbon atom takes its two empty hands and creates what's called a "double bond" with the next carbon in the chain. (Think of each school kid in the line holding *both hands* of the kid facing him. And because both his hands are now occupied, he can't hold anything else.) When there's just *one* such *double bond* in the chain, the fatty acid is called a—can you guess?—*mono*unsaturated fatty acid.

Fat Architecture

Now let's clear up all this stuff about "omegas." In fatty acids, as in real estate, there's one rule—location, location, location. Recall that if there's only *one* double bond in our little carbon atom chain, we're dealing with a *mono*unsaturated fatty acid. And if the *location* of that single double bond is on the 9th carbon counting from the end of the line, it's known as an *omega-9* fatty acid. How simple is that? The most famous source of omega-9 (monounsaturated) fat is olive oil, believed by just about everyone to be a "healthful" fat.

*Poly*unsaturated fatty acids simply have *more than one* double bond (hence the name "poly," which means "many"). Those that have their *very first* double bond on the 3rd position (counting from the end of the line) are called *omega-3s*. Those that have their very first double bond on the 6th position (again counting from the end of the line) are *omega-6s*.

OK, just in case your eyes are glazing over, there really *is* a good reason to know this stuff, and it's this: omega-3s and omega-6s are *building blocks* out of which the body makes distinct compounds (called *prostaglandins* or *eicosanoids*) that have different—and opposite—effects. For example, omega-3s are the building blocks for *anti*-inflammatory prostaglandins. Omega-6s are building blocks for *inflammatory* ones.

You might think, hey, if omega-6s make inflammatory compounds, what do I need them for? Good question, and here's the answer: you need them because inflammation is a natural part of the body's healing response. Let's say you injure your foot by stepping on a nail. What happens? Your foot swells up, because the body mounts a defensive reaction to that injury. Fluid and white blood cells rush in to surround the area, hoping to destroy any pathogens or bacteria that might have gotten in the wound, in an attempt to prevent an infection. You *need* the building blocks for that inflammation response*in your body, or you wouldn't have great "defenses" against what the body perceives as an attack.

But those inflammatory and anti-inflammatory prostaglandins need to be *in balance* in order for you to have an optimally functioning body. If your "pro-inflammation" factory is working overtime and your "anti-inflammation" factory is understaffed, you're in deep doo-doo. And that's exactly what's happened to most people eating a Western diet, which now has a ratio of about 20:1 in favor of omega-6 to omega-3. (The ideal ratio is between 1:1 and 4:1).

You can't swing a rope without hitting an omega-6 fat—they're everywhere in our diet. Corn oil, soybean oil, vegetable oil, safflower oil, canola oil—all high in omega-6s. Those of us who have been taught the mantra "saturated fat *bad*, vegetable oil *good*" might think for a minute about consuming huge amounts of "unsaturated" vegetable oils without an appropriate amount of anti-inflammatory omega-3s to balance that intake.

You might think inflammation is no big deal, but you'd be making a huge mistake. Most of us are walking around with low-grade inflammation in our bodies that flies below the radar. Inflammation damages our vascular and circulatory systems and contributes to virtually every degenerative disease known to humankind, from heart disease to Alzheimer's, from cancer to diabetes. Not for nothing did Time magazine do a cover story called "Inflammation: The Silent Killer." There's a good deal of emerging evidence, by the way, that controlled-carb diets—even those higher in saturated fat—actually *lower* inflammation in the body.[1]

Here's something else to think about: we've done such a good job of demonizing saturated fat that it's effectively been replaced in our kitchens (and in fast-food restaurants) with the supposedly more healthful "vegetable" fat, most of which is stunningly high in omega-6s. The problem is that omega-6s are "unstable" fats. When used (and reused) for frying as they are

---

*In fact, one particular omega-6 fat—linoleic acid—is actually an essential fatty acid, meaning that it's required for health but your body can't make it, so you must get it from your diet.

in most fast-food restaurants, they actually get badly damaged and create carcinogenic compounds. Researchers at the University of Minnesota have shown that when unsaturated (omega-6) vegetable oils are heated at frying temperature (365° F) for extended periods—or even, for goodness' sake, for a half hour—toxic compounds will form. One in particular—HNE—is associated with a number of very bad chronic diseases that you really don't want to have.[2]

Saturated fats—because they are highly *stable*—do *not* create these toxic compounds when heated to high temperatures. Many people who really understand fat chemistry will tell you that they would much prefer deep frying in real lard (not Crisco!) to reused canola oil any day of the week. It's far less damaging to the body. (My favorite oil for cooking at high temperatures in a wok or frying pan is Barlean's organic coconut oil.)

In addition to creating toxic compounds when heated repeatedly, vegetable oils used by fast-food restaurants often contain *trans-fats*, probably the most damaging fat on the planet (and one whose dangers dwarfs the supposed dangers of saturated fat). Up until very recently, foods like margarine were loaded with the stuff. Kind of ironic, isn't it, when you think that the whole reason for the popularity of high omega-6 vegetable oil products like margarine was the desire to eliminate the "dangerous" saturated fat from our diet—talk about the "law of unintended consequences"!

So we have nothing to fear from a higher percentage of fat in our diet, particularly when it's "good" fat—by which I mean fat that has *not* been damaged by repeated high heat, fat or oil that is *not* highly refined (like some cooking and vegetable oils) and *all* man-made trans-fats. Some cold-pressed unrefined omega-6s in the diet are fine, omega-9s are fine, omega-3s are better than fine, and—yup—*saturated fat is fine too*, especially when it comes from whole natural foods such as eggs, coconut, organic butter, and the like.

Now, here's an interesting factoid about fats: the only fatty acid that the body actually *makes* is palmitic acid—a saturated fat! Then it takes that palmitic acid and gets to work on it with a system of enzymes. It adds carbons, thus *lengthening* the chain—these enzymes are called *elongases* (they elongate the chain). It also *removes* pairs of hydrogens from some of the carbons that are saturated, thus creating new double bonds. The enzymes that do this are called *desaturases* (by removing some of the hydrogen passengers, they turn that saturated fat into an unsaturated one.) Through this system of elongases and desaturases, the body—starting with saturated fat—winds up with a whole menu of fatty acids to serve different purposes. (We also get a variety of different fatty acids directly from our diet—like, for example, omega-3s directly from fish or flaxseed.)

If saturated fat were inherently so bad for us, why would it be the very fat our body makes naturally from food?

Saturated Fat and Heart Disease: What's the Real Connection?

In the context of today's conventional wisdom, it almost sounds ludicrous to put that question out there, so deeply accepted is the idea that saturated fat and heart disease are married forever in some metabolic Universe of Bad Things. But more and more researchers are asking that identical question, and the ones who are looking honestly at the data are not so convinced that the conventional wisdom is right. In 2008, the American Society of Bariatric Physicians, in conjunction with the Metabolism Society, presented an entire two-day conference in Arizona named "Saturated Fat and Heart Disease: What's the Evidence?"

I attended that conference, in which some of the smartest researchers investigating this issue participated; and I can sum up the answer to the question "What's the Evidence?" for you in two words: Not much. (You can read an excellent report on this conference written for the general public by About.com's official guide to low-carb diets, Laura Dolson. The article is called "Saturated Fat: Not Guilty" and can be found at http://lowcarbdiets .about.com/b/2008/04/14/saturated-fat-not-guilty.htm.)

I'm sure you're thinking right about now, "*What about all those studies I've read about that 'link' saturated fat consumption with heart disease?*" Well, to unpack the problems with those studies is a bigger project than I can take on in this book. But let's consider just a few of the issues worth thinking about before you buy—hook, line, and sinker—the idea that saturated fat is always "bad."

First—and this is an incredibly important point—the "fate" of saturated fat in the body varies significantly, depending on what else is eaten. "Saturated fat is a completely neutral fat," says my friend Mike Eades, MD. "It burns like any other fat." If you're eating a high-carb diet, the effect of saturated fat may indeed be deleterious, but *if you're eating a low-carb diet, it's a whole other ballgame.* "If carbs are low, insulin is low and saturated fat is handled more efficiently," said Jeff Volek, PhD, RD, one of the major researchers in the area of diet comparisons. "When carbs are low, you're burning that saturated fat as fuel, and you're also making less of it."

One recent study tested what happens when you take obese patients and put them on a high-saturated-fat diet—but without starch. The researchers took 23 patients with atherosclerotic cardiovascular disease and put them on a high-saturated-fat diet, but one in which all the starch had been removed. Here's what happened: body weight decreased, body-fat percentage decreased, total triglycerides decreased. The researchers concluded that a high-saturated-fat/starch-avoidance diet resulted in weight loss after 6 weeks *without adverse effects on serum-lipid levels.*[3] I suspect the results would have been very different indeed if the participants had been eating a lot of carbs along with that saturated fat.

The Paradox

Remember, when you're dealing with a diet in "free-living" humans—as opposed to lab rats—you have four dietary variables (at least) to deal with: total calories, percent protein, percent carbs, and percent fat. *It is impossible to change one without changing the others.* So whenever you "test" a diet that's *high* in one of those elements, it's by definition also *lower* in another (and vice versa).

Let's say, for example, that you have a 1,500-calorie diet made up of 70% carbohydrates, 15% fat, and 15% protein. If you now raise the fat intake by 20% (from 15% to 35%), keeping overall calories and protein the same, you've automatically *lowered* the carb intake by the same 20% (from 70% of the diet to 50%). That lowering of carb intake may produce—in certain populations—a very beneficial effect, lowering both insulin levels and triglyceride levels (and possibly increasing HDL in the process). In such a scenario, it would be entirely possible to say that an *increase* in fat (even saturated fat!) was associated with a *lowered* risk for heart disease.

And that's exactly what one study showed. Research by epidemiologist Dariush Mozaffarian, MD, at Harvard found that a "higher saturated fat intake is associated with *less* progression of coronary artery disease." What? Saturated fat *good* for you? In research done at Harvard? How can this possibly be explained?

Well, some folks at the prestigious *American Journal of Clinical Nutrition* wondered the same thing. They wrote a fascinating editorial in the November 2004 issue titled "Saturated Fat Prevents Coronary Artery Disease? An American Paradox." The authors posed the not-unreasonable question, "*How can this paradox be explained?*"

How, indeed. Since, as the authors point out, it's an article of faith that saturated fat raises LDL cholesterol and *accelerates* coronary artery disease, how are we to account for a study that shows the exact opposite?

The answer that keeps emerging from the research is this: the metabolic fate of saturated fat—what it actually *does* or *does not do* in the body—depends largely on what *else* is eaten. Eat way fewer carbohydrates and way less sugar, and how much saturated fat you eat may not matter so much.[4]

This is the explanation most scientists who are now researching low-carb diets believe accounts for their findings that higher saturated fat aren't a problem, as *long as people are not eating high amounts of carbohydrate.* But once you're eating a ton of carbs, all bets are off. If you're eating the standard Western mixed diet, high in sugar, high in processed carbs, high in fast food, and hugely high in calories, then yup, adding more saturated fat is a really bad idea. Added to a high-calorie, high-carb diet, saturated fat won't be burned as "fuel" and will tend to get stored on your hips. In the context of that kind of diet, the "low-fat" folks are probably right.

But a much *better* approach would be to cut out the sugar and processed carbs! In that case, the amount of saturated fat you're consuming probably wouldn't matter so much. Remember that in the early part of the twentieth century, the percentage of the American diet was much higher in saturated fat, and we had much lower rates of heart disease. Of course, we also consumed less food in general, fast food hadn't been invented, we ate much less sugar, and we moved around more. The point is that it's not saturated fat that's the demon here.

A second reason that saturated fat has been demonized, in my opinion, is that much of the research on diet and disease has lumped saturated fat together with trans-fats. Trans-fats weren't even a health issue until relatively recently, and for decades researchers didn't distinguish between the two when doing studies of diet patterns. Why does this matter? Because man-made trans-fats really are the spawn of Satan. They clearly raise the risk for heart disease and stroke, and, according to Harvard professors Walt Willett and Alberto Ascherio, are responsible for 30,000 premature deaths a year,[5] so obviously a study that lumps trans-fats together with saturated fat is going to show some nasty associations. The question is: are those nasty health effects caused by the trans-fats, or by the saturated fats?

I think it's pretty clear that it's the trans-fats; and if you separate the two and look at their effects on the body as two distinct entities, you're going to see some very big differences. If you lump them together—as many researchers did before we knew what we know now—saturated fats are likely to be tainted by the negative actions of trans-fats.

Even the cholesterol-raising effect of saturated fat may be influenced by the presence of trans-fats. One study showed that palmitic acid (a saturated fatty acid) had no effect on cholesterol when the intake of omega-6 is greater than 4.5% of calorie intake, but if the diet contained trans-fats, the effect was completely different—LDL went up and HDL went down.[6] (How much this even matters is a whole different question. Still, it's important to point out that the combination of saturated fat and trans-fats has a different effect than saturated fat alone.)

The third reason saturated fat has such a bad reputation is that much of the saturated fat people consume comes from really crummy sources. Fried foods are not a great way to get fat in your diet. Neither are processed deli meats nor hormone-treated beef. But the saturated fat from healthy animals (like grass-fed beef or lamb) or the saturated fat in organic butter or in egg yolks is a whole different story.

I've never seen one convincing piece of evidence that saturated fat from *whole-food sources* like the ones I just mentioned has a single negative impact on heart disease, health, or mortality, especially when it's part of a diet high in plant foods, antioxidants, fiber, and the rest of the good stuff you can eat on a controlled-carbohydrate eating plan!

The Big Reason Saturated Fat Has Been Demonized: The Cholesterol Connection

And finally, the zinger—the *major* reason saturated fat has been demonized over the years is this: *cholesterol.* The perception that saturated fat *always raises cholesterol* is enough to scare anyone exposed to conventional health "wisdom," and is so embedded in the national (and international) consciousness that it would take more than a crowbar to pry it lose from our belief system.

The truth about saturated fat raising cholesterol is this: Sometimes it does. And sometimes it doesn't.

And the bigger truth—hold on to your hats—is this: *it may not even matter.*

The Cholesterol Controversy

When we focus on cholesterol, we're *not telling the whole story.* In fact, we're not even telling the most *important* part of the story, and—according to many—the part of the story we *are* telling may actually be virtually irrelevant.

Here's why.

You don't really *care* what your cholesterol level is; what you *care* about is your risk for *heart disease.* And you've come to believe they're essentially the same thing. The only reason you even *know* your cholesterol level is that it has become embedded in your consciousness (as it was in mine) as an *important marker for heart-disease risk*. In fact, for many people, it is *synonymous* with heart disease risk. (Doubt that? Try this party trick: ask five friends to say the first thing that comes to mind when you say the term "risk for heart disease." Case closed.)

But here's the thing: Fully half of the people with heart disease have perfectly "normal" cholesterol levels. And half the people who have what's considered "elevated" cholesterol have perfectly normal hearts.

As long ago as 1994, a study published in the conservative and august *Journal of the American Medical Assocation* demonstrated a complete lack of association between cholesterol levels and coronary-heart-disease mortality in persons over 70 years old. It also demonstrated a complete lack of association between cholesterol levels and mortality from any cause in that same population.[7] Since we already know that the rate of heart disease in 65-year-old men is many times that of 45-year-old men, does it make sense that cholesterol suddenly "stops" becoming a risk factor when you get older? It makes *more* sense that it wasn't that big of a risk factor in the first place! As a terrific article in Chris Kresser's blog Medicine for the 21st Century points out, this is akin to suggesting that smoking causes lung cancer in young men, but somehow stops doing it in older men![8]

Consider also a classic study conducted in France over a four-year period from March 1988 to March 1992 and published in the journal *Circulation* in 1999.[9] The study—called the Lyon Diet Heart Study—looked at 605 patients who had already had a first heart attack. These folks were *not* in great shape—they had classic risk factors, high cholesterol, many were smokers, the whole ball game. Half of the 600 or so subjects were given the standard advice about eating a "prudent" diet (lower fat, lower cholesterol) and the other half were given instructions on following what we call the "Mediterranean diet"—high in olive oil, vegetables, fruits, and so on. (Neither group was given the standard treatment for high cholesterol, a statin drug.)

Are you ready for the results?

Those following the Mediterranean diet had a 72% decrease in coronary events and a 56% decrease in overall mortality.

The results were so stunning that the study had to be stopped in the middle so that everyone could go on the diet program that had produced such outstanding results.

But that's not even the best part. Get ready for the kicker:

Though people were dying at less than half the rate expected, and were having coronary events at about one-quarter the rate expected, *their choles-terol levels hardly budged.*

Did you get that? An almost 75% decrease in heart disease *without a budge in cholesterol levels!*

Now let's fast forward to a drug study completed in 2006, the widely publicized ENHANCE trial. If you were following the news in 2008, you couldn't have missed this one, because it made the front pages of the newspapers and all of the television news shows. Here's what happened.

A combination cholesterol-lowering medication called Vytorin had been the subject of a huge research project, the results of which were finally coming to light and being given enormous negative attention. One of the many reasons for this negative attention—besides the actual results, which I'm going to share with you in a moment—was the fact that the companies jointly making the drug (Merck and Schering-Plough) waited almost 2 years before releasing the results of the study.

No wonder. The results stunk. Which was the *other* reason this drug test made the front pages. The new "wonder" drug *lowered cholesterol just fine.* In fact, it lowered it *better* than a standard statin drug. So you'd think everyone would be jumping for joy, right? Lower cholesterol, lower heart disease—let's have a party for the shareholders!

Not quite. Although the people taking Vytorin saw their cholesterol plummet just fine, they actually had *more* plaque growth than the people taking the standard cholesterol drug. The patients on Vytorin—low cholesterol and all—actually had almost twice as great an increase in the thickness of their arterial walls, a result you definitely don't want to see if you're trying to prevent heart disease.

So their cholesterol was wonderfully lowered and their risk for heart disease went up: shades of "the operation was a success, but the patient died."

Taken together—and there are countless other examples—I think we might be able to at least *question* the widely accepted dogma that *cholesterol is what we need to be focused on when it comes to heart disease.*

But wait! If cholesterol is not the huge deal everyone thinks it is, then it's reasonable to ask the question: so, why are we so afraid of saturated fat? After all, isn't the big "rap" against saturated fat that it raises cholesterol? If that's not as big a deal as we thought, why are we so afraid of saturated fat?

Now you're beginning to get it.

Fact is, according to a ton of research by Jeff Volek, PhD, RD, and others, saturated fat *sometimes* raises cholesterol and sometimes doesn't. And then there's the question of exactly what "kind" of cholesterol it does raise.

Size Matters

Most people are familiar with the concept of "good" cholesterol (HDL) and "bad" cholesterol (LDL). Problem is, that concept is woefully out of date, as "yesterday" as last month's headline in People magazine. There are several different subtypes of HDL cholesterol and several different subtypes of LDL. The subtypes of LDL have different effects on the body and are far more interesting to us than the overall LDL number, even though that's the number that most people focus on.

LDL cholesterol—the unfortunately named "bad" kind—actually comes in *several* "flavors"; it is not one homogenous substance that is "bad." There are LDL molecules that are "large" particles, and there are LDL molecules that are "small" particles. The large particles—think of them as big fluffy cotton balls—are fairly harmless. The small ones—think of them as hard little BB gun pellets—are not.

What often happens on a high-saturated-fat diet is that LDL goes up—*but this is not the whole story*. When scientists look at the *actual particle sizes* of that LDL cholesterol, they find that higher saturated-fat intake (in the context of a low-carb diet) usually results in a significant shift to *more* of the harmless big fluffy particles and *fewer* of the much more dangerous little ones.

Let's say, for the sake of argument, you are a person with an overall cholesterol of 200, 130 of which is LDL and 50 of which is HDL (the remainder is other stuff that we're not going to go into right now and isn't germane to the discussion). Furthermore, let's hypothesize that your LDL of 130 is actually ½ the harmless stuff (the big fat fluffy particles) and ½ the bad stuff (the BB gun pellets). You go on a low-carb (higher-fat) diet and— boom—your cholesterol is now 230 and your doctor is having a fit, furiously scribbling a prescription for statin drugs and reading you the riot act.

Not so fast.

What may have happened—in fact, what most *often* has happened—is that your HDL has gone up (good) and your LDL has gone up also, but something even better has happened as well, something that flies beneath the radar unless your doctor knows to check for it: the proportion of "good" (fluffy cotton balls) and "bad" (little BB pellets) cholesterol has shifted *dramatically*. You might now have an HDL of 60 and an LDL of 150, but 100 of that LDL is now the big harmless fluffy particles and only 50 of it is the bad stuff. Your total number (and even your LDL) has gone up, but *the overall lipid profile has improved substantially.*

And we haven't even begun to talk about triglycerides.

Triglycerides, which don't get nearly as much attention as cholesterol, are a far greater risk factor for heart disease than cholesterol is.[10] (They're also a significant risk for strokes.)[11] And triglyceride levels always come down on a low-carb diet. Always. Not sometimes; *all* the time. (Which makes sense—the body takes all that excess sugar and packages it into triglycerides, so the less sugar in the diet, the less triglycerides in the blood.)

Furthermore, according to a Harvard study published in *Circulation*,[12] the ratio of triglycerides to HDL cholesterol is a much better predictor of heart disease than cholesterol is. Also, according to many experts (including the Metabolic Syndrome Institute), that ratio can serve as a good "surrogate" marker for insulin resistance. Personally, if you show me a person with a ratio of 2 (triglycerides to HDL) who doesn't smoke, works out, isn't overweight, and has low markers of inflammation (CRP and homocysteine, for example), I'll bet you my life savings he's not going to have a heart attack, and I don't care what his cholesterol numbers are.

But that's just me.

Now let's reexamine the effects of this mythical low-carb diet on our mythical patient whose doctor is furiously prescribing statins.

PRE–LOW-CARB DIET	POST–LOW-CARB DIET
Triglycerides 175	Triglycerides 100
TOTAL CHOLESTEROL: 200	TOTAL CHOLESTEROL:240
HDL: 50	HDL: 60
Triglyceride-to-HDL ratio: 3	Triglyceride-to-HDL ratio: 1.66
LDL cholesterol: 130	LDL cholesterol:150
LDL "fluffy" particles: 65	LDL "fluffy" particles: 110
LDL "small" particles: 65	LDL "small" particles: 40

Post–low-carb diet, this guy should be taking that blood test home and jumping for joy. His lipid profile is vastly improved. By every measure, he's doing way better than he was before the diet.

But his cholesterol went up.

To which I say: so what?

There are currently tens of millions of Americans on cholesterol-lowering medications. As of 2006, two of the five top-selling drugs in America were cholesterol-lowering medications, and they collectively rang up sales of over 18 billion dollars. Even without throwing in the annual budget of the National Cholesterol Education Program, it's safe to say that well over 20 billion dollars a year rides on the effort to get Americans to lower cholesterol and fat. Current guidelines are to reduce saturated fat to 7% of the diet,[13] and there's a movement afoot to recommend lowering it even more. The American Academy of Pediatrics now recommends cholesterol screening for some children as young as 2, and treatment with statin drugs to lower cholesterol for some children as young as 8.[14]

Are we likely to see a moratorium on the demonization of fat and cholesterol and a move toward eliminating the real health-robbers in our diet, like sugar and processed carbs? Not bloody likely, and probably not anytime soon. As the author Upton Sinclair put it: *"It is difficult to get a man to understand something when his salary depends upon his not understanding it."*

The bottom line is that if you're eating a very-low-carb diet, I don't think you have much to worry about if it contains a relatively high amount of saturated fat (see chapter 8, "My Big Fat Diet"), and you certainly don't have anything to worry about if it contains a nice mix of fats from omega-3s, 6s, 9s, and saturated fat. If you're downing six or seven meals of fast food a day with an average daily intake of 3,500 calories (or more!), adding more saturated fat *is* going to have a negative effect—you can count on it. Added to a high-calorie, high-carb diet, saturated fat is *not* a great thing. It won't be burned as "fuel" and will tend to get stored on your hips. If that's the kind of diet you're eating, the "low-fat" folks are probably right.

But a much better approach would be to cut out the sugar and processed carbs (and lower your calories to boot), in which case the amount of saturated fat you're consuming probably wouldn't matter half as much.

Now, before we wrap this up, let's be clear about one thing: I'm *not* saying you should go out and start drinking oodles of saturated fat. (I *am* saying you shouldn't be terrified of it, but that's a different statement.) The important thing to remember is this: *the metabolic effect saturated fat has on your body—its "fate," if you will—depends entirely on what else it's consumed with.*

In 2000, Walter Willett, MD, PhD, arguably the world's most respected nutritional epidemiologist, chairman of the Department of Nutrition at the Harvard School of Public Health, and the lead researcher on the Nurses' Health Study and the Health Professional Follow-Up Study, was interviewed by Harvard's World Health News. This is what he said:

"We have found virtually no relationship between the percentage of calories from fat and any important health outcome."[15]

Amen to that.

CHAPTER 6

The Biggest Myths about Low-Carb Diets

Over the years, there have been many criticisms leveled at low-carbohydrate diets. Some of these have been repeated so often that they are now taken as gospel, even though some have never been closely examined; while others have long ago been proven false, although they continue to be repeated as if the research debunking them had never happened. Some of these beliefs are based on complete misunderstandings of biochemistry and physiology, and some on an astonishing distortion of the program being criticized. (For example, one supposedly reputable health information website criticized the Zone on the basis of the "fact" that "the Zone diet contains less than 1,000 calories," which is patently false.)

Some of these beliefs are nothing less than cultural "memes," a term meaning an idea that takes on a life of its own and is passed down from generation to generation, like the ideological version of a gene. These memes are rarely examined—they just "are." Examples of memes are tunes, catchphrases, or basic foundational beliefs—i.e., things "everybody knows" (like "the world is round," "birds fly," and "saturated fat causes heart disease"). Some memes are useful and true, but some are in dire need of reexamination and should ultimately be dumped in the cultural wastebasket.

You'd think "science," with its reliance on experiment and validation and objective measurement, would be immune to the vagaries of beliefs and prejudices. However, you'd be sadly wrong. Scientists are first and foremost people, and they can be just as shockingly petty and proprietary and stubborn as the rest of us. And entrenched beliefs and theories don't die easily. The history of science is littered with theories that lasted 50 or 100 years or more before people finally came to accept that they weren't valid.*

And the prevailing medical and dietetic beliefs can be summed up in six words: low-carb diets will hurt you.

It's going to take a while for popular opinion on that to shift, but let's take on a few of the most commonly held assumptions here and see where it takes us. At the very least, perhaps some of what I'm about to say will give you pause next time you hear one of these myths repeated with great authority as if it was gospel truth.

MYTH #1: You "Need" Carbs

When I do live workshops and talks, I often do the following demonstration: I tell everyone in the audience to pretend they are on the show Survivor and we're going to divide the room into two teams. Everyone in the room is going to be on a desert island for one year. Then I draw an imaginary line in the middle of the room and make everyone to the left of the line "Group One" and everyone on the right of the line "Group Two."

Then I say the following:

"Everyone in Group One will be fed absolutely nothing but protein and fat for one year. You will get zero carbohydrates in your diet. Everyone in Group Two will be fed nothing but carbohydrates for one year. You will get zero protein and zero fat."

Then I pause for the punch line, which is this:

"Everyone in Group Two will be dead within the year. Everyone in Group One will be doing just fine."

---

*Two recent examples come to mind. One, when Kilmer McCully, MD, of Harvard first hypothesized that homocysteine was at least as great a risk factor for heart disease as cholesterol, he was literally ridiculed out of his lab at Harvard. Twenty-five years later, homocysteine tests are routinely performed; homocysteine is widely recognized as a risk factor for heart disease, stroke, and Alzheimer's; and McCully is back at Harvard. Second example: when Jonas Folkman, MD, proposed angiogenesis as a mechanism by which cancer cells were able to thrive, he too was ridiculed, laughed at, and ostracized from the scientific community. (Establishment medicine, contrary to popular belief, does not like mavericks.) Angiogenesis is now widely accepted, and Folkman—now dead—is recognized and acclaimed as the brilliant and innovative pioneer that he was. Doctors, unfortunately, do not always take kindly to those who question their most cherished assumptions (see, for example, how the brilliant scientists who populate the International Network of Cholesterol Skeptics are treated by the conventional medical establishment, most of it documented on their website, http://www.thincs.org—it's not pretty).

The fact is—hold on to your seats now—there is no physiological need for carbohydrates in the human diet.[1]

None.

Now, before you throw this book down and decide that I'm completely crazy for making such an outrageous statement, take a look at what the august and esteemed Institute of Medicine of the National Academies has to say about this in its reference manual, *Dietary Reference Intakes: Energy, Carbohydrate, Fiber, Fat, Fatty Acids, Cholesterol, Protein, and Amino Acids.*" In case you don't want to bother looking it up, here's what it says on page 275:

"*The lower limit of dietary carbohydrate compatible with life apparently is zero, provided that adequate amounts of protein and fat are consumed.*"[2]

The Institute of Medicine goes on to say: "There are traditional populations that ingested a high fat, high protein diet containing only a minimal amount of carbohydrate for extended periods of time (Masai), and in some cases for a lifetime after infancy (Alaska and Greenland Natives, Inuits, and Pampas indigenous people) (Du Bois, 1928; Heinbecker, 1928). There was no apparent effect on health or longevity. Caucasians eating an essentially carbohydrate-free diet, resembling that of Greenland natives, for a year tolerated the diet quite well (Du Bois, 1928)."

You've probably heard that the brain requires a minimum 120 grams of carbs a day in order to function. Actually, that's technically inaccurate—it does indeed need 120 grams of glucose (sugar) to function, but it can make that glucose perfectly well from certain amino acids (found in protein) and from the glycerol backbone of triglycerides. Let's not confuse dietary carbs with glucose. They're not the same thing.

OK, now that we've got that out of the way, let me back up a minute.

The fact that there is no dietary need for carbohydrates simply means we can survive without them. It does not mean—and I am not saying—that we shouldn't eat them (see myth #2).* I'm simply pointing out a basic fact in biology. Our bodies will and can run on ketones[3]—quite nicely, thank you very much—and whereas we will die without protein and fat, we will not die without carbohydrates. However, we would not die without hot and cold running water, nor without indoor plumbing. Nor without someone to cuddle with every night. That doesn't mean we shouldn't have them.

I do think it's curious that groups like the American Dietetic Association continue to recommend that the lion's share of our calories come

---

*And I don't mean to imply that the Institute of Medicine thinks we shouldn't eat them either. They're simply saying that we appear to be able to survive quite well without them, pointing out: "The amount of dietary carbohydrate that provides for optimal health in humans is unknown."

from the one macronutrient we could actually survive without! But don't get me started.

BOTTOM LINE

Although carbohydrates like fruits, vegetables and beans provide an array of important nutrients, dietary carbohydrates are not physiologically necessary in the human diet.

MYTH #2: In a Low-Carb Diet, You'll Be Missing All the Vitally Important Nutrients that You Get from Carbs

Well, this myth would have some validity *if* low-carb advocates actually suggested cutting out all carbs.

But they don't.

Not a *single advocate* of controlled-carb eating thinks we should eat a no-carb diet. Carbs—from vegetables and fruits and legumes—provide fiber, phytochemicals, and a wealth of nutrients, vitamins, and minerals. Controlled-carb does *not* mean no-carb, and I am certainly *not* advocating a no-carb diet for anyone. A no-*junk* diet: you bet. A low-sugar diet, absolutely. But a no-carb diet? Not on your life.

What's more, you can eat a ton—and I mean a *ton*—of vegetables and even fruits, and still be on the "low" end of the carbohydrate spectrum.

Consider this: you could eat—*on a daily basis*—the following carbohydrate foods and still be consuming *under* 140 grams of carbohydrate, which is *less than half* of what most Americans now consume:

- 5 cups of spinach = 5.45 grams carbs (3.5 fiber)
- 2 cups cooked broccoli = 22.4 grams carbs (10.1 fiber)
- 1 cup of raspberries = 14.69 grams carbs (8 fiber)
- 1 medium apple= 25.13 grams carbs (4.4 fiber)
- 20 grapes = 17.74 grams carbs (0.8 fiber)
- ½ sweet potato = 11.8 grams carbs (1.9 fiber)
- ½ bowl of oatmeal= 13.5 grams carbs (2 fiber)
- ½ cup of Brussels sprouts= 5.54 grams carbs (2 fiber)
- ½ cup of blueberries = 10.72 grams carbs (1.8 fiber)
- 2 medium carrots =11.68 grams carbs (3.4 fiber)

Considering that most people in America aren't even getting 5 (let alone 7 or 9) servings of fruits and vegetables, and considering that the above list represents roughly *16 servings*, you can see that I picked a pretty extreme menu. But even so—16 servings of carb foods and you're still *under* 140 grams (138.63 to be exact, but who's counting?).

But wait: it gets better.

Most people in the low-carb world don't count fiber as part of their "carbohydrate" intake, since it has absolutely no effect on blood sugar. They subtract fiber from total carb count, and call what's left either "net carbs" or "effective carbs," which is pretty much the way it should be. The above 16 servings gives you a whopping 37.9 grams of fiber, one of the most important nutrients for health on the planet. (The average American gets between 4 and 11 grams, and every major health organization recommends between 25 and 38 grams.)

If you subtract those 37.9 grams of fiber from the overall carb total of 138.63, you are left with about 100 grams of carbs a day. That might be enough to make the American Dietetic Assocation apoplectic, but who cares? I defy anyone on the planet to show me how a diet that includes the above 16 servings of fruits and vegetables, *plus* plenty of protein (grass-fed meat, wild salmon) and fat like olive and coconut oil, nuts, avocados, and even a glass of red wine and a bite of dark chocolate, is "unhealthful." Show me. Please. I'll be right here waiting.

And I'll be waiting a hell of a long time.

Now, some people in the low-carb world would not consider 140 grams of carbs a "low-carb" diet, and, to be sure, for some people—particularly the very insulin-insensitive, or those with metabolic conditions in which every single gram of carbohydrate must be counted—this might be too high. But let's talk for a minute about the general reader: you, perhaps. A diet that reduces carbs to that very reasonable amount, and at the same time front-loads it on vegetables and fruits, is going to represent an improvement that's literally light-years ahead of what most folks are currently eating. It's going to extend your life, increase your energy, stabilize your weight, and improve your health.

Killer Carbs

Ever wonder why you're hungry for more after you eat a high-carb snack or meal?

Research by Zane Andrews, MD, and his team at Monash University in Australia identified key appetite-control cells in the human brain.* These appetite-control cells are attacked by free radicals after eating, but the attack is bigger and stronger following a meal rich in sugar and carbohydrates.

"The more carbs and sugars you eat, the more your appetite-control cells are damaged," said Andrews, the lead researcher on the study. The result? You eat more.

The forces that compel you to eat and the forces that tell the brain "Hey, this dude is full!" are constantly at war. When your stomach is empty, it triggers the release of a hunger hormone called ghrelin. When you're full, a set of neurons known as POMC's (proopiomelanocortins) kick in.

Free radicals normally created in the body attack both the "hunger" neurons and the "antihunger" neurons, but the "hunger" neurons are naturally protected. This tips the scale in the direction of hunger and cravings.

And carbs create the most damage of all.

According to Andrews, people in the age group of 25 to 50 are most at risk. "The neurons that tell people in that crucial age range not to overeat are being killed off."

Yet another reason to limit your sugar and processed carbs if you don't want to be the victim of constant cravings.

*Monash University, "Killer Carbs: Scientist Finds Key to Overeating as We Age," Science Daily (August 21, 2008). http://www.sciencedaily.com/releases/2008/08/080821110113.htm.

MYTH #3: Low-Carb Diets Induce Ketosis, a Dangerous Metabolic State

I will admit that in the last few years—between the publication of previous editions of this book and now—the subject of ketosis has faded somewhat from center stage. Once an important feature of low-carb diets (since Atkins promoted it as part of his original diet), ketosis is no longer a "required" part of any low-carb diet, unless that diet is being studied scientifically or used therapeutically (it's a mainstay of dietary treatments for childhood epilepsy,* for example, and is still very effective for weight loss in recalcitrant cases).

So although ketosis was once the focal point of the arguments against low-carb diets, it no longer is. It's now widely accepted that most people—if not all—do not *have* to be in ketosis in order to lose weight; conversely, you can be in ketosis and *not* lose weight. Nonetheless, I include this section simply to dispel many of the remaining myths about ketosis, and also perhaps as an object lesson in which we can see how a misunderstood concept can persist stubbornly for years.

And the best way I know to illustrate this is to tell you a story. Follow me on this, and you will understand more about ketosis than half the doctors in America.

Back in the 1990s, a lot of restaurants in New York City served a delicious fish that nobody would order. In fact, the presence of this fish on the menu caused more than a little distress in some circles and led to some heated exchanges between customers and restaurant managers. Animal-rights activists—who were frequently baby boomers with enough disposable income to keep the restaurants afloat—were the most vitriolic in their condemnation of the establishments that served this fish, but the outcry from "regular" folks was not much more muted.

The fish was dolphin.

You can, I'm sure, see the problem.

No one wanted to patronize an establishment that was so heartless as to serve up Flipper for the gastronomical whims of its customers.

Quite understandable.

Problem was: "dolphin" *isn't* "Flipper."

Dolphins were, and are, quite ordinary but tasty fish that look exactly like fish: they bear not even a passing resemblance to the bottle-nosed dolphins that delight us at Sea World and with whom they happen, by some weird taxonomical screw-up, to share the same name. In fact, they aren't even the same *species* (one being, of course, a fish, while the other is a mammal). Plus, the dolphin (fish) does not perform adorable tricks and does not appear to have much rapport with the average human being.

But go tell that to the table for four in the back where the kid is crying and the parents are threatening to never come back to this restaurant, ever.

---

*I recently interviewed Eric Kossoff, MD, medical director of the Johns Hopkins ketogenic diet program. Dr. Kossoff has been using both the ketogenic diet and his own version—the Modified Atkins Diet—in his treatment of epilepsy for years. "Most doctors now know it's an effective therapy," he told me. He also mentioned that he has an adult patient who has been on the ketogenic diet for 27 years. "His cholesterol is better than mine," he said.

Waiters explained, probably as many times as they had to say, "Hi, I'm Jason and I'll be your server for today," that dolphin was not *dolphin*. Yes, they did in fact share the same name, but one was a *fish* and one was the lovable marine *mammal*, and the dish on the menu, sir, was not Flipper.

Didn't matter.

No matter how many times this conversation was repeated in restaurants throughout the city, and probably throughout the country (though I can personally attest only to the number of times I heard it in New York City), it fell on deaf ears.

So restaurant owners did a smart thing.

They changed the name of the fish.

"Dolphin" now became known as "mahi-mahi," which is the Hawaiian name for dolphinfish.

End of problem.

Which brings us to ketosis.

Ketosis: Friend or Foe?

It is very difficult to read about—or write about—low-carbohydrate dieting without dealing with the term *ketosis*. If you've been around low-carb diets at all—if you've experimented with them, talked about them to your friends, read about them, read *warnings* about them—you've surely heard of ketosis. You've probably heard that it's some kind of metabolic state that accompanies these diets and that you should avoid it—and those "high-protein" fad diets that produce it—at all costs. Several years ago, in a column at iVillage. com, I wrote the following, which is still true today:

> Ketosis is so misunderstood and maligned that I really feel it's worthwhile to go into it in some detail. For those of you who are new to this, ketosis is something that happens in the body when you eat very, very few carbohydrates. Since there's very little sugar coming in, your body burns fat for fuel almost exclusively—this is called "being in ketosis." Many popular diet programs have made use of this "metabolic advantage," most famously the Atkins program, and dietitians (and doctors) have been screaming about how dangerous it is ever since, although they can never seem to tell us why. It's been popular among dieters because, among other things, even the most metabolically resistant people usually lose weight on a ketogenic diet, and many people, after an initial adjustment from a sugar-burning to a fat-burning metabolism, feel great, with increased energy and a noticeable sense of well-being.

Atkins himself wrote rhapsodically of ketosis in the first and second editions of his New Diet Revolution, calling it "one of life's charmed gifts . . . As delightful as sex and sunshine, and it has fewer drawbacks than either of them." It was Atkins who gave ketosis the nickname "the metabolic advantage."

So how can something so harmless and benevolent (and so conducive to weight loss) be widely considered one of the most dangerous states the body can be in? (If you doubt that this is the prevailing opinion, try asking your mainstream doctor what he or she thinks of it. Or ask a dietitian.)

The reason is quite simple, actually. For the better part of 30 years, mainstream medicine, dietitians, and most of the critics of the low-carb diet have completely confused two conditions, as different from each other as the dolphin (fish) and the dolphin (Flipper). One of those conditions is ordinary, benign, dietary ketosis, of which we're speaking here. The other is a life-threatening condition called diabetic ketoacidosis (more on this in a minute). Getting the mainstream to understand the difference has been harder than getting the kid at the table to understand that the restaurant really isn't serving cooked Flipper.

Atkins, in the last edition of New Diet Revolution, pretty much gave up the 30-year fight to get the medical establishment to understand the difference; he stopped using the term ketosis. He switched to the term lipolysis (fat breakdown). Only time will tell if the name change is as successful as the switch to mahi-mahi has been.

The Real Deal on Ketosis

So what is this thing called ketosis, and why should we care?

Note: I'm going to go into a little biochemistry here. I'll try to make it painless, though I understand that, for many, the term *painless biochemistry* is an oxymoron. If you want to skip the next few paragraphs, believe me, I won't be offended. If, however, you'd like to *skewer* the next person who tells you how dangerous your low-carb diet is because of ketosis, you might want to read the next few hundred words.

Your body has three main sources of fuel: carbohydrates (glucose), proteins (amino acids), and fats (fatty acids). These are broken down and combined in different ways—fats and carbs to produce energy or to be saved as fat; protein to build up tissues, bones, muscles, enzymes, and the like. Remember that the whole purpose of a low-carb diet is to make your metabolism more of a fat-burning machine than a sugar-burning machine. As Lyle McDonald, one of the best-known authorities on the ketogenic diet, says, "Ketosis is the end result of a shift in the insulin/glucagon ratio and indicates *an overall shift from a glucose- (sugar-) based metabolism to a fat-based metabolism.*" (Emphasis mine.) In other words, the whole idea is to get your body to switch fuels from primarily carbs, its preferred immediate source of energy, to primarily fat.

Carbs, or sugar, are the first source of energy used by the body, with fats providing the best *long-term* source of energy. Yet high levels of carbohydrate produce, for many people, higher levels than desirable of the hormone insulin, and fat cannot be "burned" or "released" to any significant degree in the presence of insulin. So for someone with a weight problem, high carb intake will provide all the fuel they need for living (and probably plenty for storage as fat in addition) and will raise insulin levels enough so that fat isn't released or burned.

Normally, carbs are broken down into glucose, and then pyruvic acid, and then a substance called acetyl CoA. Fats are broken down into their component parts—fatty acids and glycerol—then *further* broken down (by a process called beta-oxidation) into two carbon fragments that *also* combine to make acetyl CoA (see the illustration on the following page).

On a "normal," high-carb diet, two things happen to the acetyl CoA. First, some of it gets broken down in the liver into ketone bodies. It's important to remember that this is a *normal* part of metabolism. You are making ketone bodies right now while you sit reading this book. The liver is *always* producing ketone bodies. As McDonald says, "Ketones should not be considered a toxic substance or a by-product of abnormal human metabolism. Rather, ketones are a normal physiological substance that plays many important roles in the human body." (This, of course, did not stop Jane Brody of the New York Times—one of the biggest apologists for the high-carbohydrate/low-fat diet in America—from calling ketones "toxic compounds that can damage the brain" and "pollute the blood.")

So the liver makes ketones—which are essentially by-products of fat metabolism (specifically the breakdown of acetyl CoA)—*all the time.*

What's the *other* thing that happens to the acetyl CoA?

Well, on a diet with plenty of carbohydrates, the acetyl CoA combines with a by-product of *carbohydrate* metabolism called *oxaloacetic acid.* When acetyl CoA combines with oxaloacetic acid, it enters an energy-production cycle called the Krebs cycle. (This is what is meant by the old saying "Fat burns in a flame of carbohydrate." Without the carbohydrate necessary to produce the oxaloacetic acid, the acetyl CoA cannot gain admission to this energy cycle and be burned.)

So those are the two pathways that acetyl CoA (which, you remember,

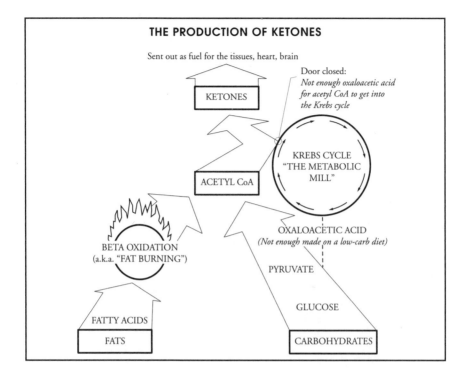

is produced by *both* fat breakdown and carbohydrate breakdown) can take when there's carbohydrate in the system.

But what happens when there isn't?

What happens when you go on a very restricted carbohydrate diet and there is not enough carbohydrate (glucose) coming down the pike to produce the oxaloacetic acid necessary to take the acetyl CoA into the Krebs cycle? Well, the acetyl CoA *accumulates* in the liver. And the liver promptly breaks it down into ketones (also known as ketone bodies—if you really want to get technical, there are three of these ketone bodies, and their names are acetoacetate, beta-hydroxybutrate, and acetone; it's the release of the acetone that gives you that "fruity" breath). The major determinant of whether the liver will produce a significant or negligible amount of ketone bodies is the amount of sugar (liver glycogen) that's around. In a low-carb diet, there's not a lot. So all of the acetyl CoA has to be broken down into ketones, and these ketones—products of *fat* breakdown—are now being made in sufficient quantities that you can detect them in the urine. The "normal" level of ketones in the blood is about 0.1 mmol/dl; mild ketosis is 0.2 mmol/dl. Ketogenic diets typically produce between 5 and 7 mmol/dl (see the chart on the following page).

COMPARISON OF KETONE CONCENTRATIONS UNDER DIFFERENT CONDITIONS	
Metabolic State	**Ketone Body Concentration (mmol/dl)**
mixed (regular) diet	0.01
ketosis	0.02
fasting 2–3 days	1
after exercise	up to 2
fasting 1 week	5
ketogenic diet	5–6
fasting 3–4 weeks	6–8
ketoacidosis	8+
diabetic ketoacidosis	up to 25

Note: Ketone body concentrations are higher when fasting than during a ketogenic diet due to the slight insulin response from eating.

Reprinted from Lyle McDonald, *The Ketogenic Diet: A Complete Guide for the Dieter and Practitioner* (Kearney, Neb.: Morris Publishing, 1998), by permission of the author.

After data from G.A. Mitchell et al, "Medical Aspects of Ketone Body Metabolism," *Clinical and Investigative Medicine* 18 (1995):193–216, and A. M. Robinson et al, "Physiological Roles of Ketone Bodies as Substrates and Signals in Mammalian Tissues," *Physiological Reviews* 60 (1980): 143–87.

Please remember: these ketones are benign products of normal metabolism, and the fact that you can actually see their presence in the urine (by the use of ketone test strips) simply means that your body is breaking down fat for energy in measurable, significant amounts.

So, how did ketone bodies get such a bad rap?

There are two reasons.

Ketosis and Diabetic Ketoacidosis

To understand the primary reason keytones have been vilified, we have to look at the type 1 diabetic. As you may remember from earlier discussion, insulin is responsible for getting sugar *out of the bloodstream* and *into the cells*, thus keeping blood sugar (glucose) within a tightly controlled range. Insulin also keeps fat from being broken down, which is why it needs to be in balance with its sister hormone, glucagon. Glucagon is responsible for releasing fat into the bloodstream, where it can be broken down and used for energy. Insulin is responsible for *storing* it.

The type 1 diabetic cannot make insulin.

With no insulin, two things happen, neither of them good. One, blood sugar rises to very dangerous levels. Two, with no insulin to put the brakes on glucagon, fat is broken down and released into the bloodstream faster than it can possibly be used, and the production of ketone bodies is seriously ramped up. In addition, these ketones *cannot* be used by the body tissues like they can in normal dietary ketosis. This is because there's tons of glucose around, which is the preferred fuel, so the ketones just keep accumulating at an alarming rate. This state is called *diabetic ketoacidosis*, and it is indeed very dangerous and life-threatening to an untreated type 1 diabetic. Remember, a ketogenic diet produces, on average, 5 to 7 mmol/dl of ketones, and does it in the presence of *normal to low* blood sugar. The untreated type 1 diabetic will produce ketones in the range of 25 mmol/dll (350 to 600% higher than normal!) and will do it in the presence of *extraordinarily high and dangerous* levels of blood sugar. There is absolutely no comparison between the two states. The person *without* uncontrolled type 1 diabetes has a number of normal feedback mechanisms that will always keep the ketones in a safe range, mechanisms that *do not exist* with the untreated type 1 diabetic. Diabetic ketoacidosis *cannot happen* when there is even a small amount of insulin around, as there *always* is in those not suffering from type 1 diabetes, even when the person is on a ketogenic diet.

The second reason ketosis has gotten a bad rap is a reversal of a medical fact. Ketosis is one of the metabolic adaptations to starvation. When you're starving, the body uses ketones for fuel. Starving is bad. Therefore, people who didn't think about it very clearly reversed the order and assumed that since ketosis is one of the *reactions* to something bad, ketosis *itself* must be bad. That's like assuming that umbrellas cause rain. Ketosis in

COMPARISON OF DIETARY KETOSIS WITH DIABETIC KETOACIDOSIS			
	Normal Diet	**Ketosis**	**Diabetic Ketoacidosis**
blood glucose (mg/dl)	80–120	~65–80	**300+**
insulin	moderate	low	**absent**
glucagon	low	high	**high**
ketone production (g/day)	low	115–180	400
ketone concentrations	0.1	4–10	
blood pH	7.4	7.4	**<7.3**

Reprinted from Lyle McDonald, *The Ketogenic Diet: A Complete Guide for the Dieter and Practitioner* (Kearney, Neb.: Morris Publishing, 1998), by permission of the author.

starvation is very, very different from ketosis in the ketogenic (high-fat or high-protein) diet. Why? In starvation, the body is *breaking down muscle* in the absence of dietary protein. In the low-carb diet, dietary protein is plentiful and prevents the loss of muscle that occurs with true starvation. The loss of body protein is actually what causes death from starvation. When you supply sufficient protein in the diet, this simply doesn't happen.

Are Ketones Dangerous?

Hardly. They're a perfectly good source of energy. Drs. Donald and Judith Voet, authors of a popular medical biochemistry textbook, say that ketones "serve as important metabolic fuels for many peripheral tissues, particularly heart and skeletal muscle."[4] And a recent paper coauthored by a number of distinguished researchers, including one from Harvard Medical School, stated that ketones provide an efficient source of energy for the brain and that mild ketosis—the kind you achieve on a low-carb diet—could have a wide range of benefits for conditions ranging from Alzheimer's to Parkinson's.[5]

KETONES FOR ALZHEIMER'S?

In Alzheimer's disease, some brain cells have difficulty metabolizing glucose, the primary source of energy for the brain. Deprived of fuel, some of these valuable neurons may die.

KETONES TO THE RESCUE

Ketones are such good fuel for the brain that a Colorado biotech company called Accera developed an oral liquid that helps the body produce more of them.* The drug—brand name Axona—is marketed as a potential adjunct treatment for Alzheimer's.

Ketones are a wonderful alternative fuel for the brain, which functions quite well on them after a brief period of adaptation. The patients enrolled in the Ketasyn trial showed significant improvement in memory and cognition.

*http://www.drugresearcher.com/Emerging-targets/Brain-energy-boost-slows-Alzheimer-s

A ketogenic diet should not be used by three groups of people: (1) uncontrolled type 1 diabetics (for the reasons outlined above); (2) pregnant or nursing women (not because higher levels of ketones in the blood are dangerous, but just because we don't know for sure if they have any effect on the baby); and (3) people with existing kidney disease (see myth #5 for a full explanation of the connection between protein and kidneys).

If you are not in one of these three groups—type 1 diabetics, pregnant or nursing women, or people with existing kidney disease—the ketogenic diet is *perfectly and utterly safe.*

Let's take a look at the science.

A recent study in the *Journal of Nutrition* looked at the effects of a 6-week ketogenic diet on risk factors for cardiovascular disease.[6] The study found *improvements* in triglycerides and insulin levels, plus a slight *increase* in HDL cholesterol (the "good" kind). Most importantly, the *type* of LDL ("bad" cholesterol) tended to change from the kind that's dangerous (pattern B) to the kind that's not (pattern A). Other studies have shown similar results.[7]

A recent study at the University of Cincinnati and Children's Hospital Medical Center in Cincinnati specifically looked at the effects of a very-low-carbohydrate diet on cardiovascular risk factors in fifty-three obese but otherwise healthy women. The women were placed on either a very-low-carbohydrate diet with unrestricted calories, or a low-fat diet that was calorie-restricted. The low-carb group lost significantly more weight and, more importantly, more *body fat* than the low-fat diet group. (Interestingly, after the study, both groups of women wound up maintaining their weight loss on about the same number of calories—1,300.)

This last-mentioned study is particularly interesting for a couple of reasons. One, the low-carb group *was* in ketosis, but as the authors noted, the level of ketones wasn't even close to that seen in starvation or diabetic ketoacidosis and presented no problems whatsoever. Two, the subjects on the very-low-carbohydrate diet experienced significantly more weight loss than the low-fat group *and* maintained great readings for blood chemistries and cardiovascular risk factors *while consuming more than 50% of their calories as fat and 20% as saturated fat.* Current standards for healthful eating include reducing total fat intake to less than 30% of total calories and decreasing saturated fat to less than 10%, which is supposed to both lower cholesterol and decrease the risk of obesity. These subjects accomplished the same thing while eating a heck of a lot more fat—and saturated fat— than the current standards, *plus* they lost more weight in the bargain. The authors wisely conclude that "this study provides a surprising challenge to prevailing dietary practice."[8]

Finally, ketogenic diets have been used as treatments for childhood epilepsy for more than 70 years. They are currently used at seventy-eight centers in the United States alone, including Children's Hospital in Los Angeles, John Hopkins in Baltimore, the UCLA School of Medicine, Children's Hospital in Boston, the Montefiore Medical Center and Columbia Presbyterian Medical Center in New York, and the Lucille Packard Children's Hospital at Stanford, whose website states: "No patient has had serious complications."

Do You Have to Be in Ketosis to Lose Weight on a Low-Carb Diet?

No. You don't.

Ketosis is actually only a feature of some low-carb diets, and not even that many. It is stressed in the early version of Atkins; it is likely (but not mandatory) in Protein Power, the Paleo Solution, and a few others. Many other low-carb programs don't even mention it. The point is that it is not something to fear. Many nutrition experts—myself included—feel that you don't have to be in ketosis to get the benefits of a low-carb diet. You can "flirt" with ketosis, be on the cusp of ketosis, but unless you are very metabolically resistant, you may be able to get the benefits of low-carb eating without ever worrying about your ketone levels.

Perhaps the most sober and rational summary of the ketogenic diet is given by Lyle McDonald, who wrote the definitive book on the subject and accumulated the greatest number of scientific references on ketosis ever seen in one place. He says: "After years of experimenting with the [ketogenic] diet myself, and getting feedback from hundreds and hundreds of people, about the best anyone can say is that the ketogenic diet is a diet that works very well for many but not for all."

Amen.

BOTTOM LINE

Dietary ketosis is not the same as diabetic ketoacidosis. The ketosis of a low-carb diet is not the same as ketosis in starvation. Many studies have demonstrated the safety of ketogenic diets, even for children.

MYTH #4: Low-Carbohydrate Diets Cause Calcium Loss, Bone Loss, and/or Osteoporosis

This criticism of low-carb (or high-protein) diets is based on the fact that higher levels of protein result in higher levels of calcium in the urine, leading some people to the erroneous conclusion that protein causes bone loss. But a tremendous number of recent studies are showing something quite the opposite.

Want Strong Bones? Eat More Protein!

The Framingham Osteoporosis Study investigated protein consumption over a 4-year period among 615 elderly men and women with an average age of 75. The amount of protein eaten daily ranged from a low of 14 grams a day to a high of 175 grams. And guess what? The people who consumed *more* protein had less bone loss! Those who ate less protein had more bone loss, both at the femoral bone and at the spine. The study also found that "higher intake of animal protein *does not appear to affect the skeleton adversely.*"[9] (Emphasis mine.)

Calcium is better absorbed on a higher-protein diet, even if there is somewhat more *urinary* calcium excretion. High-protein diets in two recent studies resulted in *significantly more* calcium absorption than the low-protein diets, which were associated with *decreased* absorption.[10] Interestingly, the actual "low-protein" diet that caused decreased calcium absorption in these studies had about the same amount of protein that the government recommends for adults! The authors concluded that this fact "raises new questions about the optimal amount of dietary protein required for normal calcium metabolism and bone health in young women." And a 2002 study in *Obesity Research* looked at a high-protein versus low-protein diet to determine whether the protein content of the diet impacted bone mineral density. It did. *Bone mineral loss was greater in the low-protein group.*[11]

In other words, without enough protein, you just ain't gonna build (and preserve) strong bones, and the definition of "enough protein" may turn out to be a lot more than we previously thought.

The Verdict on Protein: Not Guilty

So, how did protein get this bad reputation for causing calcium loss and osteoporosis? It partly stems from something in the body called the acid–base balance. All foods eventually digest and present themselves to the kidneys as either acid or alkaline (base). When there is too much acid, the body needs to buffer it, and calcium is one of the best buffering agents. Meats—along with many other foods, especially grains—are known to be acid-producing; hence the deduction that high-protein diets would cause a leeching of calcium from the bone in order to alkalize the acid content.

But here's the thing: we now know that if you take in enough alkalinizing nutrients, this doesn't happen. If you balance your high-protein foods with calcium (and potassium), you will not lose calcium from your bones! An interesting side note: you can take all the supplemental calcium you want; if you don't get enough protein, it's not going to make much difference to your bone health. The studies are very clear on this: *extra calcium is not enough to affect the skeleton when protein intake is low.*[12]

In short, it doesn't matter if there is a little more calcium in the urine as long as the body is holding on to more calcium than it's losing (i.e., is in "positive" calcium balance). And it will do that when there's plenty of protein plus calcium (and other minerals) in the diet.

BOTTOM LINE

Higher protein intakes do not cause bone loss or osteoporosis, especially in the presence of adequate mineral intakes. In fact, lower protein intakes are associated with more bone loss.

MYTH #5: High-Protein Diets Cause Damage to the Kidneys

You will often hear from ill-informed sources that a high-protein diet damages the kidneys. Not so. Consider the following: everyone knows about step classes and aerobics. They are great calorie burners, get the blood and oxygen flowing, are good conditioners of the cardiovascular system, and, with certain variations, can even be good for muscle toning. So they're a good thing, right?

Yes.

Except if you have a broken leg.

If you have a broken leg, or a sprained ankle, or shin splints, I'm going to suggest that you not take a step class until the injury heals. Under these special circumstances, the very weight-bearing that does so much good for the normal person is going to be more stress than you need during the healing phase. I'm going to tell you to stay off the leg, let it heal, and avoid putting additional stress on it at this time.

Does the fact that step class is not good for a person with a broken leg mean that the step class *led* to the broken leg?

No. And ketogenic diets do not—I repeat, *do not*—cause kidney disease. If your doctor says they do, politely ask him or her to show you the studies. (They don't exist.) Ketogenic diets are, however, *not* a good thing if you have an *existing kidney disease*, much the way a step class is not a good thing if your leg is already broken.

High Protein Causes Kidney Disease? Not.

The oft-repeated medical legend that high-protein diets cause kidney disease came from reversing a medical fact. The medical fact is that reducing protein (up to a point) lessens the decline of renal (kidney) function in people who already have kidney disease. Because restricting protein seems to be a good strategy for those with *existing* kidney failure (or even some kidney weakness), some people drew the illogical conclusion that the reverse must also be true—that large amounts of protein *lead* to kidney failure.

In any case, it is not proteins per se that cause problems, even for those who already have renal disease: it is the *glycolated* proteins. These sugar-sticky proteins, you may remember, are the result of excess sugar in the blood bumping into protein molecules. These sugar-coated proteins are called AGEs, advanced glycolated end-products. The AGEs themselves then stick together, forming even bigger collections of molecules, which are too large to pass through the filtering mechanisms of the *glomerulus*, the network of blood capillaries in the kidneys that acts as a filter for waste products from the blood. This reduces GFR (glomerular filtration rate), a measure of kidney function.

High-protein intake *does not* cause this to happen in normally functioning kidneys. In 2003, a study of 1,624 women enrolled in the Nurses' Health Study concluded that "high protein intake was *not* associated with renal function decline in women with normal renal function."[13] Another study in the *American Journal of Kidney Diseases* showed that protein intake had *no effect* on GFR in healthy male subjects.[14] And a third study in the *International Journal of Obesity* compared a high-protein with a low-protein weight-loss diet and concluded that healthy kidneys adapted to protein intake and that the high-protein diet caused no adverse effects.[15]

If you don't currently have kidney disease, a low-carbohydrate diet is actually an ideal way to help control the blood-sugar levels that can eventually lead to kidney disease. Of course, just to be safe, you should check with your doctor to make sure you don't have any undiagnosed kidney impairment; but if you don't, you're sure not going to develop it from being on a low-carb diet.

BOTTOM LINE

Higher protein intakes do not cause any damage whatsoever to healthy kidneys.

MYTH #6: The Only Reason You Lose Weight on a Low-Carb Diet Is Because It's Low in Calories

The short response to this myth is simple: *so what?*

This accusation—that low-carb diets work only because they are low in calories—is particularly amusing because it is never made against high-carb weight-loss diets that are *equally* low in calories. In fact, there is only a 121-calorie difference between the most stringent induction phase of the Atkins diet and the Dean Ornish ultra-low-fat diet. And after the first couple of weeks, when you get into the ongoing weight-loss phase of Atkins, you're actually consuming 354 calories more than you would be on the Dean Ornish diet and 165 calories *more* than you would be on Weight Watchers![16] Yet you never hear the establishment say that the Ornish low-fat diet works only because it's low-calorie!

Look, on virtually every weight-loss diet in the world, you ultimately wind up consuming fewer calories than you did while you were putting on weight. I don't care if the diet is low-fat, high-fat, low-carb, high-carb, vegetarian, Food Guide Pyramid, raw food, you name it—ultimately, they are *all* reduced-calorie diets. One of the primary reasons most of them fail is hunger. By now, we know that insulin is called the hunger hormone for a very good reason, and insulin is elevated *most* by high-carbohydrate diets. So if you have a choice of gritting your teeth and staying on a 1,200-calorie, low-fat, high-carbohydrate diet that leaves you hungry and craving sweets all the time—or of going on a diet with the *same number of calories* that allows you to eat rich, satisfying, natural foods and doesn't leave you hungry all the time, which would *you* pick?

Exactly. That's why the short answer to this myth is "Who cares?" Even if it were true that low-carb diets work only because they are low-calorie, who gives a rat's tail? If two "diets" with an equal number of calories produce equal weight loss but one is easier to stay on, why in the world wouldn't you go with it?

More Food on a Low-Carb Diet?

Because a low-carbohydrate diet is able to reduce insulin levels and is far more likely to induce hormonally balanced states than conventional high-carb diets, it is possible—though we're not 100% sure—that you may be able to consume somewhat more calories on a low-carb diet than you would on a high-carb diet and still lose weight. One dramatic study compared a low-fat diet to an Atkins-type diet in two groups of overweight adolescent boys. After three months, the low-carb group lost more than twice as much weight as the low-fat group (19 pounds for the low-carb group and 8.5 pounds for the low-fat group); the low-fat group averaged 1,100 calories a day, while the Atkins group averaged 1,803![17]

Recently, a number of studies have come out showing that weight loss is actually greater on a low-carb diet than on a conventional low-fat diet that has the same number of calories.[18] To be fair, there are plenty of studies showing that both diets produce identical weight loss. (Interestingly, there are virtually no studies that show that low-carb diets produce less weight loss!) But even in the studies that show identical weight loss, triglycerides and HDL levels almost always improve on the higher-protein diets. For example, Alain Golay, a respected researcher who is no particular advocate of low-carb diets, recently tested a low-carb (25%) diet against a typical higher-carb (45%) diet for weight loss and found that, while there was not much difference in weight loss, the low-carb group had significantly greater improvements in fasting insulin and triglycerides.[19] In another study, he pitted a low-carb (15%) diet against a higher-carb (45%) diet and again found similar weight loss but marked improvements in glucose, insulin, cholesterol, and triglycerides on the low-carb diet only; no such benefits were seen on the high-carb diet.[20] If two "diets"—high-protein/low-carb and high-carb/low-fat—are equal in calories and produce equal weight loss but the first produces significantly improved blood chemistry and lowers the risk for heart disease and diabetes, why in the world wouldn't you choose that one?

Many studies have been done comparing all kinds of different diets for weight loss; but the truth is that very few studies have lasted more than a year, leading many experts to conclude that while you can basically lose weight on any diet, we really have no idea whether any particular regimen is easier to stay on over the long haul. The action is clearly in *maintaining* weight loss, and since the lower-carb diets seem to be much more satiating, we can speculate that they may turn out to be a lot easier to maintain as a lifestyle than a diet that simply reduces fat, which is turning out to be a lot less important than previously thought. In fact, in 2002, Dr. Walter Willett, chairman of the Department of Nutrition at Harvard University's School of Public Health and one of the most respected researchers in the field, declared in two articles—one in *Obesity Reviews*[21] and one in the *American Journal of Medicine*[22]—that dietary fat is *not* a major determinant of body fat and plays virtually no role in obesity. What about calories?

Since most low-carb-diet authors do not advocate counting calories (at least at first) and because most low-carb diets are based on the premise that it is critical to control the hormonal responses to food, many people have gotten the idea that low-carb theorists think calories don't matter at all. This is simply not so. As I wrote in a previous book, calories are still on the marquee; it's just that they are not starring players anymore. Of *course* calories still count—there isn't a responsible low-carb diet writer out there who would argue the point. But controlling hormones counts *at least as much*, if not more. If I take in 1,500 calories a day from sugar and insulin-raising carbohydrates, I will find it notoriously difficult to lose any weight, since the high levels of insulin I produce are going to effectively block fat from being released from my fat cells. Yet if I take in the same 1,500 calories—or even a few more!—from a diet with fewer carbs and more protein and fat, the resulting balance between insulin and glucagon is going to be much more favorable to fat release. And I'm likely to lose a lot more weight for the same caloric price.

On the other hand, to play devil's advocate, if I take in 15,000 calories, all from fat with a little protein, producing the absolute minimum amount of insulin, I'm *still* going to gain weight. Why? Because even though the "doors" to the fat cells are now open for business, there is simply no reason for my body to *release* any of the fat inside them for fuel, because I'm already consuming way more fuel than I could possibly need.

Now, can you lose weight on a low-calorie diet that is not low-carb? Of course you can. People do it all the time. But consider the following: most weight-loss diets—of any kind—wind up being lower in carbohydrates *even if they are not "low-carb" diets*. The average overweight American man is easily able to consume 3,500 calories daily, and let's hypothetically say 65% of it is from carbs. That's a total of 2,275 calories from carbs, or 569 grams of carbohydrates a day. The National Weight Control Registry, which follows people who have successfully lost at least 30 pounds and kept it off for more than a year, has found that the average man on a successful weight-maintenance diet consumes 1,724 calories, of which 56% come from carbohydrates.[23] So our typical National Weight Control Registry man is consuming 237 grams of carbs a day, *a 59% reduction in carbohydrates from what he was eating when he put the weight on!*

The average successful *woman* on the registry maintains her weight at 1,297 calories, 55% from carbohydrates.[24] We can postulate that if she was 50 pounds overweight to begin with, she was eating *at least* 2,000 calories a day minimum (probably more), and even if only 60% of that came from carbs, that's 300 grams of carbs a day. At her present maintenance level, she's consuming 178 grams, a 41% reduction in carb intake, certainly enough to make a major impact on insulin levels.

Yes, calories count. But so do hormones, and way more than the dietary establishment believes.

BOTTOM LINE

Calories count, but so do hormones. Many studies show more weight lost on low-carb diets than on high-carb diets with the same number of calories, and more of that weight comes from fat. Even those studies that show equal weight loss invariably show better blood chemistry on the low-carb diets. Lowering fat in the diet is not the answer to obesity.

MYTH #7: Low-Carb Diets Increase the Risk for Heart Disease

In Denmark, the number of storks is positively correlated with the number of babies born.

This interesting fact was taught to me in graduate school by a wonderful psychology professor named Dr. Scott Fraser, who used it to teach a lesson about scientific studies that has allowed me to understand a great many things about research. I will pass it on to you, and you may never look at research studies in quite the same way.

So let's repeat: in Denmark, the more storks, the more babies. This positive correlation holds up year in and year out.

OK, class, what shall we conclude from this?

I hope you see what I'm getting at.

Here's what's *actually* going on. In the particular part of Denmark where the study was done, single people live mainly in the cities. When they get married and decide to raise a family, they move to the suburbs. The architectural design of the suburbs in Denmark favors angled roofs made of tar. Storks nest in angled roofs made of tar. Both storks and young married couples wanting to have children gravitate to the same area, albeit for somewhat different reasons.

A LITTLE INTERNET HUMOR

1. *The Japanese eat very little fat and suffer fewer heart attacks than the British or Americans.*

2. *The Mexicans eat a lot of fat and suffer fewer heart attacks than the British or Americans.*

3. *The Japanese drink very little red wine and suffer fewer heart attacks than the British or Americans.*

4. *The Italians drink excessive amounts of red wine and suffer fewer heart attacks than the British or Americans.*

5. *The Germans drink a lot of beers and eat lots of sausages and fats and suffer fewer heart attacks than the British or Americans.*

Conclusion: Eat and drink what you like. Speaking English is apparently what kills you.

But they are *found together*, consistently, year after year. They are *positively correlated*.

The lesson: *correlation* does not equal *causation*. When two variables are found together, it does not mean that one caused the other. Diabetes went way up during the Clinton presidency, so an increase in diabetes is positively correlated with the Clintons. Statistical studies have also noted that the number of new radio and television sets purchased correlates with an increased number of deaths from coronary disease.[25] In Stockholm, Sweden, there was a correlation between the municipal tax rate and coronary mortality, leading to the interesting proposition that if tax rates were lowered, there would be less heart disease![26]

One scholar described this as the "yellow finger" phenomenon. Men with yellow fingertips are more likely to die of lung cancer. The reason: they are smokers. That's why they *have* yellow fingers. The yellowed tips of their fingers are the result of holding twenty cigarettes a day for 20 years. Washing off the yellow will not reduce their risk for lung cancer.

This brings us to cholesterol, heart disease, and the low-carb diet.

The Birth of the Diet-Heart Hypothesis and the Demonization of Saturated Fat

When the diet-heart hypothesis—the idea that saturated fat causes heart disease—was first proposed in the 1950s by Ancel Keys (see chapter 2), very little was known about either fat or cholesterol. Cholesterol, which is actually not a fat at all but a waxy molecule classified as a sterol, is the parent molecule for all the sex hormones in the body. Without it, you would not have testosterone, the estrogens, progesterone, or DHEA, not to mention cortisol and aldosterone. Most of the cholesterol in your body is *produced* by your body. *Dietary* cholesterol has virtually *no effect* on the amount of cholesterol in your blood. Two major long-term studies, Framingham and Tecumseh, confirm this (see the following tables);[27] they show that those who ate the most cholesterol had exactly the same level of cholesterol in their blood as those who ate the least. Even Keys, the author of the diet-heart hypothesis, knew this and said, in 1991: "*There's no connection whatsoever between cholesterol in food and cholesterol in blood and we've known that all along. Cholesterol in the diet doesn't matter at all unless you happen to be a chicken or a rabbit.*"[28]

CHOLESTEROL INTAKE—THE FRAMINGHAM HEART STUDY			
	Average Cholesterol From Food	Below Average Cholesterol From Food	Above Average Cholesterol From Food
		Blood Cholesterol	
	mg/day	mmol/L	mmol/L
Men	704 ± 220.9	6.16	6.16
Women	492 ± 170.0	6.37	6.26

CHOLESTEROL INTAKE AND BLOOD LIPIDS—THE TECUMSEH STUDY			
Blood Cholesterol in Thirds	Lower	Middle	Upper
Daily Intake of Cholesterol (mg)	554	566	533

What we do know is that dietary fat has an effect on serum cholesterol. What is a lot less clear is whether it matters much. (Michael and Mary Dan Eades call "Cholesterol Madness" the most important chapter in their book "not because we believe cholesterol is such an important problem but because *everybody else does*." I'm with the Eadeses, as I discussed in more detail in chapter 5.) Fully 50% of heart attacks happen to people with completely normal cholesterol numbers.[29] The Tokelauan Islanders get 63% of their diet from the healthy saturated fat in coconuts, and, though their cholesterol levels are a bit high, they have virtually no heart disease.[30]

Fats: The Good, the Bad, and the Ugly

We know a lot more about fat than we did back in the '50s and even in the '80s, when the message was "All fat is bad." Most people are now aware that there are "good" fats and "bad" fats, and most people believe that the bad fats are saturated. Not so fast. It's turning out to be even more complicated than that. We now know that there is a type of fat far more dangerous and insidious than saturated fat: *trans-fat;* and virtually all of the data we have that "links" saturated fat with heart disease did not distinguish between *saturated* fats and *trans-fats*. Therefore, it is almost impossible to know whether or not saturated fats got the blame for something that was really being done by trans-fats.[31] Saturated fats, for example, *lower* lipoprotein(a), a risk factor for heart disease, and *raise* protective HDL cholesterol; trans-fats not only do the exact opposite but also raise LDL cholesterol![32] Many of us now believe that saturated fats have gotten the blame for damage that is actually caused by trans-fats. Virtually every low-carbohydrate diet, by definition, contains incredibly low amounts of trans-fats.

Furthermore, we also know that "saturated fat" is not a homogeneous entity. It consists of many different types of fatty acids, and some of them are downright beneficial for health. For example, lauric acid has antimicrobial and antiviral properties and is able to fight bacteria. Caprylic acid is used to fight yeast. Short- and medium-chain saturated fatty acids like those found in coconuts are actually much more likely to be burned for fuel than stored as fat, and can be a great adjunct to a weight-loss program.[33] And others, like stearic acid, have no effect whatsoever on cholesterol, except to possibly *raise* protective HDL.

Consider this, as the brilliant investigative reporter and three-time National Association of Science Writers' Science in Society Award–winner Gary Taubes did in a recent article in *Science*. A porterhouse steak cooks down to about half fat and half protein. Of that fat, 51% is monounsaturated, mostly all from oleic acid, the same monounsaturated fat found in heart-healthy olive oil. Forty-five percent is saturated, but a third of that is stearic acid, which at worst is harmless and at best raises HDL cholesterol. The remaining 4% is polyunsaturated. Thus, a porterhouse steak may actually be better for your heart—especially if eaten with a generous helping of vegetables—than a no-fat meal of high-glycemic, triglyceride-raising pasta.[34]

There's More to Cholesterol Than Just "Good" and "Bad"

Most people are aware that cholesterol comes in two "flavors," good (HDL) and bad (LDL). But most people do not know that both HDL and LDL have different subclasses, and that these subclasses behave quite differently in the body. For example, LDL cholesterol has at least five subtypes, two of which are very important for the purposes of our discussion—pattern A, which are large, fluffy, cotton ball–like molecules, and pattern B, which are small, dense molecules that look like BB gun pellets. It is these small, dense LDL molecules that cause plaque and contribute to heart disease; the fluffy LDL is fairly harmless. In recent years, studies have begun to look at the factors that affect these particle sizes.[35] We are finding out that while the traditional high-carb, low-fat diet may in fact lower *overall* LDL, it *raises* the dangerous pattern B molecules and *lowers* protective HDL cholesterol. So while your overall cholesterol number may go down, your overall risk may go *up*. Not only that: high-carbohydrate diets significantly raise triglycerides—this is inarguable and has been shown in virtually every major study comparing high-carb to low-carb diets. The combination of high triglycerides and low HDL is far more predictive of heart disease (and far more dangerous) than an overall elevated cholesterol number.[36]

In the following story, you can see cholesterol madness in action: I have a dear friend who is in great shape and exercises every day. He came to me because he and his doctor were very concerned that his cholesterol was too high. I looked at his blood tests. He had normal lipoprotein(a), a fasting glucose under 100, a fasting insulin of 5, triglycerides under 100, an HDL of 60 (giving him a triglyceride/HDL ratio of less than 2!), a cholesterol ratio itself of 3, normal C-reactive protein (a measure of inflammation), and a homocysteine (a huge risk factor for heart disease) under 7—but his overall cholesterol was 240. I wish I had those numbers! This man had a better chance of winning the lottery than he did of ever getting heart disease. He will never have a heart attack. Yet his doctor was ready to put him on a lifetime of expensive medication with potentially damaging side effects to bring down a number that *did not matter!*

You might reasonably ask at this point: if cholesterol is not as important an issue as we thought, how is it that the statin drugs (which reduce cholesterol) save lives?

Good question.

The statin drugs probably do save some lives (though the number is probably way less than you've been lead to believe, and the cost remains to be seen). However, whether they do so by reducing cholesterol is an open question. What the statins do *in addition* to lowering cholesterol is reduce *inflammation,* which *is* a cause of heart disease. What they do to cholesterol, in my opinion, is the least important thing that they do in the body. You can reduce inflammation by consuming omega-3 fatty acids and reducing consumption of grains without the possible statin drug side effects of liver toxicity and mitochondrial damage, and without the increased risk for death from other causes that is associated with cholesterol numbers that are too low.

Do Low-Fat Diets Prevent Heart Disease?

So, then, what about that famous Dean Ornish study that showed that low-fat diets reverse heart disease?

Actually, it showed no such thing. The Ornish study took forty-eight middle-aged white men with existing moderate to severe coronary heart disease. The researchers then did five—count 'em, *five*—simultaneous interventions with these men. They put them on a stress-reduction program. They got them to stop smoking. They gave them group therapy and support. They had them do daily aerobic exercise. *And* they put them on a very high-fiber diet, which also happened to be low in fat. Why anyone would conclude that it was the low-fat part of this multiple intervention that caused their improvement is a mystery. If we put those same men on a program of exercise, stress reduction, smoking cessation, group support, and meditation and included a pack of M&M's in their diet every day, would we conclude that M&M's reduce heart disease? I would argue that Ornish would have gotten the identical results—perhaps even *better* ones—using all those good interventions plus a diet loaded with fiber, absent of trans-fats, absent of sugar, containing very low amounts of vegetable fats, *and* containing plenty of good-quality protein from grass-fed animals plus saturated, monounsaturated, and omega-3 fats. We'll never know, because when five factors are involved, it is impossible to say which of them—or what combination of them—is responsible for the results.[37]

On a personal note: in researching this book, I read through literally hundreds of studies on cholesterol, fat, and heart disease. I could have rented a cot in the National Library of Medicine. I read the papers that appeared in the medical journals, I read the reanalysis of the data by scholars who questioned the cholesterol/saturated-fat hypothesis of heart disease, I studied their arguments, I read the rebuttals to their arguments, and I read the rebuttals to the *rebuttals.*

I have, I confess, come to believe—along with a growing number of health professionals—that saturated fat and cholesterol are, for the most part, innocent bystanders. They were in the wrong place at the wrong time, Your Honor, and they hung out with the wrong crowd. As I mentioned earlier, virtually every epidemiological study that linked saturated-fat consumption with increased risk of cardiovascular diseases failed to separate saturated fat from its extremely dangerous cohort, trans-fatty acids.[38] Nor did the studies implicating saturated fat distinguish the *source* of the saturated fat consumed: saturated fat from natural foods like butter, eggs, and grain-fed cattle is *not* the same as saturated fat from fries and burgers; most people in industrial nations consume their saturated fat from hot dogs, fast-food hamburgers, and processed deli meats like salami and bologna. The people consuming the most saturated fat in those studies ate few fruits and vegetables and little fiber. But they ate something like 150 pounds of sugar per year (the latest figures from the USDA from 1997, projected to soon rise to 170 pounds). And for the most part, they did not exercise. Although it is extremely convenient to blame a single factor (like saturated fat) for heart disease, the fact is that a matrix of lifestyle and dietary characteristics such as the ones just mentioned are found *together*. In my opinion, saturated fat and cholesterol are not the bad guys here.

New research is beginning to support this. When a recent study in the *British Medical Journal* factored in fiber intake, the usual association between saturated fat and coronary-disease risk practically vanished. The study concluded that the adverse effects of saturated fat and cholesterol are "at least in part explained by their low-fiber content and their associations with other risk factors." The researchers further stated that "benefits of reducing intakes of saturated fat and cholesterol are likely to be modest *unless accompanied by an increased consumption of foods rich in fiber*." The study also commented on how the inclusion of omega-3 fats in the diet had a protective effect on the heart.[39]

However . . .

I realize that this is a radical position and a hard sell to a population that has been raised on the premise that saturated fat and cholesterol are basically the children of Satan. So let me put you at ease: to do a low-carb diet, you do not have to accept the position that cholesterol and saturated fat are relatively harmless. In fact, many of the low-carb authors don't accept that position either, so you will be in good company (notable exceptions—with whom I agree—are the Eadeses, Schwarzbein, and Atkins). You can do the Hamptons Diet, in which almost all of the fat comes from monounsaturated sources. You can do the Zone, which limits saturated fat and stresses omega-3s. You can do the Paleo Diet, or the South Beach Diet, both of which are about as anti–saturated fat as you can get. Or you can do Protein Power or Atkins and just make sure you're getting a ton of omega-3s.

On virtually all low-carb diets, blood-lipid chemistries improve. That's what is important, and that is the take-home point here. Even those studies that showed identical weight loss with low-carb versus high-carb diets demonstrated this: low-carb diets beat the pants off high-carb diets every time when it comes to lowering triglycerides and raising HDL, even in those few cases where weight loss was identical.[40]

And here's the pièce de résistance. If you and/or your doctor are still concerned about the amount of fat in low-carb diets, consider the following (see the following table): if you are a male who is 40 to 50 pounds over-weight, you have probably been consuming a diet of *at least* 3,500 calories a day (probably more: one fast-food order of fries alone is 700). Let's say you've been adhering to the dietary guidelines of no more than 30% of your calories from fat, with no more than 10% of the total diet from satu-rated fat. That means you have been consuming about 1,050 calories a day from fat, of which 350 are from saturated fat.

MALE, 40 TO 50 POUNDS OVERWEIGHT: FAT INTAKE ON CURRENT DIET COMPARED WITH LOW-CARB DIET					
	Calories	% Total Fat	Fat Calories	% Saturated Fat	Saturated-Fat Calories
Current diet (follows dietary guidelines for fat)	3,500–4,000	30%	1,050–1,200	10%	350–400
Low-carb, high-fat diet	1,700	50%	850	20%	340

Now look at what happens if you go on a typical low-carb weight reduc-tion diet. You would consume in the ballpark of 1,700 satisfying, filling calo-ries. Let's give the worst-case scenario, from your doctor's point of view, and say that a full 50% of those 1,700 calories come from fat—that's 850 fat calories, definitely a high-fat diet in anyone's book. Say that 20% (twice the dietary guidelines) of your total calories comes from saturated fat (340). Even with these numbers, you would actually consume 20% *less* overall fat on a low-carb diet than you were before, when you were following the dietary guidelines. This should put both you and your doctor at ease.

BOTTOM LINE

Low-carbohydrate diets do not increase the risk for heart disease. If anything, they improve blood-lipid profiles.

CHAPTER 7

But What about the China Study?

With fair regularity, I get an e-mail or blog comment that takes me to task for recommending low-carb diets, for suggesting that humans usually do better with some animal products in their diet, for questioning the significance of cholesterol as a risk factor for heart disease, and for completely dismissing the obsolete notion that cholesterol in the diet makes a whit of difference to anything. These letters are often snarky, mean-spirited, and condescending, and more than a few of them end with the same rhetorical question: *"Didn't you ever hear of the China Study?"* The sarcastic tone is always the same, as if they were asking a heathen, *"Didn't you ever hear of a little thing called the Bible?"*

Well, yes, actually, I have heard of the China Study. Not only have I heard of it, but I've read the book *and* seen the movie *Forks over Knives*. I've also heard of the work of Joel Furhman, Caldwell B. Esselstyn, John McDougall, Neil Barnard, and all the rest of the good folks who believe, deeply in their DNA, that animal products are bad, bad, bad, and that fat should be mostly avoided (especially saturated fat!) and that a whole-foods, plant-based diet is the best answer to obesity, diabetes, cancer, and heart disease.

So yes, I'm quite familiar with the China Study. But unlike my vegan friends who treat it as some kind of final authority, I'm not at all convinced that T. Colin Campbell's book *The China Study*—or even the *real* China project on which it's based—is the be-all and end-all of nutritional research. Nor am I convinced by the pro-vegan arguments of Campbell, Furhman, or any of their rabidly fanatic followers.

Oh, heck, let me be real: I think the argument advanced in *The China Study* is basically bunk.

First, some background. Campbell's book is not the *actual* "China

Study"; it's an *interpretation of* an 894-page behemoth of a book called *Diet, Life-style, and Mortality in China: A Study of the Characteristics of 65 Chinese Countries*, authored by four researchers, of which Campbell was one. (The other three are Chen Junshi, Li Junyao, and Richard Peto.)

Diet, Life-style, and Mortality in China is an enormous book consisting of data on 367 variables measured in 65 different counties and involving no less than 6,500 adults. The book is physically imposing—about the size of the *Physicians' Desk Reference*, and weighing nearly as much. Only the first 80 pages are text. After that, you get 800 pages of pure numeric data, densely packed on the page and looking like ticker-tape printout from the New York Stock Exchange. Understand, now, that they took 367 variables and correlated each one with the other 366, generating over 100,000 data points (or associations), of which 92,000 were statistically meaningless. (The other 8,000 were statistically significant.) Any way you slice it, that's a whole lotta numbers.

The first thing to know about *Diet, Life-Style, and Mortality in China* is that it's an *observational* study, not a clinical one. The original data from *Diet, Life-style, and Mortality in China* represent thousands and thousands of *associations* between variables. An association simply means that *two things are found together*. Statisticians call such associations *correlations*.

The great danger in observational studies is to believe that *correlation* is the same as *causation*. It's not. Case in point: In certain areas of Denmark, there are lots of storks and lots of babies, meaning there's a *positive correlation* between storks and babies (the more storks that are found in a given area, the more babies there are likely to be). Yet no one seriously thinks that one causes the other. The presence of storks and babies is an *association*, but it is clearly being caused by some other extraneous factor.* We'll come back to this point later on.

The China Study is Campbell's popular book in which he basically presents his own theory that animal protein causes cancer as well as all sorts of other unpleasantries. He bolsters his antiprotein argument by using a very select group of those 8,000 associations from the original China Study that, taken out of context, could be used to promote his case. (These numbers sound all the more impressive if you haven't been trained in statistics and interpretation.) Interestingly, only 39 of its 350 pages are devoted to the *actual* China

---

*For those who are dying to know, here's the answer to the puzzle: The suburban areas of Denmark are where young couples move when they want to start families. The houses in the suburban areas of Denmark tend to have sloping roofs. Storks love sloping roofs, and tend to flock to places that have them. Hence the association between lots of storks and lots of babies.

Study. *The China Study* is Campbell's *interpretation* of the findings from that enormous study as well as a few other studies he worked on, woven together with his own personal philosophy about how we should all eat. (A more appropriate title for his book would have been *A Manifesto for Veganism.*)

As anyone who watched the political debates in the early 2010s knows, it is entirely possible to have two experts examine a hugely complex set of figures and facts and draw entirely different conclusions about what they mean. (Debt reduction and health care costs, anyone?) Campbell looked at the massive raw data accumulated in the China Study, chose certain things to highlight (it's called "cherry-picking the evidence") and connected the dots in a particular way to make a particular case. It is entirely possible to connect them in a completely *different* way and reach completely different conclusions (more on that in a moment).

Campbell—a lovely, sincere man who has made some important contributions to the field of nutrition—is proselytizing for a cause he truly believes in. Since I share his love for animals, I'm sympathetic. (Campbell is on the advisory board of the Physicians Committee for Responsible Medicine, which describes itself as "a nonprofit organization that promotes preventive medicine, conducts clinical research, and encourages higher standards for ethics and effectiveness in research," but whose opposition to the use of animal foods reflects its ties to People for the Ethical Treatment of Animals [PETA] and other animal rights groups.)

The problem is there's more than a little fuzzy math in *The China Study*, and his arguments are full of holes.

Full disclosure: Campbell's book and arguments have been brilliantly, methodically deconstructed elsewhere, point by point and statistical fallacy by statistical fallacy, by others, and I'm particularly indebted to four of them. Denise Minger has written several lengthy and cogent pieces, widely available on the Internet, that rebut Campbell point by point (see *Resources*, page 375). Her critique—a cogent, well-argued, and heavily referenced work noticeably absent of malice—went viral the moment it appeared and garnished so much attention that Campbell himself was compelled to offer a reply. The brilliant, irascible Anthony Colpo has written some damning critiques of the China Study as well, as has the always-dependable Chris Masterjohn. My friend Mike Eades, MD—whose blog at proteinpower.com never disappoints—has decimated it as well. Rather than reinventing the wheel, I'll summarize a few important points made by these four analysts, but I urge you to read their original pieces on the China Study if you want to delve into all the microscopic details. I'm deeply indebted to all four, particularly Minger, for the material that follows.

So, ladies and gentlemen, without further ado . . . here are a few selected points to consider about *The China Study*.

Cherry-Picking the Evidence: How to Lie With Statistics

To really understand the holes in Campbell's arguments, you have to know just a little about statistics and research design, and that's been one of the greatest challenges in getting people to understand the problems with *The China Study*.

Let's say you're interested in studying multivitamins and in finding out whether people who take them actually live longer. So you take a large sample of people, track them for 30 years, and see whether the vitamin users live longer than those who *don't* take vitamins. At the end of the 30 years, you have some good data to show that people who take vitamins live longer than people who don't. You would have shown a *positive correlation* between vitamin use and a longer life.

If you're trying to make the case for multivitamin use, you can just stop there. You've made your point, and it can sound pretty impressive, especially if you're only talking to the public and not to other scientists. But what you actually have on your hands is a massively worthless study.

To make the study useful, you have to ask (and answer) a few more questions: Are vitamin takers more likely to exercise? To go to the doctor? To pay attention to the nutritional labels? To avoid trans-fats? These are all things that could easily affect the outcome of your study.

The finding—that vitamin use is associated with longer life—is called an *unadjusted correlation*. It's just raw data. It doesn't answer any of the above questions, and researchers know this. That's why in most studies, they use sophisticated statistical techniques to "adjust" for the possible influence of these extraneous variables. Most commonly, researchers make "adjustments" for age, sex, history of disease, medications, body mass index, and other factors that are known to influence outcomes in these kinds of studies. By "leveling" the playing field statistically, they hope to eliminate the contribution of these factors to their data.

So back to the vitamin study. If our researchers now "adjust" for such variables as exercise, age, sickness, medications, and so on, they have a much more accurate picture of whether vitamins extend life. If, after all these adjustments, vitamin use still correlates strongly with longer life, we can be much more confident that it's the vitamins—and not, say, the regular exercise vitamin users tend to engage in—that's responsible for the results.

Back to Campbell and his unadjusted data.

When Campbell's raw data showed a positive relationship between plant food consumption and health, he quoted these *unadjusted correlations* with no problem. (They supported his beliefs that animal foods are the spawn of Satan and that we'd all be better off eating carrots.) But when making the case *against* animal foods, he suddenly switched to *adjusted* correlations. That's fine—but shouldn't the same statistical standard be used for both?

As Minger points out, had he used the same (*un*adjusted) correlations for animal food variables, he would have found only neutral or inverse correlations between cardiovascular disease and animal products. If you want to make the argument that only adjusted correlations count, fine, count me in. But then why not use them on the plant food data? Perhaps Campbell felt that if he applied the same loose standard to the plant food data as he did to the animal food data, all those glowing positive correlations between plant food and health might collapse, and his pro-vegan case might dissolve.

Then there's the problem of "cherry-picking the evidence"—quoting associations that bolster your case while conveniently ignoring those that don't.

Here's an example: One of the counties studied in the original China Study was Tuoli. Look at the diet of the Tuoli residents and you'd think the whole darn county was on the Atkins diet. Forty-five percent of their diet was fat (!), and they consumed roughly 135 grams of animal protein a day. (For comparison, the FDA recommends 50 grams a day for most Americans.) So according to Campbell's theory, these folks must be dead men walking. Yet the raw data tells a different story. According to the data in the China Study, they had low rates of cancer, low rates of heart disease, and were generally extremely healthy, more so than some of the counties that were nearly vegan.

Here's another example: Campbell makes much of associations between *animal products* and various diseases, yet fails to explore a much *stronger* correlation (r=0.67) between wheat and heart disease. Yet he's been aware of the possibility of a wheat–heart disease connection since at least 1998, when he wrote in another paper, ". . . *enhancement of coronary artery disease risk by wheat consumption may be a possibility.*"[1] Further, by Campbell's own admission, wheat flour intake correlates significantly with *greater* body weight, *and* with *lower* blood levels of the omega-3 DHA and monounsaturated fats, both of which are very heart-protective.[2]

Speaking of wheat, even a cursory glance at the data discussed in cardiologist William Davis's excellent book *Wheat Belly* would lead any thinking person to suspect that wheat is *at least* as likely a culprit in heart disease as animal foods. Yet this avenue of investigation is ignored or dismissed by Campbell.

It's an interesting omission. Campbell makes much of his correlations between animal protein and cardiovascular disease yet conveniently forgets that the data from the China Study clearly show that wheat flour has a correlation of .67 with heart attacks and coronary heart disease. Similarly, Campbell talks about the possible role cow's milk plays in causing type 1 diabetes, but he leaves out the fact that wheat gluten does the same thing.[3] (How do you manage to forget that? Simple. You don't. You just ignore it, since it doesn't bolster your case.)

Wheat flour also has a correlation of .46 with cervical cancer, .54 with hypertensive heart disease, .47 with stroke, and .41 with diseases of the blood and blood-forming organs. You could be forgiven for suspecting that this stuff wasn't discussed very much since it doesn't support Campbell's jihad against animal foods as the main driver of Western diseases.

So Campbell looks at these 8,000 associations and, incredibly, sums them up thusly: "People who ate the most animal-based foods got the most chronic disease."[4]

But—as Minger, Masterjohn, and others have pointed out—when you compare Campbell's "summary" with the actual data, the result paints a very different picture. Sugar, certain carbs, and even fiber all have associations with cancer mortality that's about seven times the magnitude of the association with animal protein. Didn't know that from reading *The China Study*, did you? I'll bet you also didn't know that the only statistically significant association between a macronutrient and cancer mortality was—get this—a slightly *negative* association between cancer mortality and total fat intake, meaning those eating the *most* fats and oils had slightly *fewer* deaths from cancer. Oh, did Campbell omit that? Imagine that!

The Protein and Cancer Argument

Campbell never really said protein *causes* cancer, though you could certainly be left with that impression from a cursory reading of his book. What he *did* say was that carcinogens *initiate* cancer, but diet can *promote* it. I have absolutely no problem with this idea, which I like to call the "Miracle-Gro" theory.

Miracle-Gro fertilizer won't magically grow plants where there are no seeds, but it *will* promote growth once the seeds are firmly planted in the ground.

So how did Campbell come to focus on protein (and animal products in general) as the big promoter of cancer?

Glad you asked.

It all started with Campbell's early studies on rats (and ended with him becoming the poster child for veganism). You see, cancer is often induced in rats by feeding them *aflatoxin,* a nasty chemical found in peanuts. Researchers found that once cancer was induced, a diet of 20% casein (a protein in milk) *promoted* the cancer, while a diet of only 5% casein did not. What's more, when the same rats were fed plant protein (instead of casein), it didn't seem to matter how much they ate—plant protein, in any quantity studied, did not promote cancer in the same way as casein did. From this, Campbell concluded that animal protein was a likely suspect in the development of cancer.

So how exactly does protein promote cancer, you ask? Certain liver enzymes convert aflatoxin into a really nasty substance that Campbell believes initiates the formation of cancer. Feed a rat lower amounts of protein, he says, and you lower the activity of this enzyme; feed it a lot more protein and you up the activity of this enzyme. Hence the conclusion that protein is associated with cancer.

Sounds plausible (almost) until you realize that in this experiment, sugar (sucrose) was eaten along with the protein. But in experiments when *starch* was used (instead of sugar), the impact of the protein was far less. So protein and sugar *together* may produce an effect, but protein with *starch* produces much less of one. "Who knows whether or not it's even the protein that has the effect and not the sugar?" asks Mike Eades. "It can't be shown from this study."

Campbell generalizes from casein to all animal-food protein. But this conclusion is hardly warranted by the data. Another component of milk protein—whey—actually has a *protective* effect against colon cancer.[5] Was that mentioned? Nope. Why would it be? It doesn't support Campbell's anti–animal products agenda.

And as far as plant protein *not* contributing to the promotion of cancer, that may have more to do with adaptation than it does with anything else. Rats on farms like to hang out in hay and grain, which are two of their favorite foods. Both hay and grain are common places for the growth of the fungus that produces aflatoxin. Eades suggests that over multiple generations, rodents have clearly adapted to this combo of plant protein and aflatoxin. "In my opinion," writes Eades, "making a huge issue of the fact that rats didn't get cancer after dosing with aflatoxin irrespective of how much plant protein they ate is pretty disingenuous."

Campbell even ignores his own previous findings in his quest to demonize all animal products. In an earlier experiment, he studied three groups of carcinogen-exposed rats.[6] All three groups were fed about 20% protein and 20% fat, but the protein and the fat came from different sources. One group was fed casein (a protein from milk) plus corn oil (which is high in omega-6 fat). The second group was fed fish protein and corn oil, while the third group was fed fish protein plus fish oil (which is high in omega-3 fats).

So what happened? There were significant increases in precancerous growths (known as *preneoplastic lesions*) in the casein/corn oil group and the fish protein/corn oil group. (Was it the protein? Or was it the corn oil? I'm betting on the corn oil, but we'll never know.) Point is, the *third* group—fish protein plus fish oil—had a completely different result. The fish oil, in Campbell's own words, "had a dramatic effect both on the development in the number and size of preneoplastic lesions." What's more, "no carcinomas . . . were observed in the F/F (fish protein/fish oil) group, whereas the F/C (fish protein/corn oil) group had an incidence of 3 per 16 with 6 total carcinomas."

Here's the conclusion, in Campbell's own words:

"[A] 20% menhaden oil diet, *rich in omega-3 fatty acids*, produced a *significant decrease* in the development of both the size and number of preneoplastic lesions when compared to a 20% corn oil diet rich in omega-6 fatty acids. *This study provides evidence that fish oils*, rich in omega-3 fatty acids, *may have potential as inhibitory agents in cancer development*."[7] (Emphasis mine.)

Let's remember that Campbell's whole theory is that nutrients from animal-based foods *increase* tumor development while nutrients from plant-based foods *decrease* tumor development.

As Minger wryly notes, "Last time I checked, fish oil ain't no plant food.

"Why does Campbell avoid mentioning anything potentially positive about animal products in *The China Study, including evidence unearthed by his own research?* For someone who has openly censured the nutritional bias rampant in the scientific community, this seems a tad hypocritical."

The Protein and Heart Disease Problem

Campbell loves to quote Dean Ornish and Caldwell Esselstyn, two doctors who have gotten some impressive results in reversing heart disease with plant-based diets. Yet he conveniently omits the equally impressive research of George Mann on the heart-healthy Masai who practically live on milk, meat, and blood, or the extensive research of Weston Price, who studied fourteen different primitive cultures, many of which were absolutely thriving on high intakes of animal foods.

What's even more interesting is that the China Study itself contains data that—at the very least—questions the central thesis of Campbell's book *The China Study*.

Let me explain.

You see, different regions of China have vastly different rates of heart disease mortality. Out of every 100,000 deaths, Fusui—one of the counties studied—has a measly 1.5 deaths due to heart disease while Dunhuang—another county studied—has 184. (For reference, out of every 100,000 deaths in the United States, 106 are attributed to heart disease.) When you compare the five counties with the highest heart disease rates (Dunhuang, Longxian, Tulufan, Yongning, and Jiangxiang) with the five counties with the lowest heart disease rates (Fusui, Qiyang, Cangwu, Mayang, and Linwu)—some very interesting contrasts show up.

But they're not exactly what you'd expect if you buy Campbell's theory.

Compared to the high heart disease regions, the heart-healthy regions had *higher* intakes of animal protein, animal fat, saturated fat, and dietary cholesterol.

The healthier regions also consumed less fiber, less plant protein, less vegetable oil, and less wheat flour.

Again, correlation doesn't prove causation, but still it's impossible to ignore the fact that some regions in China consume an awful lot more animal foods than the average Chinese while having extremely low rates of heart disease. Nor the fact that out of all the counties studied, Longxian—the county that consumed the absolute *lowest* amount of animal foods—had the *next-to-highest* rate of heart disease mortality. Did I say "impossible to ignore"? Sorry. It's not impossible at all—Campbell ignored it just fine.

A side note: Denise Minger created a series of visually compelling and instructive graphs comparing the five counties that had the healthiest hearts with the five counties with the highest rates of heart disease. Taking data from the actual China Study,[8] she compared the two groups on such metrics as total animal fat intake, total animal food intake, total saturated fat intake, percent of calories from animal protein, percent of protein from animal foods, and so on.[9] If Campbell's interpretation of the raw data were correct, we'd expect to see a clear relationship between animal protein consumption and heart disease. Instead, we see nothing of the sort.

The Mortality/Overall Health Problem

Another thing Minger did was to look at the mortality differences between the five counties that ate the most animal foods and the five counties that ate the least. Counties were all over the place in terms of protein consumed, with animal protein consumption ranging from almost zero to nearly 135 grams a day. So, if Campbell's theory is true, you'd expect to see some huge differences in health risks between the counties that were practically vegan and the counties that were practically Atkinsian. Especially since, according to Campbell, "*even relatively small amounts of animal-based food*" increase the risk of disease.

Minger painstakingly graphed the mortality rates (deaths per 1,000 inhabitants) from cervical cancer, breast cancer, stomach cancer, leukemia, lymphoma, brain and neurological diseases, diabetes, stroke, heart attacks and coronary artery disease, and deaths from all cancers for each of the five "near-vegan" counties and each of the five "near-Atkins" counties.[10] It's a set of graphs worth looking at, but I'll summarize them in three words: not much difference. Overall mortality rates for both sets of counties are quite similar, with the high-animal-food counties coming out more favorably in death from all cancers, heart attacks, brain and neurological diseases, lymphoma, and cervical cancer. Though, as Minger correctly points out, this little 10-county sample doesn't carry a ton of scientific clout because of its small sample size, it sure blows some serious holes in Campbell's "summary" of the important points:

"*People who ate the most animal-based foods got the most chronic disease . . . People who ate the most plant-based foods were the healthiest and tended to avoid chronic disease.*"

As Jon Stewart might say, "Hmm . . . not so much."

OK, you say, you don't trust Minger, who by her own (incredibly modest) self-description is just "some girl with a blog." How about Harvard researchers? Here's what the two lead researchers on the Nurses' Health Study had to say about the original China Study. As you can see, they interpreted the data quite differently than Campbell did in his book *The China Study*:

"A survey of 65 counties in rural China, however, did not find a clear association between animal product consumption and risk of heart disease or major cancers."[11]

The Protein/Calcium Problem

In an article in the Cornell Chronicle, Campbell claimed that animal protein "*almost certainly contributes to a significant loss of bone calcium while vegetable-based diets clearly protect against bone loss.*"[12]

But the actual study on which he based this comment—"Dietary Calcium and Bone Density among Middle-aged and Elderly Women in China,"—a paper on which *Campbell himself was one of the authors*—tells quite a different story.[13] Here's what Campbell and his coauthors wrote in that very paper:

> The results strongly indicated that dietary calcium, especially from dairy sources, increased bone mass in middle-aged and elderly women by facilitating optimal peak bone mass earlier in life . . .
> Nondairy calcium . . . showed no association with bone variables after age and/or body weight were adjusted for. . .
> . . . calcium from dairy sources was correlated with bone variables to a higher degree than was calcium from nondairy sources, probably resulting from the higher bioavailablity of dairy calcium"[14]

Protein and calcium have an interesting symbiotic relationship when it comes to bones. Protein works great for strong bones when you're taking in enough calcium. But high-protein intakes can work against you when calcium intake is low. So it wouldn't be entirely surprising if a higher protein/ weaker bone connection showed up in areas of China like Changle, which, on average, took in the highest amount of nondairy animal food but *also* took in the least amount of calcium. Was it the protein? Or the combination of protein *with* a low-calcium intake?

What's more, a number of studies have shown the exact opposite of what Campbell claims is a universal truth regarding protein and bones. One study investigated the diet of a cohort of women from the Iowa Women's Health Study and followed them up for 1–3 years. In this study, a clear association was found between increased dietary protein intake—*especially from animal sources*—and a reduced risk of hip fracture.[15]

The Framingham Osteoporosis Study also looked at protein intake and bone loss in elderly people. "Lower protein intake was significantly related to bone loss," wrote the researchers, with "persons in the lowest quartile of protein intake (showing) the greatest bone loss." The researchers' conclusion was pretty clear: "Even after controlling for known confounders including weight loss, *women and men with relatively lower protein intake had increased bone loss*, suggesting that *protein intake is important in maintaining bone or minimizing bone loss in elderly persons.*"[16] (Emphasis mine.)

Then there was the Rancho Bernardo Study, which studied a cohort of 970 men and women between the ages of 55 and 92. They found a "positive association between animal protein consumption . . . and bone mineral density," which was statistically significant in women. But for both sexes a *negative* association between vegetable protein and bone mineral density was observed.[17]

And finally, if there were any more doubt, the results of a study from the Agricultural Research Service of the USDA should put the issue to bed. The title says it all: "Controlled High Meat Diets Do Not Affect Calcium Retention or Indices of Bone Status in Healthy Postmenopausal Women." The researchers' conclusion: "Calcium retention is not reduced when subjects consume a high protein diet from common dietary sources such as meat."[18]

So, not only do Campbell's *own* findings and studies directly contradict his conclusions, but so do several other independent studies that show absolutely no negative effect on bones or bone-mineral density from a diet that is high in animal protein. Quite the contrary.

It's instructive at this point to mention an absolutely stunning paper in the *American Journal of Clinical Nutrition*,[19] but first, a word of background. Nearly 80 years ago, it was shown that ingestion of protein increases the amount of calcium excreted in the urine. But most of this work was done with isolated protein feedings, and it wasn't at all clear whether the same thing would happen using real protein-containing foods. Robert P. Heaney, MD, the author of the paper I'm about to discuss, tried to test this notion using real people consuming real food. He did some early research showing that in free-living middle-aged women, the more protein they ate, the more calcium they excreted in their urine. "This study," he writes, "cited extensively since its publication, contributed to the widespread impression that protein is harmful to bone."

However, as Heaney points out in his paper "Protein Intake and Bone Health: The Influence of Belief Systems on the Conduct of Nutritional Science," that impression is absolutely incorrect.

The first thing he mentions in his paper is that taking a little extra calcium offsets the slight loss of calcium in the urine from higher protein intakes. So, at very *low* levels of calcium intake, protein may indeed have a negative effect on calcium balance. But this effect disappears as soon as calcium intake is adequate. "In brief," he writes, "if protein exerts a negative effect, it is only under conditions of low calcium intake."

Further debunking the idea that protein has a negative effect on bone strength, he states: "Since our study was reported, an impressive body of literature has proven that protein tends to have a positive effect on bone overall." Two randomized controlled trials showed that increased protein intake dramatically improved outcomes after hip fracture,[20] and subsequent work showed that protein supplements reduce bone loss at the contralateral hip in patients with upper-femoral fracture.[21]

Heaney—who, let's remember, did some of the original research upon which most of the "protein is death to bones" propaganda was based—essentially repudiates this interpretation of his work. "A ferment in the larger society has arisen out of opposition to the use of animal products," he writes. "Although only a tiny proportion of the general public or the nutritional science community holds this view, *the zeal of these groups and their eagerness to exploit any evidence that suggests harmful effects of animal products have had a disproportionate effect both on public consciousness and on the agenda of nutritional science itself.*"[22] (Emphasis mine.)

Think he might've been talking about the Campbell-Barnard-Furhman contingent?

Finally, he concludes by pointing out that there is exactly zero evidence that primitive humans had low intakes of either total protein or of animal protein. "That, coupled with the generally very robust skeletons of our hominid forbears, makes it difficult to sustain a case, either evidential or deductive, for overall skeletal harm related either to protein intake or to animal protein. Indeed the balance of the evidence seems to indicate the opposite."[23]

The Attribution Problem

Pitchers often throw sand over their left shoulders, thinking it brings them good luck. Rain men think their dances bring on the rain. Medicine men in primitive cultures often believe that disease is caused by demonic possession. This judgment about what causes what is called *attribution*, and it refers to the way humans construct the world and assign meaning to events they observe. There's even a whole theory in psychology (the Attribution Theory) that seeks to explain how we attribute *cause* to the events around us.

We humans are remarkably bad at attribution, which is to say that we are often clueless about causes. The point of science is to remove this natural human defect by applying all the tools—statistical and otherwise—of objective assessment, independent of our private beliefs or values. Unfortunately, it rarely works that way, even in science. Particularly when there is a massive amount of data—such as in the China Study—it is very easy to fall victim to what's called "confirmation bias," the tendency to interpret data according to something you already believe is true. Example: If you firmly believe your house is inhabited by ghosts, you will tend to hear every creak in the attic as "proof" of what you already "know."

Campbell—and his like-minded colleagues—are not people of ill intent. Far from it. They genuinely believe we'd all be healthier if we eschewed all animal products from our diet. But like all humans, they're not exempt from confirmation bias, letting those strong beliefs color the way they interpret the world.

Campbell isn't alone in reading masses of data and connecting just the dots that form the picture he wants to paint while leaving the rest of them alone. Neal Barnard (head of the radically vegan Physicians Committee for Responsible Medicine), John McDougall, Dean Ornish, Caldwell Esselstyn and Joel Furhman have all advocated programs that eschew meat and animal products. Ask any one of them what makes their programs "successful," and they will undoubtedly focus on the elimination of those terrible animal foods that "everyone knows" cause heart disease. But a closer look at their programs tells a more nuanced story.

Ornish's original "reversing heart disease" study put men on a very-low-fat vegetarian diet, but it *also* employed anger management, stress reduction, low-sugar diets, smoking cessation, and exercise. Ornish may *attribute* his results to his low-fat diet, but it's impossible to know for sure. Esselstyn may believe that his (almost) zero-fat program at the Cleveland Clinic gets good results because of the elimination of saturated fat, but let's remember that his program *also* eliminates pro-inflammatory vegetable oils and refined grains, both of which are way more of a problem than saturated fat. Even the rabidly vegan Barnard advises readers to keep vegetable oils to a minimum and to favor low-glycemic foods. And McDougall's vegetarian program strongly recommends cutting back on four demons in the American diet: refined flour, refined cereals, soft drinks, and vegetable oils.

Though these fine gentlemen may well believe that animal foods are the real villains in our diet, we'll never know if the elimination of all that other crap (including refined, pro-inflammatory vegetable oils and sugar) was the real driver behind whatever positive results they've achieved with clients. Personally, I think that if you eliminate sugar, wheat, dairy, and high-glycemic processed carbs, it wouldn't much matter whether you ate a pound of grass-fed meat a day. But since all these guys are *already convinced* it's the animal foods, fat, and cholesterol that are causing all the damage, they simply assume that the "rest of the stuff" is just the icing on the cake.

The truth is "that other stuff" may be the cake itself.

Miscellaneous Untruths

In his quest to demonize animal foods while portraying plant foods as the savior of the human race, Campbell makes incredible and fully disprovable statements like "Folic acid is a compound derived exclusively from plant-based foods such as green and leafy vegetables,"[24] or "Eating foods that contain any cholesterol above 0 mg is unhealthy."

Point of information, Your Honor: chicken liver contains nearly four times the folate of spinach. A look through the USDA database[25] or a search for folic acid on Nutridata clearly shows that the foods highest in folate are meats like duck, goose, and turkey. (Pan-fried beef liver, for example, has 260 mcg of folate per 100 gram serving; spinach has 194.) And the idea that *eating* cholesterol raises *blood levels* of cholesterol is so far past its expiration date that it's hard to find even conservative nutritionists who still believe this. Even Ancel Keys, the man most associated with the "diet-heart hypothesis"—the idea that fat in the diet causes heart disease—didn't believe this nonsense. In 1997, he wrote: "*There's no connection whatsoever between the cholesterol in food and cholesterol in the blood. And we've known that all along. Cholesterol in the diet doesn't matter at all unless you happen to be a chicken or a rabbit.*"

Campbell makes the same mistake everyone else does in equating a blood marker (cholesterol) with a disease (heart disease). They're hardly the same. Even a study Campbell himself worked on concluded, "Within China, neither plasma total cholesterol nor LDL cholesterol was associated with CVD (cardiovascular disease). The results indicate that geographical differences in CVD mortality within China are caused primarily by factors other than dietary or plasma cholesterol."[26]

That same study uncovered some associations that Campbell would probably like to forget, since they hardly support his thesis. Wheat flour and salt were *positively* correlated with cardiovascular disease, *positively* correlated with HHD (hypertensive heart disease) and *positively* correlated with stroke. And the total amount of polyunsaturated fatty acids in red blood cells— especially the pro-inflammatory omega-6 fats so prevalent in vegetable oils—was *also* positively correlated with coronary heart disease and hypertensive heart disease.[27]

THE BOTTOM LINE

The bottom line is that The China Study represents a point of view, not incontrovertible fact. It's a collection of carefully selected associations threaded together to support a particular point of view. As Minger and others have shown with painstaking detail, you could easily use a different collection of carefully selected associations from the very same database and arrive at an entirely different set of conclusions. Campbell ignores the substantial amount of data—both in the China Study and elsewhere—showing benefits for animal-based foods, and conveniently excludes all of the data that indicts plant foods as causative of disease (wheat flour for one).

Campbell has responded to the critical blogosphere on a couple of occasions. Quick summary of his rebuttals: "These people aren't professional researchers and besides they have an 'agenda.' I'm a trained scientist. You should trust me, not your lying eyes."

It's a profoundly lame rebuttal. As Minger points out, "It doesn't require a PhD to be a critical thinker, nor does a laundry list of credentials prevent a person from falling victim to biased thinking."

CHAPTER 8

My Big Fat Diet: The Town That Lost 1,200 Pounds

*I*f you're interested in weight loss—or even if you're not—the headline is virtually guaranteed to grab your attention: "The Town That Lost 1,200 Pounds!"

That's exactly what readers first saw when they picked up the March 16, 2008 Sunday edition of the Canadian newspaper *The Province*. Here's how reporter Lena Sin started the story:

> His town was shrinking, and Greg Wadhams was determined to shrink with it. So on a cold December night in 2006, the 55-year-old commercial fisherman sat down to say goodbye to the past. He devoured a spread of chicken chow mein, fried rice and deep-fried prawns to triumphant delight. Then, with the final bite, he bade farewell to his favorite foods.
>
> Intrigued? Read on.

Greg Wadhams lives in the small fishing village of Alert Bay, off the northern tip of Vancouver Island in British Columbia. Most of the inhabitants of this sleepy town (population 1,500) are members of the 'Namgis First Nations people—the Canadian counterpart to what we would call American Indians. Obesity and diabetes are rampant here, about 3 to 5 times greater than the national average. Understanding why this is so can teach us a lot about diabetes and obesity—and about the value of low-carb diets.

The 'Namgis have always been fishermen. But the local fishing industry was collapsing. Wild salmon supplies were diminished, largely because sea lice from the increasing number of salmon farms were making their way into the oceans and killing thousands of the wild fish. Fuel prices had made it difficult, if not impossible, for local fishermen to regularly travel out and back to their usual fishing sites. Meanwhile, supermarkets had sprung up, and convenience foods were everywhere. Paralleling the experience of the formerly lean Pima Indians on the Arizona reservations—now among the most obese and diabetic people in the world—the 'Namgis had begun to consume vast amounts of packaged convenience foods, sugar, and other supermarket "staples."

The disastrous effects of this Canadian version of the "Standard American Diet" were even more pronounced with these First Nations people. Genetically, they are perfectly well adapted to a world in which food is hunted, fished, gathered, and plucked. They are supremely *ill*-equipped—as are most of us—to deal with a food supply that comes mostly from the 7-Eleven.

Jay Wortman, MD, a researcher from the University of British Columbia, had more than a passing interest in what was happening on Cormorant Island, which consists primarily of the village of Alert Bay. Several years ago, he had noticed that he was gaining weight. His blood pressure was rising, and he was constantly tired and thirsty. A vigorous guy who exudes good health from every pore, he slowly realized that he was exhibiting all the classic symptoms of type 2 diabetes.

"I stopped eating sugar and starch just to get my blood sugar down," Wortman said when I interviewed him. While he did not intend this dietary change to be a treatment for diabetes, a curious thing happened. "Cutting out sugar and starch literally reversed all my signs and symptoms of diabetes," he told me. His blood pressure normalized and his energy came back.

He began to wonder if similar dietary changes could make a difference to the First Nations people of Alert Bay.

With funding from Health Canada and the University of British Columbia, he decided to find out.

Wortman—along with colleagues Mary Vernon, MD, Eric Westman, MD, and nutritional biochemist Stephen Phinney, PhD—designed a 1-year study to see what would happen if the First Nations people returned to their "native" aboriginal diet. "People here traditionally got their calories mostly from protein and fat," Wortman told me. "If you 'reverse-engineered' their traditional diet, you would come up with something that looks—in modern parlance—like the Atkins diet." Wortman enrolled about 100 people in his study and got to work.

One of the first things he did was to go into people's homes and perform an exorcism on their kitchen. Gently but firmly, he removed all starch, cereals, rice, popcorn, flour, pasta, sugar, and breads. Gradually the participants got the idea. Burgers were served, but without the buns. Fries were banished. Salads came without croutons. Butter and cream were back on the menu.

The First Nations people traditionally got a large percentage of their calories from eulachon grease—a rich monounsaturated fat extracted from a little smelt-like fish (the eulachon) that was a staple of the native diet. In the "old" days, they ate tons of the stuff; but they had effectively banished it from their diet, believing all fat was bad. Eulachon grease—back on the table! Ditto with any kind of fish and traditional inland aboriginal foods like deer and roast elk. Salmon was cooked on an open fire and generously dipped in eulachon oil. Potatoes, bye-bye. "We supplemented the traditional diet with 'market foods' like bacon, cheese, and all the vegetables you could buy," said Wortman, "but the main thing was the avoidance of starch and sugar, because these were not components of the traditional diet."

And then a funny thing happened.

People who had struggled with weight for years started to shed pounds—lots of them. Jill Cook, a school principal who had struggled with weight all her life and who had previously managed to drop all of 7 pounds on a strict 4-month Jenny Craig routine, lost 58 pounds (not to mention 9 inches off her waist and 7 off her chest). Art Dick, a tribal chief who had been on a ton of medications for diabetes, was able to get off 75% of his meds within 4 days of starting the program. Andrea Cranmer lost 22 pounds and went from a size 16 to a size 12. The aforementioned Greg Wadhams lost 40 pounds and no longer requires drugs to treat his diabetes. "Our forefathers sure must've known something we didn't know, because when you eat [this] way you just feel good!" he told *The Province.*

While this might sound like the stuff of which infomercials are made, it all went into the database of the rigorously designed study. "The average weight loss was 7.5 kg (16.5 pounds) over 3 months, 11 kg (24.2 pounds) over 6 months," Wortman reports. "We saw a change in diabetes symptoms in as little as 3 days. Triglycerides went down about 30%—better than any drug we have. People lost weight, their lipid profile improved, their blood-sugar control got better, their A1c [a long-term measure of blood sugar and a risk factor for diabetes] went down," he told me. "All the things we hoped would happen seem to be happening."

As well as some things that were unexpected.

"There was a real change in attitude," Wortman told me. People started feeling good. "All my mental, emotional, spiritual, and physical aspects are finally feeling like they're in some kind of unity together, and that's so cool," said Andrea Cranmer. "What we didn't anticipate was the tremendous impact on the mental health of the community," Wortman told me. "People were happier. They spontaneously started forming support groups. It became a community affair."

So here's the question: how can a diet so filled with fat and protein—foods that the traditional health establishment tells you are "bad" for you—and lacking the cornerstone of mainstream dietary recommendations (grains, carbohydrates, cereals)—produce such impressive results in so many people?

A couple of reasons suggest themselves—besides the obvious one (that the mainstream dietary recommendations are for the most part bone-headed).

First, there's more and more evidence that saturated fat has a profoundly different fate in the body when it's consumed in the context of a very-low-carb diet. This is a critically important point, and one that has been made by a number of researchers, notably Jeff Volek, PhD, RD, of the University of Connecticut, who has done some of the most extensive and comprehensive research on low-carb diets. "Saturated fat is relatively passive," Volek told me. "[The thing that] controls what happens with saturated fat in the diet is the carb content of the diet. If carbs are low, insulin is low and saturated fat is handled more efficiently. It's burned as a fuel.

"In contrast," he continued, "when carbs are high, insulin is high. Then you're *inhibiting* the burning of saturated fat and potentially making a lot more of it, so you tend to see harmful atherogenic effects."

According to Volek—and many others—you can't really talk about saturated fat without considering the background levels of carbohydrate. "What happens with saturated fat is completely dependent on whether you're on a low-carb or a high-carb diet," says Colette Heimowitz, M.Sc, a nutritional scientist and coauthor of The Atkins Advantage. "Despite ingesting more saturated fat on low carb, the amount in the plasma (blood) is significantly less. Fat oxidation ('fat burning') is increased and fat synthesis (making new fat) is decreased."

So why do so many studies seem to show negative health effects of saturated fat intake? "All those studies are in the context of mixed diets," Heimowitz explained. "When you're on a high-carb diet, your saturated fat should probably be exactly what's recommended—no more than 10% of total calories, ⅓ of your fat. But when you're on a very low-carb diet, it's a whole different story."

Whenever I'm asked to explain this seeming paradox, the example I use is house paint. Pick your favorite color—mine is red—and then consider how it looks when you put it on a nice clean white surface. Now imagine that same color mixed with another one—say purple, or blue or green. Some of those combinations produce really hideous results. How the color "behaves" depends completely on what it's mixed with (if anything). By itself it's gorgeous, but mixed with a noncomplementary color . . . not so much.

"Although people on a high-fat, low-carb diet eat more saturated fat, their blood levels (of saturated fats) actually go down," explains Stephen Phinney, PhD, the nutritional biochemist who worked with Wortman on the Alert Bay study.[1] While the exact reason for that paradox is still being investigated, "the interim answer appears to be that when you take carbohydrates out of the diet, it causes less interference with the body's natural ability to handle fats and that the saturated fats are burned and not retained."

And what about the "side effect" of the dietary experiment, the fact that well-being improved and people seemed—well, happier?

One hypothesis has to do with inflammation. "When you have insulin resistance and metabolic syndrome, you have high inflammatory levels," Wortman reflected. "You have poor energy and you just feel crappy and you're irritable." Not so coincidentally, when you go on a low-carbohydrate diet, many of the pro-inflammatory foods in your diet are eliminated.

Research comparing the metabolic effects of low-fat and low-carb diets on inflammatory markers (such as TNF-alpha and interleukin-6) confirms this inflammation connection. A study by Jeff Volek and his associates published in the January 2008 issue of the scientific journal *Lipids* concluded that "a very low carbohydrate diet resulted in profound alterations in fatty acid composition and reduced inflammation compared to a low fat diet."[2] Richard Feinman, PhD, professor of biochemistry at SUNY Downstate Medical Center and one of the researchers involved in the study, comments: "The inflammation results open a new aspect of the problem. From a practical standpoint, continued demonstrations that carbohydrate restriction is more beneficial than low fat could be good news to those wishing to forestall or manage the diseases associated with metabolic syndrome."[3]

Another hypothesis has to do with oxidative stress, the technical name for what happens when nasty rogue molecules called "free radicals" attack and damage cells and DNA. Oxidative stress is known to be a significant component of aging, and it figures prominently in a host of diseases including atherosclerosis. "Inflammation might be one way the body has of responding to oxidative stress," Wortman suggests. Research has shown that a ketogenic (very-low-carbohydrate diet) "up regulates" (or turns on the production factory) for glutathione (GSH), a powerful antioxidant in the body, helping to protect DNA from damage.[4]

Could all these metabolic mechanisms help account for why the people of Alert Bay seemed so energized and felt so darn good? Who knows? Weight loss has so many overlapping dimensions—social, interpersonal, metabolic, hormonal—that it's hard to sort out what's responsible for what. One thing that's clear is that people lost a ton of weight, felt better about themselves, and—as a "side" benefit—seemed more connected and supportive as a community.

The "town that lost 1,200 pounds" also seemed to have gained an awful lot in the process of losing.

CHAPTER 9

Twenty-three Modern Low-Carb Diets and What They Can Do for You

Each of the original seventeen programs I reviewed in the first edition of *Living Low Carb* was selected for one of three reasons: it was extremely popular, it was extremely good, or it had gotten a lot of attention by the media. By the time the later editions of *Living Low Carb* came out, the list had been expanded to thirty-eight diets.

In this edition, I've greatly reduced the number of programs reviewed. Many of the diets discussed in previous editions aren't around anymore. Others were just retreads of previous diets and virtually no one bothers with them. Some—like the terrible Scarsdale Diet—were included just for their historical value. But some programs have passed the test of time and deserve discussion, if only because many people still follow them.

Readers of past editions may wonder why so many of the diets reviewed in this chapter have such high ratings, since I've never been shy about panning a diet, and many programs in past editions received a rating of either zero or one star. In this edition, I've just dumped the losers. As a result, most of what remains—plus some new programs that have cropped up since the last editions—are pretty darn good.

What draws a person to a particular program probably comes down to feelings. Diets are "brands," much like clothing lines, and their creators and spokespeople have specific voices. Sometimes one voice speaks to you more than another, even if the two are saying the same thing. There's nothing wrong with that. My purpose here is to give you a good sampling of the diet books on the market and to evaluate them in terms of what we've learned about weight loss in the past decade. Your job is to read and sample and then use your gut to tell you which program makes sense for *you*.

And if you turn out to be wrong . . . just pick another! Or make your *own* program (with the help of chapter 12). The point here is that virtually all of the diets discussed in this edition share a similar orientation, even if there are significant—okay, sometimes vast—differences in the specifics. But all of these diet authors know that sugar is the problem, "carb intolerance" is real, and that counting calories and running on the treadmill just ain't gonna cut it.

And if there's one thing that all low-carb diet authors understand, it's that food has a hormonal effect. That's the basis of all low-carb diets, and that's one major reason why they work.

JONNY'S FAVORITES

Having reviewed more diet books than I care to remember, I'm often asked about my personal favorites. So—since you asked—I'll tell you. Remember, these are just the ones that speak loudest to me *personally*.

Both *The Paleo Solution* and *The Primal Blueprint* stand out as the best and most user-friendly of the new diets. I love them both, although, interestingly, they are least like conventional diet books, low-carb or otherwise. Unlike most diet books, they offer exemplary overall eating programs with minimal day-by-day guidance. Both of them, although they differ in presentation and style, are nothing short of terrific. If you put Robb Wolf (*Paleo Solution*), Mark Sisson (The *Primal Blueprint*), and me in a room and told us to discuss our eating and nutrition philosophy, I doubt we'd find much to disagree on.

For a more structured program that takes you by the hand and gives you a step-by-step action plan for breaking cravings and addictions, I'm partial to *Unleash Your Thin*. Full disclosure: I can't be objective about this program, since I wrote it—but I honestly believe it incorporates the best of all the low-carb programs that went before it while adding some new dimensions (such as guided meditation).

For the "classics," I continue to have the highest regard for *Protein Power, Atkins,* and *The Zone* (even though the Zone is not a low-carb diet). Atkins, the Eadeses, and Sears were pioneers, and it's just hard to improve on what they did.

One thing will become abundantly clear from reading these reviews: all low-carb diets are not the same! When I give a program a rave review, I've spelled out exactly why that is; and when I have reservations, I've told you what they are—it's always up to you to decide if you agree with me or not. With very few exceptions, the programs have *something* to recommend them; and even in those cases where I've given a less-than-glowing overall review, I've tried to represent fairly the strengths of the program as well as detailed reasons for my reservations.

As you will see, the outlines and discussions of these diets are detailed enough that you should be able to get a very good idea of what the program entails and decide whether it is a good match for you, or at least determine whether you'd like to explore it further by reading the book on which it's based.

So that you can get a sense of the program at a glance, I've given you the "In a Nutshell" description; after that, there's a much more detailed explanation of the diet itself, followed by "Jonny's Lowdown." The programs are "rated" between one and five stars, but be sure to read the explanation in the Lowdown to see how I chose the rating. Understand that the ratings are my own opinions, based on the information I've shared with you in the discussion, and they reflect my personal biases. (I'm pretty sure that my biases are the correct ones, though I suppose that everyone else thinks theirs are correct as well!) That, as the saying goes, is what makes a horse race. Or a political election. Or even a diet plan.

Happy reading!

1. *The Atkins Diet*—Robert Atkins, MD
2. *The All-New Atkins Advantage*—Stuart Trager, MD, and Colette Heimowitz, M.Sc
3. *The Biggest Loser*—Maggie Greenwood-Robinson, PhD, et al.
4. *The Carbohydrate Addict's Diet*—Rachael Heller, MA, M.Ph, PhD, and Richard Heller, MS, PhD
5. *The Diabetes Diet and the Diabetes Solution*—Richard K. Bernstein, MD
6. *The Dukan Diet*—Pierre Dukan, MD
7. *The Fat Flush Plan*—Ann Louise Gittleman, PhD, CNS
8. *The Fat Resistance Diet*—Leo Galland, MD
9. *The Hamptons Diet*—Fred Pescatore, MD
10. *The Low GI Diet Revolution*—Jennie Brand-Miller, PhD, et al.
11. *The Paleo Diet*—Loren Cordain, PhD
12. *The Paleo Solution*—Robb Wolf
13. *The Primal Blueprint*—Mark Sisson

14. *Protein Power*—Michael Eades, MD and Mary Dan Eades, MD
15. *The Rosedale Diet*—Ron Rosedale, MD
16. *The 6-Week Cure for the Middle-Aged Middle*— Michael Eades, MD and Mary Dan Eades, MD
17. *The Schwarzbein Principle*—Diana Schwarzbein, MD and Nancy Deville
18. *The South Beach Diet*—Arthur Agatston, MD
19. *South Beach Recharged*—Arthur Agatston, MD and Joseph Signorile, PhD
20. *The UltraSimple Diet*—Mark Hyman, MD
21. *Unleash Your Thin*—Jonny Bowden, PhD, CNS
22. *Women's Health Perfect Body Diet*—Cassandra Forsythe, MS
23. *The Zone*—Barry Sears, PhD

1. THE ATKINS DIET

ROBERT ATKINS, MD

WHAT IT IS IN A NUTSHELL

An easy-to-follow, specific dietary plan in four distinct stages. Stage one is "induction": a very low-carb (20 grams or less) approach to jump-starting weight loss. You move through the four stages, adding more carbs in specific increments until you find the level of carbohydrate consumption at which you can continue to lose weight gradually and consistently. You stay at that level of carb consumption until you are within a few pounds of your goal, and then you transition into a lifetime maintenance plan.

About the Atkins Diet

The Atkins diet was introduced in 1972 with the first edition of Dr. Atkins' *New Diet Revolution* and immediately became an object of scorn and disdain by the conventional medical establishment. Why? Because it went completely against the accepted dietary truths of the time. In many ways it still does, though cracks in the cement are beginning to show, and the dietary establishment is finally becoming less certain that its nutritional commandments are actually true. As you may remember from chapter 2, the conventional wisdom that Atkins opposed included the following:

- To lose weight, you must eat a low-fat, high-carbohydrate diet.
- High-fat diets cause heart disease.
- Low-fat, high-carbohydrate diets prevent heart disease.
- All calories are the same.

Dr. Robert Atkins, a cardiologist and something of a visionary, was the first to bring to popular attention the influence of the hormone insulin on weight loss and to introduce the notion that *controlling insulin effectively is the key to losing weight.* By now, if you've read chapters 2 and 3 of *Living Low Carb,* you are familiar with the central role that insulin control plays in virtually every carbohydrate-restricted diet and the reasons it occupies center stage. But in 1972, virtually no one in America who wasn't either a diabetic or a doctor had heard of insulin, let alone understood its role in weight gain and obesity. And it was not until much later that the public began to get a glimmer of insulin's role in heart disease, hypertension, and aging.

Atkins explained that insulin causes the body to store fat, that some people are metabolically primed to put out more insulin than others in response to the same foods, that sugar and carbohydrates were the prime offenders when it came to raising insulin, and that elevated levels of this hormone invariably resulted in increased body fat. He argued that it is not *fat* in the diet per se that makes you fat, but rather *sugar*—even more precisely, fat *in combination* with high sugar—and the resulting insulin that leads to weight gain. Atkins took serious issue with the idea that fat causes heart disease and claimed that his diet would actually *improve* blood-lipid profiles, measurements that show up in blood tests as risk factors for heart disease.

What is the actual diet that stirred such passionate controversy? Well, the Atkins diet is, and always has been, a four-stage affair, but most people think of it as synonymous with the first stage, "induction." During induction, you eat all the fat and protein you want, but you limit carbohydrates to 20 grams per day—an extremely low level of carbohydrate consumption equal to about 2 cups of loosely packed salad and 1 cup of a vegetable like spinach, broccoli, Brussels sprouts, or zucchini. At stage one, there is absolutely *no* rice, potatoes, cereal, starch, pasta, bread, fruit, or dairy products other than cheese, cream, and butter.

To anyone who has read a diet book in the last 10 years that wasn't written by low-fat guru Dean Ornish or his followers, this list of prohibited foods sounds pretty familiar. But you have to realize that in 1972, banning these foods for even 2 weeks was the nutritional equivalent of suggesting that every school and office in the country burn the American flag. These foods were the holy grail of the low-fat religion. Bagels were the breakfast of choice for health-conscious Americans. Oils, fats, butter, cheese, cream, steak, and the like were considered heart attacks on a plate, and here Atkins was making them the centerpiece of his eating plan.

The establishment thought him quite mad.

If this weren't enough, Atkins spoke in downright loving terms of something called ketosis, which he termed "the metabolic advantage" and compared to sunshine and sex. For Atkins, being in ketosis was the secret to unlocking your fat stores and burning fat for fuel. Ketosis was the desired goal of the induction phase. Being in ketosis was a virtual guarantee that you were accessing your stubborn fat stores and throwing them on the metabolic flame, using your fat, instead of your sugar, for energy. A big part of the program involved checking your urine for ketones, which are the by-product of this kind of fat breakdown.

The problem was that mainstream medicine considered ketosis to be not only undesirable but dangerous, a metabolic state to be avoided at all costs. For the most part, they still do—see chapter 6 for a full explanation of why the common belief that ketosis is dangerous is wholly without merit. The emphasis on ketosis, coupled with the recommendation to eat unlimited amounts of fat, was enough to make Atkins a complete pariah in the medical establishment, and it is only now, more than 35 years after the publication of the original book and nearly a decade after his death, that we are beginning to see a slow turnaround in that evaluation.

Briefly, ketosis works this way: when there is not enough carbohydrate (sugar) coming into the body and when sugar stores (glycogen) have been essentially used up, the body is forced to go to its fat stores for fuel. Furthermore, because there isn't enough sugar to get fat into the usual slow-burning energy production cycles of the body (known as the Krebs cycle), the fat has to be broken down in another pathway, with the result that *ketones*—byproducts of this incomplete fat burning—are made and used freely for energy by most of the tissues, including the brain and the heart. Forced to run on a fuel of fat, the body drops weight as the fat is burned off.

The advantages of this plan are twofold. First, the severe restriction of carbohydrates and sugar in the diet immediately brings down your level of insulin, the hormone that is released in response to carbohydrates (and to some extent protein). By dialing down insulin production, you are forced to burn your own fat, a situation Atkins referred to as biologic utopia. Since insulin is a "storage" hormone, less *insulin* means less *fat storage*. Dietary fat has no effect on insulin, so, Atkins reasoned, even if there *is* a lot of fat coming into the diet, there's not enough insulin to drive the "fat-storing" machinery.

Second, going into ketosis was a way of "tripping the metabolic switch" from a sugar-burning metabolism to a fat-burning one. Excess calories cause weight gain only when you're eating a lot of carbohydrates, said Atkins. Dump the carbohydrates, and the fat in your diet is not a problem. He also claimed, to the sputtering frustration of his detractors, that you could consume *more* calories on his program and *still* lose weight, precisely because the fat-storing hormone, insulin, remained at low levels.

Atkins argued that obesity exists when the metabolism is not functioning correctly, but that metabolic disturbances have little to do with the fat we eat; rather, they are caused by eating too many carbohydrates. According to Atkins, if you've been overweight for a long time, it's a virtual certainty that your body has problems processing sugar.

Atkins also believed that the biggest reason people gain back weight lost on a diet is hunger, and that hunger is just about inevitable when you go on a reduced-calorie, high-carbohydrate, low-fat diet. On his program, hunger was virtually eliminated, as were cravings and blood-sugar instabilities. There are good physiological reasons that the appetite is suppressed on a low-carbohydrate diet rich in protein and fat—for example, the release of the hormone CCK (which tells your brain you are full) and the possible suppression of a substance in the brain called neuropeptide Y, which stimulates appetite.

The rules of his induction phase are straightforward and simple. You do not count calories. You *do* not count protein. You do not count fat. You do count grams of carbohydrate, and you can have up to 20 grams a day in the form of *either* 2 cups of loosely packed salad and 1 cup of uncooked vegetables chosen from a specific list *or* 3 cups of salad. Period. As mentioned earlier, you can't have starches, grains, sugar, fruit, or alcohol. You cannot eat nuts, seeds, or "mixed" foods (combinations of protein and carbohydrate) like beans, chickpeas, or legumes. It is also suggested that you avoid the artificial sweetener aspartame (Equal) and caffeine, the latter because it can lead to low blood sugar and stimulate cravings.

Weight loss in the induction phase is fairly quick and dramatic. Much, but not all, of the weight loss is water and bloat, largely because insulin's message to the kidneys is to stockpile salt (and therefore water) is no longer being sent. But the induction phase is only meant as a jump-start. Though Atkins felt it was perfectly safe to stay in the induction phase for a month or so, he encouraged dieters to progress to stage two, which he calls ongoing weight loss, or OWL.

The key to the success of OWL is finding what Atkins calls your *Critical Carbohydrate Level for Losing,* or CCLL. (Some version of this has been adapted by virtually every low-carbohydrate diet that uses the concept of "stages.") Here's how it works. After completing the initial induction phase, you slowly add back carbohydrates at a very specific rate of 5 grams *per week* (the amount of carbs in another cup of salad, half an avocado, or six to eight stalks of asparagus, for example). This would put you at 25 grams of carbs per week. If you continue losing, in the next week you go up to 30 grams. You continue this progression upward until your weight loss stalls, and then you cut back to the previous level. That level is what Atkins calls your CCLL.

The rules for OWL are simple: you still eat as much protein and fat as you want (stopping when you're satisfied, of course); you increase carbs by no more than 5 grams per week; you add one new food group at a time to see if it has any negative impact on cravings or symptoms (such as headaches, bloating, and so on); and you continue this way until you are close to your goal weight.

When you are 5 to 10 pounds from your goal, you move to stage three, "premaintenance." During premaintenance, you up your carbs by another 10 grams per week (typical 10-gram portions are ½ cup of almonds, filberts, or macadamia nuts; ¼ cup of yams or beans; and 1 cup of strawberries or watermelon). Again, you're looking for the level of carbohydrate consumption that will let you keep losing, albeit at a much slower rate. If you overshoot that level and stop losing completely or even start gaining, you drop back down a level. Simple.

Atkins stresses the importance of the premaintenance stage, but I imagine it's the one most people resist the most. Here's why: when you're within spitting distance of your goal, you are naturally tempted to keep doing what you're doing until you get there. Atkins wants you to actually *slow the weight loss down* during premaintenance to less than a pound a week for 2 to 3 months. Premaintenance is seen as a kind of driver's ed for lifetime maintenance. You're using this time to learn and master new habits of eating that will last the rest of your life. You need to do a great deal of experimenting and tweaking, as the difference between your Critical Carb Level for *Losing* and your Critical Carb Level for *Maintaining* is likely to be very small. Finally, when you do arrive at your goal, you increase the carbohydrate level—again in measured increments and very gradually and carefully—until you find the level that allows you to stay exactly at that weight. Now you're in stage four, "maintenance"; the number of grams of carbohydrate you're consuming is your Critical Carb Level for Maintaining, and that's what you continue eating to stay at your goal weight.

Atkins spends a lot of time discussing metabolic resistance to weight loss, which he defines as the inability to burn fat or lose weight. He identifies four major causes of metabolic resistance, which are discussed at length in chapter 20 of his *New Diet Revolution*. Obviously, excessive insulin and insulin resistance is one of the causes (see chapter 3 for a full discussion on insulin resistance). Prescription drugs or hormones are another, and an underactive or malfunctioning thyroid is another. The last is yeast.

Atkins' discussion of yeast is useful reading for everyone who has had trouble losing weight. I believe yeast is a far more common factor in weight-loss problems than was previously thought. Atkins explains that yeast overgrowth is commonly found in conjunction with a sensitivity to mold, and that the combination may easily suppress metabolism. Dr. Alan Schwartz, medical director of the Holistic Resource Center in Agoura Hills, California, has said that yeast creates its own food source by literally demanding sugar to feed on (i.e., cravings), a theory that would dovetail nicely with Atkins's. Yeast, a living organism, also produces waste products and toxins, which can weaken the immune system and lead to food intolerances, another obstacle to weight loss. While the mechanisms are not completely understood, it's a good bet that Atkins was right about the yeast connection. Fortunately, the Atkins diet—at least the induction phase—virtually eliminates all of yeast's favorite foods, and the classic antiyeast diet looks a lot like Atkins's induction.

Atkins identifies what he calls three levels of metabolic resistance: high, average, and low. How easily your body responds to carbohydrate restriction defines your level of metabolic resistance. He suspected that most people with a high level of metabolic resistance would wind up with a maintenance level of somewhere around 25 to 40 grams of carbs a day. Those with a low level of resistance would be in the 60-to-90 gram range, and regular exercisers would be at 90-plus grams of carbohydrate per day.

Atkins has been one of the most misunderstood diet authors and has been the target of more attacks than any other low-carb proponent, probably because his was the first and the most commercially successful of the plans and also, to the constant chagrin of the establishment, because he simply wouldn't go away. While some of the larger criticisms of the Atkins diet are applicable to all low-carb diets and have been dealt with in depth in chapter 6, some are specific to Atkins and are briefly addressed here.

One of the sources of misinformation about Atkins came because many people confused the *induction* phase with the whole program. Atkins was very clear that induction was for a limited time only. A common criticism of Atkins is that he doesn't allow you to eat vegetables and fruits. Actually, he said no such thing. Atkins was a nutritionist, and a very good one at that—he did not want you to miss the incredible nutritional benefits of the phytochemicals found in vegetables and fruits, which you add back to the program in the subsequent stages of his plan. He never said you couldn't eat vegetables and fruits. He *did* say you couldn't eat junk carbohydrates.

Another problem with the public's (and medical establishment's) perception of Atkins's program is that it was based solely on the first (1972) edition of his book. In that edition, where Atkins first put forth the radical proposition that cutting carbohydrates was the key to controlling insulin, he didn't pay as much attention to what you were *allowed* to eat, concentrating instead on the foods you were not allowed. Atkins in 1972 was like the doorman at an exclusive club who is given the order "*don't let in anyone wearing sneakers!*" and, as a result, is so focused on the ground that he doesn't realize he is letting in all kinds of other riffraff that just happen to be wearing shoes. Atkins revised the book twice (in 1992 and 2002), and with each edition he became more outspoken about the need to emphasize omega-3 fats, eliminate trans-fats, and include plenty of vegetables and fiber in the diet. But he could never shake the 1972 image as the diet doc who lets you eat pork rinds and lard.

Finally, it bears mentioning that the fully developed Atkins program is a three-pronged approach to health that involves not just carbohydrate management (he later called the diet a "controlled-carbohydrate approach to eating"), but also exercise and nutritional supplementation. In his New York clinic, only a small percentage of patients came in solely for weight loss. Atkins should be remembered for his marvelous work in the field of complementary and integrative medicine as well as for his pioneering work on diet.

The Atkins Diet as a Lifestyle: Who It Works for, Who Should Look Elsewhere

While his last book, *Atkins for Life*, is a pretty good template for healthy living that almost anyone could benefit from (and is not wildly different from the Zone or the last stage of the Fat Flush Plan), the Atkins diet proper is likely to be most successful with, and most appreciated by, those who really have a fair amount of weight to lose and have had a great deal of difficulty getting it off. People with only 10 to 15 pounds to lose could certainly do the program, but the exacting and cautious approach to adding carbohydrates back 5 grams at a time is likely to be overkill for them.

In the next decade, I believe we will have a much better understanding of the nascent concept of metabolic typing, but even now it appears that there are some types who do very well on higher-protein, higher-fat diets and some who do not. Obviously the protein types are going to fare well on this diet and not find it nearly as difficult and restrictive as those with a different sort of metabolic blueprint.

JONNY'S LOWDOWN ★★★★★

Rereading the Atkins opus for the zillionth time in preparation for this book, I was once again struck by the disparity between what he actually said and what people think he said. The Atkins diet was never an "all-protein" diet; in fact, a recent statistical analysis put the induction phase at 35% protein and the maintenance phase at only 25%![1] He stressed vegetables, talked about fiber, went to great lengths to emphasize individual responses and the need for customizing, and thought that both exercise and nutritional supplements were absolutely vital for optimal health. The later version of his book—as well as the breezier Atkins for Life—*is heavily referenced with a superb bibliography of scientific studies.*

Atkins's only real mistake was in portraying ketosis as identical to fat loss and making it seem as though calories didn't matter at all. He kind of boxed himself into a corner on this one. Ketosis doesn't cause fat loss; it is simply the by-product of fat burning. Yes, ketosis occurs when you are burning fat for fuel, but you will dip into stored fat only if you are not getting enough fuel from the diet. If your diet is 10,000 calories made up of 90% fat and 10% protein, you will most certainly be in deep ketosis, but you will gain weight like crazy.

I don't think everyone who needs to lose weight must go on Atkins, but it is certainly a viable option and likely to be quite helpful for people with carb addictions, resistant metabolisms, significant insulin problems, and a fair amount of weight to lose. It deserves every one of its five stars.

2. The All-New Atkins Advantage

Stuart Trager, MD and Colette Heimowitz, M.Sc

WHAT IT IS IN A NUTSHELL

A modern update and expansion of the Atkins diet suitable for all sorts of people. More user-friendly than the original. Benefits from the addition of terrific exercise and motivational sections.

About The All-New Atkins Advantage

The All-New Atkins Advantage was written by Stuart Trager, MD and Colette Heimowitz, M.Sc, and is subtitled *The 12-Week Low-Carb Program to Lose Weight, Achieve Peak Fitness and Health, and Maximize Your Willpower to Reach Life Goals.* It's a tall order, but the book does an awfully good job of delivering on its promise.

Trager is a board-certified orthopedic surgeon; but what's particularly interesting about him—from a low-carb-diet point of view—is that he's an Ironman athlete. And not just any Ironman athlete (not that there's such a thing as an "ordinary" Ironman!): he's an eight-time Ironman and a top-ten finisher at the Ultraman World Championship. Meet him in person and he's a wiry, muscular guy who looks like he could pull a tugboat across the

San Francisco Bay. Why is this interesting? Because Atkins—and low-carb diets in general—are frequently perceived as being antithetical to energy and athletic performance.

If this were true, someone forgot to tell Trager, or, for that matter, his coauthor, Colette Heimowitz, a highly respected nutritionist and educator who serves as vice president for education for the newly re-formed Atkins Nutritionals, and is herself a walking example of how to look 15 years younger than your age without surgery. Both Trager and Heimowitz credit the Atkins Nutritional Approach for helping them achieve peak fitness and health.

This book, therefore, is an interesting departure from the standard Atkins diet, since it's authored by two people who clearly don't have a weight problem, and who have adapted the principles of what was once known only as a "weight-loss diet" to people wanting to lose a few pounds and get in great shape. In other words, almost all of us.

The five principles of the All-New Atkins Advantage Program are as follows:

- Higher protein (especially at breakfast)
- Good fat (meaning no trans-fats!)
- Low sugar (plenty of vegetables and low-sugar fruits like berries)
- High fiber (at least 25 grams a day)
- Adequate vitamins and minerals

According to the authors, following just these five principles will give you a huge advantage in attaining your goals from the point of weight management and the point of better health. It's hard to disagree with that.

One thing that distinguishes *The All-New Atkins Advantage* from previous Atkins books (especially the original) is the emphasis on motivation and fitness. There are some good motivational tips, taken right out of the contemporary life-coach playbook, including relaxation techniques, journaling, and exercises to change negative thinking. Stretching exercises are recommended and clearly illustrated, as are weight-training exercises. The exercise prescription is a tad conventional (cardio 2–4 times a week, strength training 2–3 times, stretching frequently); but if you follow it, you will see results. Later in the program, you also incorporate a "fitness challenge," such as seeing how long it takes you to walk a mile. It's a pretty comprehensive program, well written, visually appealing, and user-friendly.

The four stages of Atkins are explained well and clearly and perhaps in a more approachable (and flexible) way than in the previous books, certainly more so than in the original *Atkins Diet Revolution*. The whole look of the program—though not necessarily the fundamentals—has been modernized and updated.

As with the "original" Atkins, the program begins with the "induction" phase. That's the very first stage of Atkins, the one where you "induce" weight loss with a mere 20 grams of carbs a day. (It's this stage which many people wrongly assume to be the whole Atkins diet.) As in the "original," you add back 5 grams of carbs a week.

In this book, they've made the process of adding back carbs in 5-gram increments ridiculously easy. There are weeklong meal plans for each level of carb intake, beginning with 7 days' worth of meals and snacks that contain no more than 20 grams of carbs per day total, followed with a week's worth of 25-gram plans, and so on up to the 80-gram-per-day level, which presumably would be for people well into the 3rd phase ("premaintenance") or 4th phase ("maintenance").

Truth be told, by the time this book was written, Atkins had become a nutritional-products company, so there's more than a little hawking of Atkins products (bars and shakes) incorporated into the suggested menus. This isn't necessarily a bad thing, because the products are good ones, among the best of the "low-carb" bars and shakes. They have no trans-fats, a fair amount of fiber, no sugar, and a decent amount of protein, plus they taste pretty good. Plus, if you wanted to, you could do the program without any products, since the menus that incorporate them are merely suggestions.

The book has a nice clear description of what they call "The Atkins Carbohydrate Ladder." These are carbohydrate foods in the suggested order of reintroduction into your menu. The first rung on the ladder is salad and other low-glycemic vegetables like asparagus and spinach. The next rung is seeds and nuts, followed by berries. Next level is legumes, and the one after that is fruits other than berries (apples, oranges, grapes). Next comes starchy vegetables (sweet potatoes), and last is whole grains.

In keeping with the whole "individualized" approach to the New Atkins Advantage, the authors explain that there's no "right" or "wrong" about which foods you must include in the carbohydrate ladder as you begin reintroducing carbs during phases 2 to 4 of the eating plan. "The question of how high you can climb on the ladder—and when you will do so—will depend entirely on your metabolism and your activity level. Some people can climb quite high—and those individuals will be able to enjoy legumes, whole grains, and starchier vegetables in later phases of the program," they write. "A few lucky individuals can even enjoy some of these foods in Ongoing Weight Loss (OWL—or phase 2). Others may find that in Lifetime

Maintenance, they cannot or rarely tolerate items at the top of the Carbo-hydrate Ladder. *The point is that everyone needs to ascend gradually in order to find out what he or she can tolerate without instigating weight gain or cravings."* (Emphasis mine.)

The All-New Atkins Advantage as a Lifestyle: Who It Works for, Who Should Look Elsewhere

This program is likely to work for many people, but like the original Atkins, it's especially good for people who are terribly insulin-resistant and have a lot of weight to lose. These people seem to benefit the most from the rigorous first stage of induction. The later stages—particularly the maintenance phase—sound to me like a pretty good way to eat in general, and should have broad appeal to a wide range of people, including those who are very fit and active.

If you're not one who does well with very careful monitoring of carb levels in 5-gram increments, you're likely to find this frustrating. If you like things spelled out for you and are good at sticking to a program, you'll probably find this very appealing.

JONNY'S LOWDOWN ★ ★ ★ ★ ★

A breezier, friendlier, more-inclusive version of Atkins with an expanded reach, likely to appeal not only to those who have a lot of weight to lose but to active, fit people who feel better on lower carb intakes. There's a lot more recognition of individual differences and a lot less rigidity than in the original. The addition of the exercise program plus motivational and life coaching tips makes this a far more comprehensive program than the original Atkins diet.

3. THE BIGGEST LOSER

MAGGIE GREENWOOD-ROBINSON, PhD, ET AL.

WHAT IT IS IN A NUTSHELL

The diet and exercise program designed by the creators of the hit television show The Biggest Loser. *Surprisingly smart, effective, and easy to follow.*

About The Biggest Loser

I'll admit it—when I first heard the idea for the new television show *The Biggest Loser*, I thought it was a terrible idea for a television show. Weight loss as a spectator sport? That's like watching paint dry.

Once the show had its debut in 2006 and I actually saw it, I revised my opinion—I now thought it was not only a terrible idea but also that it sent a terrible message to the general public. First of all, people were losing 17 pounds a week, a completely ridiculous amount that could never be sustained and was only happening because some of them were weighing in at over 400 to begin with. Second of all: by the second week, folks were being "kicked off the island" if they "only" lost something like 12 pounds. Third of all, humiliation and embarrassment were key parts of the "entertainment," and I thought the whole thing was pretty disgusting.

Well, that shows you how good I am at predicting television hits.

The show's been a runaway success and has given birth to a number of spin-off cottage industries such as the book being reviewed here. Which, needless to say, I expected to hate.

I was wrong.

I still think some of what you see on television is unrealistic. But I've since tempered my opinion and come to realize that there things about the show that many people find inspiring and motivating, not the least of which is the sense of community and accountability that's encouraged, and that is so much a part of any successful weight-loss program. And as for the book— well, it's surprisingly good. One might almost say terrific.

The Biggest Loser: The Weight Loss Program to Transform Your Body, Health and Life turns out to be one of the best of the fitness and diet books around. Although it's short on technical information (which you probably don't need anyway), it's a real example of a program that has incorporated what we've learned about controlled-carbohydrate eating into a really smart plan that many people will find very useful. Here's how the authors characterize the diet:

> *The Biggest Loser* diet is a calorie-controlled, carbohydrate-modified, fat-reduced diet geared to help you burn pound after pound of pure fat—and do so without deprivation or loss of energy. What's more the diet is high in protein. Protein has a hunger-controlling effect on the body—which is why higher-protein diets are so effective for weight loss and fat burning.

They got that right.

Let's look at the specifics. First thing that got my attention was the calorie formula. I've long said that the "formulas" for how many calories you need are ridiculously overinflated. In the "old" days when I was the iVillage.com "Weight Loss Coach," I'd hear from women all the time who were telling me they were following the guidelines for their weight and height that they found on various Internet sites and could never lose weight. When I questioned them further, I'd invariably discover that they were eating way too many calories. Typically the "guidelines" would tell a 150-pound woman to eat over 2,000 calories a day. No wonder she wouldn't lose weight. Remember, even in low-carb, calories do count.

The calorie formula for the "Biggest Loser" program is—hold on to your horses—present weight times 7 (for weight loss).

Now I can almost hear you gasping "That's so little!" Well, yes, it's pretty low. But consider that for years nutritionists like me have been using the "target weight times 10" formula for weight loss, and consider that this formula uses your present weight—not your target weight—so they're not far apart. For example, let's say you were 180 pounds and your target was 130. By my formula, (target weight x 10), you'd be aiming for 130 x 10 calories or 1,300 calories. By their formula (present weight x 7), you'd be aiming for 180 x 7 or. . . (drum roll, please) . . . 1,260 calories. Pretty similar, and, in my opinion, pretty on the money. (By the way, you'd be amazed at how much good food you can eat for that number of calories).

Note that these formulas do break down a bit at the extremes of weight. For example, if you're 110 pounds and want to be 100 pounds, the formula isn't that great. But most people following "The Biggest Loser" are not going to be fighting the last 5 or 10 pounds on what is already a tiny body. For most people the formula is fine, and a refreshing change from the bloated calorie formulas that predominate in magazines and on the Internet.

The second thing I liked about the Biggest Loser program was the questions it asks you to answer. To wit: "Why do you want to lose weight?" (By the way, this isn't a dumb question. It gets you thinking about goals, motives, and what's really important to you.) Or: "What can I do this week to increase my energy?" All good stuff, all part of the kind of program that is about more than just following a diet.

And speaking of diet, it's pretty darn good.

They have something called "The Biggest Loser Pyramid"; and let me tell you, it's a heck of a lot better than the USDA version, even the new supposedly "improved" USDA pyramid (http://www.ChooseMyPlate.gov).

At the base of the pyramid are fruits and vegetables—4 servings daily.

Next up, protein—3 servings a day. Next up, whole grains, 2 servings a day. And finally at the tippy top, a "discretionary" 200 calories to be "spent" on things like fats, oils, spreads, sugar-free desserts, reduced-fat foods, or condiments and sauces.

OK, it's not perfect. We could do with more vegetables, some people could lose the grains, we probably don't need the sugar-free desserts—but look, this is not a strict "low-carb" plan: it's a smart, sensible plan for the masses that is a huge—repeat huge—improvement over most of the dietary advice that's routinely given. And it still manages to incorporate some of the principles of low-carbing.

I particularly like the list of foods to avoid, which include everything that would be a low-carber's nightmare: white bread, white pasta, white potatoes, pastries, potato chips—you get the idea. And a lovely mention of the entire category of "appetite-stimulating foods," the definition of which everyone reading this book already knows from experience!

There's a terrific section called "how to structure your meals." Example: for breakfast, ½ protein serving, 1 whole grain serving, 1 fruit. For dinner, ½ protein serving, ½ whole grain serving, and 3 vegetable servings. That kind of thing. Since a lot of the questions I routinely get on my website have to do with practical tips like how to put a meal together, I think this section of the program addresses a big need, and does it quite well.

The exercise section, needless to say, is exemplary.

The Biggest Loser as a Lifestyle: Who It Works for, Who Should Look Elsewhere

Since the greatest successes on "The Biggest Loser" have been with people who are seriously overweight, it's likely that the seriously overweight will be exactly the group this book will appeal to. That's the market the show has staked out. Of course, the usual caveats apply—many people who are seriously overweight have many other "co-morbid" conditions, such as high blood pressure. I would not suggest undertaking this rigorous an exercise program without clearing it with your health practitioner. Remember that on the TV show, everyone has medical clearance and there is a doctor around at all times.

JONNY'S LOWDOWN ★★★★

I like this book a lot. Strict "low-carbers" may find fault with the fact that it's hardly an orthodox low-carb plan, but it's a perfect example of what I wanted this book to highlight—diet and nutrition programs that weren't necessarily "strictly' low carb in the "old school" sense, but had nonetheless adapted successfully many of the principles of healthy low-carb eating. This book fits the bill perfectly.

Particular kudos for the highly motivating quotes from successful participants on The Biggest Loser television show, which should serve to inspire many a reader. And more kudos still for paying attention to the psychological and motivational aspects of weight loss. You can't go wrong with this book.

4. The Carbohydrate Addict's Diet

Rachael Heller, MA, M.Ph, PhD and Richard Heller, MS, PhD

WHAT IT IS IN A NUTSHELL

Those with a sense of humor call this plan "Atkins with dessert." You eat two protein-and-vegetable meals a day and one "reward meal," during which you can eat anything you like. On most variations of the plan, there are no snacks.

About the Carbohydrate Addict's Diet

The Hellers are pretty much responsible for adding the term *carbohydrate addict* to the popular lexicon. They define carbohydrate addiction as follows: "a compelling hunger, craving or desire for carbohydrate-rich foods; an escalating or recurring need or drive for starches, snack foods, or sweets." Sound familiar? It does to a lot of people. Rachael Heller certainly recognized herself in that description. And she discovered the principles upon which the diet is based quite accidentally, through a fortuitous experience in her own life.

At the time of her discovery, Rachael weighed 268 pounds. She had had a weight problem all her life, weighing more than 200 pounds by the age of 12 and more than 300 pounds by age 17. She spent the better part of 20 years on diets, on liquid fasts, in Overeaters Anonymous, you name it. She became a psychologist largely because she wanted to learn about the psychological causes of overeating. Her own eating was, to put it mildly, out of control.

One day, because a medical test that had to be done on an empty stomach was postponed from the morning to late afternoon, Rachael found herself not being able to eat until early evening. At dinner, she ate everything in sight, then got on the scale the next day and found, to her astonishment, that she had lost 2 pounds. Equally important—and somewhat surprising—was that on the day of the test, when she *didn't* eat breakfast or lunch, she *also* wasn't particularly hungry. She tried the same routine the next day—no breakfast, no lunch, no hunger, big dinner—and boom, off came another pound.

She continued to experiment and add refinements to the diet (which thankfully included putting breakfast and lunch back into the mix), and ultimately lost 150 pounds, which she has kept off to this day. It was out of this experience that the Carbohydrate Addict's Diet was born and the theory behind why it works was developed.

As with many low-carbohydrate diets, the theory centers on the activity of insulin, but with a slightly different twist. As we know from elsewhere in this book, there are many people who oversecrete insulin in response to food (particularly carbohydrates), and many who eventually become *insulin-resistant*, meaning that their cells no longer "pay attention" to the insulin in their bloodstream. This leaves them with elevated levels of blood sugar and of insulin (a situation that can easily precede diabetes and certainly precedes other health problems). We also know that elevated insulin *prevents* fat burning and *encourages* fat storage. The Hellers hypothesize one more chain in this link, which is critical to the understanding of the carbohydrate "addict." According to the Hellers, too much insulin in the bloodstream prevents the rise of the brain chemical serotonin. (Make sure you read Jonny's Lowdown for a discussion: in my opinion, this is a misreading of the science.) Serotonin is the neurotransmitter that is intimately connected with feelings of satisfaction (antidepressants like Prozac and Zoloft work by basically keeping serotonin hanging around in the brain). If serotonin levels fail to rise, which is what the Hellers hypothesize in this scenario, the carb addict will not feel satisfied and will attempt to satisfy the gnawing hunger by again consuming carbs, which of course will spark another release of insulin, and the cycle will start again. "The repetition of this cycle," say the Hellers, "forms the physical basis of what we call carbohydrate addiction."

Meanwhile, of course, the carb addict will get fatter and fatter.

According to the Hellers, a normal person can eat a carbohydrate-rich meal and be satisfied for 4 or 5 hours, whereas carb addicts, with their impaired carbohydrate-insulin-serotonin mechanisms, might feel hungry again in a couple of hours, or even less, and find themselves with a craving for more sweets.

Another premise central to the development of this diet was this: it isn't only the amount of carbs you eat that matters; it is how *frequently* you eat them. (Therein lies the reason that Rachael felt less hungry when she didn't eat until dinnertime on those first few days of experimenting.) The Hellers believe that any weight-loss diet that prescribes three or more small meals each day that contain anything more than minor amounts of carbohydrates will ultimately fail with the carbohydrate addict. In the Hellers' view, hyper-insulinemia (high levels of insulin) is the best explanation for recurring cravings and hunger and the body's tendency to store fat.

In summary, the following applies to the carbohydrate addict:

- For the amount of carbs consumed, too much insulin is produced.
- The constant excess of insulin eventually leads to insulin insensitivity.
- Serotonin (a feel-good brain chemical) does not rise enough to cause the addict to feel satisfied and to produce the signal to stop eating, so the addict continues to eat carb-rich food.
- Production of insulin rises with each subsequent carb intake.
- Greater and greater amounts of carbs may be consumed with no increase in satisfaction.

The Hellers use the addiction model throughout their book. In the patients they have worked with, they identified three levels of addiction, characterized by an escalating need for carbs and sweets as you move up the "ladder." In level 1, you are simply interested in eating all the time, craving basically wholesome foods but lots of them; in level 2, there is an increased desire for carbs, especially breads and baked goods; and in level 3, there is a much greater reliance on snacks and sandwiches as staples of the diet, with a high contribution from cakes, candies, potato chips, popcorn, cook-ies, pies, and the like. This is also accompanied by more and more compul-siveness.

Addiction "triggers" can come from emotional events, day-to-day events, or food. Examples of emotional triggers include unexpressed anger, anxiety, depression, a sense of being out of control, excitement, and frustra-tion. Examples of daily-life triggers are stresses of any kind, PMS, illness, or a change in home life. Finally, food triggers are all the things dieters com-monly report as deadly and that you would expect to be on a list like this: bread and other grain products, fruit, sweet desserts, snack foods, all kinds of pasta, french fries, and, of course, sugar.

Carbohydrate addicts have the greatest difficulty controlling their eat-ing when they consume carbohydrates several times a day. According to the Hellers, when the *number* of carb meals (or snacks) is reduced, eating becomes far more controlled and there is a dramatic decrease in cravings. So here's the program they recommend:

- Two low-carb meals per day (which they call "complementary" meals)
- One "reward" meal per day

Complementary meals are defined as high in fiber, low in fat, and low in carbs. They are basically made up of protein and vegetables (with no fat added). The protein can be either 3 to 4 ounces of meat, fish, or fowl or 2 ounces of cheese. You can have 2 cups of vegetables or salad, but you can't use the vegetables on the "higher-carbohydrate" list. The vegetables on that list have more than 4 grams of carbs per serving, and you *can* eat them, but only at the reward meal. (Some of the vegetables on the Hellers' list don't belong there, such as broccoli, which actually has only about 2 grams of effective carbohydrate* per serving, and avocado, which is not even a vegetable and, in any case, doesn't contain 4 grams of effective carbohydrate.) Other "high-carb per serving" vegetables not to be eaten during the complementary meals include potatoes and corn.

Reward meals, which happen once a day, usually at dinnertime, are made up of anything you like. Quantities are not limited. There are only three rules.

1. The meal must be equally balanced, in thirds, among protein, vegetables, and starch (or dessert).
2. The meal must be consumed within one hour of starting.
3. You can go back for seconds on this meal, but if you do, you have to eat equal amounts from all three categories.

There is a one-hour time limit for the reward meal because of the Hellers' understanding of what is called the biphasic release of insulin (more about this in Jonny's Lowdown). Insulin is released in 2 phases (hence the term *biphasic*). The 1st phase occurs within minutes of consuming carbs: the pancreas releases a fixed amount of insulin regardless of how much carbohydrate is being consumed at the time. The 2nd phase of insulin release—according to the Hellers but to no one else in the field—takes place about 75 to 90 minutes after eating and is dependent on how much carbohydrate

---

*To get the "effective" (or "net") carb content of a food, you simply look at the label and subtract the number of grams of fiber from the total number of carbohydrates. What's left is the net amount of carbs, which is all you need to count.

you actually ate at the meal. If the "initial jolt" of insulin release in phase 1 wasn't enough to handle the carb load, the 2nd phase shoots out more. Thus, they maintain, you want to consume your entire reward meal within 60 minutes to prevent that "second surge" of insulin production.

Alcohol is not prohibited on this diet, but it needs to be consumed as part of the reward meal. Artificial sweeteners are not permitted, and for a very good theoretical reason: it is hypothesized that insulin release might be subject to conditioned responses, much like salivation was conditioned in Pavlov's dogs, whose mouths watered when they heard a bell that had been rung every time dinner was served. The Hellers put forth the very interesting hypothesis that artificial sweeteners somehow trick the body into releasing insulin, probably because they taste sweet and because the body becomes used to secreting insulin when the taste buds and the brain notice the sweet stuff coming in. In addition, the sweetness keeps the addictive cycle going and keeps you wanting more.

Snacking is not allowed between meals (except on a variation called Plan A, which allows one "complementary" snack per day). The Hellers explain that "one piece of fruit eaten other than during the reward meal can reverse the whole metabolic process that is emptying your fat cells. That apple or banana or whatever can be the difference between weight loss and weight gain."

There is a seventeen-item quiz you can take to determine whether this diet is for you. It's called the Carbohydrate Addict's Test, and it is also available in a shortened form (a ten-question "Quick Quiz") on the website (http://www.carbohydrateaddicts.com). Your score identifies you as having "doubtful addiction," "mild carbohydrate addiction," "moderate carbohydrate addiction," or "severe carbohydrate addiction." The Hellers claim that they have refined the quiz so that it now identifies 87% of carb addicts and gives a "false positive" (i.e., mislabels a "normal person" as an addict) only 4% of the time. They also point out that their diet was not designed to address the eating patterns or problems of those with "doubtful addiction."

The Carbohydrate Addict's Diet as a Lifestyle: Who It Works for, Who Should Look Elsewhere

This program has a huge following and has helped many people. I suspect that those who score highest on the Carbohydrate Addict's Test are the best candidates for this diet. There are many people for whom the idea of giving up their favorite foods, even if it's not for the rest of their lives and even if it will result in demonstrably improved health and a great deal of weight loss, is simply too great a sacrifice to contemplate. This program has great appeal to people who feel that way and who find enormous comfort in the fact that they're never more than 24 hours away from any food they choose to eat. On the other hand, there are many people who are simply too carb-sensitive or sugar-addicted to be able to handle trigger foods in any amount, even if it is only once a day. If this is you, you should look for a more carb-restricted plan.

JONNY'S LOWDOWN ★★★

I have absolutely no doubt that there is such a thing as carbohydrate (and sugar) addiction, but I'm not at all sure that the mechanisms behind it are fully understood. The Hellers are very sincere, very kind people who have helped thousands of people, but the theory behind the program is, depending on where you stand, either really weak or completely false. While it seems pretty clear that there are both insulin and serotonin abnormalities in the obese, it's not at all clear that high levels of insulin depress levels of serotonin, as the Hellers hypothesize—in fact, the majority of the evidence points to the opposite response.

Current thinking is that it works like this: insulin not only removes sugar from the bloodstream, but also removes amino acids (protein). Tryptophan, the building block of serotonin, is a little runt of a molecule that is constantly competing with the other amino acids for "elevator space" into the brain, where it can be converted to serotonin. As Kathleen DesMaisons, PhD, author of The Sugar Addict's Total Recovery Program and an expert on addictive nutrition, colorfully explains, it's as if a bunch of big bodybuilders and a little runty guy are standing around the gym, waiting for the bench press. All of a sudden a really great-looking chick walks into the gym and all the bodybuilders gravitate to her, leaving the bench press empty for the runty guy. Insulin functions in the body like the great-looking chick: it temporarily removes the competition, letting tryptophan get up into the brain.[2] Hence, it is thought that more insulin increases serotonin, not lowers it.

The Hellers predict that the more insulin you have hanging around, the less serotonin in the brain, giving rise to all those terrible cravings. A 2002 article in the Journal of Clinical Epidemiology[3] suggested exactly the opposite. It found that insulin sensitivity (which would mean lower levels of insulin) was positively related to suicide and accident rates—the authors postulated that accidents and suicide are frequently associated with lowered serotonin. In this model, less insulin goes with less serotonin. The Hellers, remember, postulate the opposite: for them, insulin resistance (higher levels of insulin) equals less serotonin. Calvin Ezrin, MD, author of Your Fat Can Make You Thin, explains the mechanism rather well and shows why high levels of insulin lead to higher levels of serotonin, not lower ones.[4]

The two-shot, biphasic theory of insulin release seems to be completely misunderstood by the Hellers. According to Dr. David Leonardi, who lectures worldwide on diabetes and is the medical director of the Leonardi Medical Institute for Vitality and Longevity in Denver, insulin is indeed released in 2 phases, but there is not a 75- to-90-minute gap between the two.

"If you eat a bunch of carbohydrates in fifteen minutes, believe me, you're not going to have to wait sixty minutes to get that second phase of insulin release," he says, raising questions shared by many about the theory behind the one-hour time limit on the reward meal.[5]

Finally, I'm not comfortable with the short shrift exercise gets in this program. The Hellers are entirely right that exercise alone is not a great weight-loss method, but it's vital to both maintaining weight and to raising metabolic rate.

But sometimes a program works well even if it is not for the reasons its designers believe. The Hellers have come up with something that works for a lot of people, even if they're not 100% correct about why.

---

5. THE DIABETES DIET AND THE DIABETES SOLUTION

RICHARD K. BERNSTEIN, MD

WHAT IT IS IN A NUTSHELL

A definitive program for treating diabetes with a low-carb diet by one of the most respected thinkers in the field. Bernstein is a type I diabetic who developed this program for himself and his patients. The Diabetes Solution is much more detailed and technical; The Diabetes Diet is kind of like the CliffsNotes version of what you need to know.

About the Diabetes Diet and the Diabetes Solution

Diabetes and obesity are so often found together that people working in the field have coined a new term that conflates the two: diabesity. About 80% of type 2 diabetics are overweight, about 80% of diabetics are insulin-resistant, and insulin resistance is the core symptom of metabolic syndrome (one feature of which is abdominal obesity). Given that, it's easy to see how the two conditions can become entangled. For most of the diet-book authors discussed in this book, the low-carb diet is the treatment of choice for diabetes *and* obesity.

It certainly is for Richard Bernstein, MD. "The diet presented in these pages was originally designed as a diabetes diet," writes Bernstein. "[A]nd as effective as it has been for countless diabetics, it is much more than that. Indeed, as more information has become available over the last two decades on the *toxic nature of a high-carbohydrate diet*, it has never been clearer that the *benefits of this diet are nearly as profound for those who do not have diabetes as for those who do.*" (Emphasis mine.)

From time to time, I get interviewed by magazines, newspapers, and television shows about "the right diet" for all manner of things—to treat yeast, acne, obesity, diabetes, you name it. Interestingly, the prescription is almost always the same—get the sugar out. As Bernstein himself pointed out in the previous paragraph, you don't have to have diabetes to benefit substantially from the Diabetes Diet. If you *do*, this book is a major find. If you don't, it's still loaded with incredibly important information that may help prevent you from getting it. At the very least, following the guidelines found within will most assuredly help you lose weight.

Richard Bernstein was diagnosed with diabetes at age 12 the year I was born—1946. From that day forward, he's made understanding diabetes—its causes, prevention, and treatment—his life's work. For as long as I've been in the field of nutrition, he's been the "go-to" guy for diabetes and blood-sugar management, and he's pretty much an icon in the low-carb community for reasons that will become apparent shortly.

Bernstein's path from patient to healer tells us a lot about the diabetes establishment. When he became a successful business executive and engineer, a career in medicine was the last thing on his mind. But after conscientiously following "doctor's orders" for more than two decades, he found his health failing badly. His own discoveries on how to manage his blood sugar—and the complete lack of interest in those discoveries from the "medical establishment"—prompted him to enter medical school at age 45 so that he could publish his findings and eventually treat other diabetics.

"What if I, a physician, told you, a diabetic, to eat a diet that consisted of 60 percent sugar, 20 percent protein and 20 percent fat?" he asks in the book. "But this is just the diet to which I was subjected for many years. The ADA (American Diabetes Association) made this recommendation to diabetics for decades." According to Bernstein—and virtually every other knowledgeable author and doctor who writes and promotes a low-carb diet and therefore bucks the "establishment"—the real dietary problem for diabetics is fast-acting or large amounts of carbohydrate, which result in high blood sugars requiring large amounts of insulin to contain them. The key to controlling and managing diabetes—and, as we'll see, to controlling and managing weight—is in controlling blood sugar.

And there's no better way to do so than with a low-carb diet.

This flies in the face of "conventional" wisdom and advice, which—as you may have guessed by now—is anything but "wise." "With some important exceptions carbohydrates have the same effect on blood glucose levels that table sugar does," Bernstein writes. "The ADA has recently recognized officially that, for example, bread is as fast-acting a carbohydrate as table sugar. But instead of issuing a recommendation against eating bread, its response has been to say that table sugar is therefore okay, and can be 'exchanged' for other carbohydrates. To me, this is nonsense."

The Diabetes Diet is actually a consumer version of Bernstein's more comprehensive and still-classic work, *The Diabetes Solution*. If you want a really detailed explanation of diabetes (both type 1 and type 2) and want to understand this disease and all its treatment options in great depth, *The Diabetes Solution* is the go-to book. *The Diabetes Diet* is the CliffsNotes version—it tells you just what to do and gives you just enough information to understand why you are doing it. For the vast majority of people, *The Diabetes Diet* is all you'll need to control blood sugar, lose weight, and prevent (or treat) diabetes.

Let's get right to the actual diet plan first, which is actually pretty simple once you understand the thinking behind it. Bernstein calls it the 6–12–12 plan. His basic approach is to first set carbohydrate amounts for each meal. Breakfast contains 6 grams of carbs, lunch and dinner 12 grams each. "What I'm advocating is really as easy to conceive as the old meat, potatoes, vegetable, salad picture—just leave out the potato," he explains.

If you're wondering why the carb allowance at breakfast is lower, it's because of something Bernstein calls the "Dawn Phenomenon." Bernstein suggests that for reasons not entirely clear, the body "deactivates" more circulating insulin in the early morning hours than at other times of the day. When there's not enough insulin, your body makes sugar from protein (a process called gluconeogenesis) and your blood sugar goes up. Nondiabetics will simply make more insulin to handle the increased blood sugar, but type 1 diabetics can't (and, according to Bernstein, many type 2 diabetics also show signs of the same phenomena). That's why he halves the amount of carbs allowed in the early part of the day. Whether the Dawn Phenomenon is a problem for nondiabetics is not addressed—the much more common approach among many nutritionists is to actually allow a bit *more* carbohydrates in the early part of the day as opposed to, say, at night.

If you're diabetic, I'd recommend following Bernstein's prescription. If you're not, you could experiment.

Snacks are fine, with a caveat. "For many people with diabetes, snacks should be neither mandatory nor forbidden," Bernstein explains. "Snacks should be a convenience, to relieve hunger if meals are delayed or spaced too far for comfort." Because many diabetics take fast-acting blood-sugar–lowering medications before meals, it may be necessary to take that medication before snacks as well.

Even if you're not on medication, his advice about snacks applies to anyone wanting to control blood sugar: "Be sure your prior meal has been fully digested before your snack starts (this usually means waiting 4–5 hours)," he cautions. "This is so that the effects upon blood sugar will not add to one another." The same rule applies to snacks as to meals: carb limit of 6 grams during the first few hours after arising, and 12 grams of carbs afterwards, whether it's in a meal or a snack.

There's a list of all the "really good" low-carbohydrate vegetables, a portion of which have about the same effect on blood sugar as 6 grams of carbohydrate, and the list will come as no surprise to anyone familiar with low-carb diets. It's the same list of standbys—from artichokes to zucchini—that you'll see in many plans, often under the heading "Free Foods."

But Bernstein has some important points of disagreement with many "traditional" low-carb plans, and they're very much worth reading and thinking about. For one thing, he's very aware of the issue of carbohydrate addiction, and for that reason alone, there are no "treat" days here. "Many low-carb diet plans ignore the reality that much of overweight and obesity is directly related to carbohydrate addiction and constant snacking," he writes. He correctly points out that many dietitians and doctors don't really understand carb addiction at all. "Treat days are a little like having a smoker go all week without a cigarette and then saying 'go ahead and have a cigarette on Saturday.'" In Bernstein's view, for people with a history of overeating "treats," it's much simpler just to give up the treats than to have the self-discipline to eat only one small portion of sweets or starches on a treat day. I couldn't agree more.

The second big difference between Bernstein and many traditional low-carb plans—including, by the way, Atkins—is that there are no "phases," and that's not by accident. As we've seen throughout this book, many low-carb plans begin with a highly restricted regimen and then allow you to gradually reintroduce more carbs as you progress. For Bernstein, this approach is fraught with problems. "Just as you start to lose weight nicely, you change your diet," he says. "Many low-carb diets might as well add the caveat that after phase one, you're going to quit the diet because suddenly you're back to the same old stuff that got you into trouble in the first place."

There's a genuine difference of opinion here, and neither side is "wrong." We've seen lots of studies over the years where people lose weight at a nice clip in the early stages of carb restriction, only to gain quite a bit of it back. Talk to a lot of the docs and researchers off the record and you start to hear the same story—people keep eating the higher-fat higher-protein diet they lost weight on, but add back the foods that caused the problem in the first place. They figure that bacon and eggs are fine—why not add a little toast and potatoes, since they've already lost the weight? This defeats the whole purpose and causes the regain so commonly seen in low-carb diet studies.

"The amount of carbohydrate that you ought to eat will remain constant for life," says Bernstein. "For purposes of weight loss, or if you significantly increase or decrease your physical activity, protein amounts can be adjusted, but that's about it." Though it sounds like tough love, in this respect the Bernstein diet is much simpler to follow.

On the other side of this argument are those who feel that judiciously and carefully adding small amounts of carbs back while monitoring your weight and health is perfectly fine to do. The problem may be that some people just can't do it. It's an open question that has no "right" answer other than "*it depends on the person, the situation, and the individual metabolism.*"

Bernstein also has a slightly different take on protein than many of the other low-carb-diet authors. While he's hardly antiprotein, he doesn't feel it should be unlimited. "A certain amount of protein does get converted to blood sugar by the body, and that will raise insulin and build fat," he points out.

The Diabetes Diet and the Diabetes Solution as a Lifestyle: Who It Works for, Who Should Look Elsewhere

Without a doubt, this is the program I'd use if I were diabetic. And for good measure, I'd buy the companion book, *The Diabetes Solution*, which goes into even more detail about things that can be of enormous help to any diabetic.

But this program is also great for weight loss. It's definitely a little strict—think Atkins Phase 1, but indefinitely. (There are a number of distinctions between the Bernstein program and the Atkins Phase 1, but you get the idea). If you're the type who would rather pull the Band-Aid off all at once and be done with it, you'll probably resonate to this book. There's no "treat day," no cheating, and it's tough love all the way. But it works.

If you can't fathom the idea of protein, fat, and vegetables making up your diet for pretty much the rest of your life, you might want to look at some of the other programs. If you're not diabetic or not seriously overweight—and if you're not what we might call "metabolically resistant"—you may be able to tolerate a bit more generous a carb allowance than the one in The Diabetes Diet.

And if you simply want to make some basic healthful changes to your diet and move in a more low-carb direction, this book is probably not for you.

JONNY'S LOWDOWN ★ ★ ★ ★ ★ (ESPECIALLY IF YOU'RE DIABETIC)

A very good no-nonsense program by the guru of low-carb approaches for diabetes. Yes, it's strict, and yes, it could be even be considered "hard," but there's a big upside: once you commit to it, it's easy to do, and it will pretty much knock your cravings out of the ballpark. And it will control your blood sugar, whether you're diabetic or not.

Whether it's necessary to go this drastically low-carb forever is an open question. A lot of studies show disappointing weight regain after an initial success using carb restriction, and I suspect that's because people simply start adding back carbs way more than they should. If you had high blood pressure and medication controlled it, would you stop taking the treatment and expect your blood pressure to stay low? Low-carb diets—in Bernstein's view—are the treatment for diabetics (and perhaps for anyone with an insulin related weight problem). For him, there's no going back—the carb level of the diet is pretty much fixed, and that's that.

---

6. The Dukan Diet

Pierre Dukan, MD

WHAT IT IS IN A NUTSHELL

A low-carb plan with some interesting twists and novel recommendations. The diet itself is divided into 4 phases, all built around protein as its centerpiece, with each phase having a very specific purpose. Though choices are limited during the 1st phase (when you drop the most weight), the plan allows you to add back foods like bread and starches in very controlled ways once you've moved into the 3rd phase. The final, 4th phase of the plan is different from all other 4-phase plans (like Atkins, for example) in that there is a built-in mechanism for preventing rebound weight gain.

About the Dukan Diet

The Dukan Diet was created by Pierre Dukan, MD, a medical doctor specializing in human nutrition since 1973. It was first published in France, where it has been at the top of the bestseller list since 2006. It then became an Internet phenomenon as a community of millions of people started exchanging their ideas on websites, forums, and blogs devoted to the Dukan method. The book was introduced across the pond in 2011 with a brand new American edition. I expect it will get a lot of attention.

Dukan started his work in the weight-loss field as a young doctor practicing general medicine in Paris. One of his patients happened to be obese and asked Dukan how to lose weight. "All I knew about nutrition and obesity (in those days) was what my teachers had passed on at medical school, which amounted to simply suggesting low-calorie diets and miniature-sized meals so tiny that any obese person would laugh and run a mile in the opposite direction," writes Dukan.

Dukan—not unlike Dr. William Harvey who had treated our friend the British undertaker William Banting in the 1850s (see chapter 2)—went on pure instinct and prescribed an all-meat diet for his obese patient.

Five days later, he had lost 12 pounds. After 20 days, his weight had dropped an incredible 22 pounds. His blood tests were all perfectly normal. "This is how the first phases of the Dukan diet were born," writes Dukan.

Over the years, Dukan noticed that the vast majority of dieters inevitably lose the war against weight. This led to the creation of additional phases whose sole purpose was to protect the gains made in the first phases. (More on that in a moment.)

According to Dukan, the program takes into account everything that is essential for the success of any weight-loss program:

1. It offers overweight people trying to lose weight a system with specific instructions that get them on track, with stages and objectives, leaving no room for ambiguity or deviation.
2. The initial weight loss is substantial and sufficiently rapid to launch the diet and instill lasting motivation.

3. It is a low-frustration diet. Weighing food portions and calorie counting are banned, and it allows you total freedom to eat a certain number of popular foods.
4. It is a comprehensive weight loss program, an integrated whole that you can either take or leave.

Let's take a look at the specifics of the program.

Phase 1: The "Attack" Phase or "The Pure Protein Diet"

The "Attack" phase is simple: pure protein. That's it. You can eat meat, fish, poultry, whole eggs, and nonfat dairy products. (The recommendation to eat nonfat or low-fat versions of high-protein foods is one of the main reservations I have about the plan. We'll get into that later on.) The Attack phase can last for as little as a day or can go for as many as 10. Most people do it for between 2 to 7 days. (The number of days you stay on it has a lot to do with how much you need to lose.) Weight loss is rapid, which can be very motivating.

The Attack phase also contains three other "prescriptions," but they're easy to follow. You should drink at least 1½ quarts of water or mineral water. You should go for one (compulsory) walk a day for 20 minutes. And you should eat the "oat bran galette."

What's that, you ask? Well the third prescription for the Attack phase involves a daily dose of 1½ tablespoons of oat bran, which you can add to your milk or yogurt. But Dukan recommends eating it as a light and easy pancake, which he calls "the oat bran galette."

Phase 2: The "Cruise" Phase or "The Alternating Protein Diet"

On the "Cruise" phase, you alternate one day of protein only (just like in the 1st phase) with a day of protein plus vegetables. You can add any nonstarchy vegetables, raw or cooked. (Dukan has a suggested list in the book under the heading "100 Natural Foods that Keep You Slim.") According to Dukan, this alternating cycle works like the "injection-combustion cycle of a two-speed engine, burning up its calorie quota."

You stay on the Cruise phase without a break until your target weight is reached. "The alternating protein diet is still one of the diets least affected by resistance induced by previous attempts at weight loss," writes Dukan.

During the Cruise phase, the daily oat bran requirement increases to 2 tablespoons, and the recommended exercise goes from 20 minutes of walking to 30.

Phase 3: The "Consolidation" Phase or "The Transition Diet" (5 Days for Every Pound Lost)

The purpose of this stage is to get you eating a wider variety of foods again, while specifically avoiding the traditional "rebound" effect experienced by so many people after losing a lot of weight.

Dukan believes that gradually including a wider range of foods that are richer and more gratifying but in very limited quantities will allow your body's metabolism to adjust to your new weight and stabilize your weight loss.

Dukan makes a decent case for this reintroduction, pointing out that many people regain weight very quickly because they go from the "diet" to their old way of eating. His notion was that if you reintroduce the "nondiet" foods in a very controlled and structured way, you have a lot less chance of experiencing the explosive weight gain that comes from just going "off" the program completely.

One novel thing here is that the length of time you stay on this "Consolidation" phase is determined by how much weight you lost in the previous two stages. You stay on this 3rd phase for 5 days for each pound you've lost so far.

In the Consolidation phase, you add 2 slices of bread and 1 portion of fruit and cheese into your daily diet, along with up to 2 servings a week of starchy carbs (or grains) and 2 "celebration" meals. There's a specific order and structure to this reintroduction. Since you already know the length of your Consolidation phase (the number of pounds you lost times 5), you now divide the total Consolidation phase into two halves. In the first half, you're allowed one serving of starchy foods a week; in the second half, you can have two servings. "This approach avoids the risk of you starting to eat sugar-rich foods too suddenly," says Dukan.

Similarly, the 2 "celebration" meals are phased in during this period. During the first half, you can have one celebration meal a week, and you can up it to two during the second half.

The celebration meal deserves some explanation, as it could easily be confused with the "reward meal" in the Carbohydrate Addict's Diet. It's very different. At each celebration meal, you can eat whatever food you want and especially whatever food you've missed during the weight-loss period. But there are some very important caveats. Number one: never have second helpings of the same dish. Number two: when you can have 2 celebration meals a week (during the second half of this phase), never have them back-to-back. Third, everything is allowed but only one of each: 1 starter, 1 main dish, 1 dessert, and 1 glass of wine. All in "reasonable" quantity—but only one of each.

The Consolidation phase has another critical feature, which it shares with all the other phases (including the next and final phase coming up). During the entire Consolidation phase you eat "pure protein" a day a week. This is the same diet you ate exclusively during the Attack phase, and on alternate days during the Cruise phase.

During Consolidation, you also continue with the 2 daily tablespoons of oat bran a day, and with daily walking, though Dukan says you now can lower your walking time to 25 minutes if you so choose.

Phase 4: The "Stabilization" Phase

The Stabilization phase assumes you have now reached your target weight (which you should have done before starting Phase 3) and have kept it consistently, give or take a pound, throughout the long Phase 3 Consolidation period. So this phase is more like a "return to the real world" phase, and as such, is much less defined than the three previous phases.

This phase simply gives you more leeway to introduce more foods.

Dukan believes that the Consolidation phase allowed your body to adjust to the new weight and stop "defending" the old one by holding on to every excess calorie and gram of sugar. In other terminology, one might say your weight has now reached a new "set point."

Dukan suggests you adopt the basic foods you ate during the Consolidation phase as your new "baseline" and just add back new foods judiciously and carefully, always monitoring to see your reaction. There is also a non-negotiable one-day-a-week commitment to "pure protein," the same diet you ate daily during Phase 1. And finally, you must continue with 3 tablespoons of oat bran for the rest of your life.

The Dukan Diet as a Lifestyle: Who It Works for, Who Should Look Elsewhere

When I was a kid and Elvis Presley was first putting out records (that's 33 rpm records, folks), one of them had the legend written across it: "50,000 Elvis Fans Can't Be Wrong!" Of course, 50,000 was a lot back then, pre-Internet, but I couldn't help thinking of that legend when trying to answer the question "Who would the Dukan diet work for?" Why? Because it's sold over 3.5 million copies in 14 different languages and is the subject of hundreds of message boards and websites populated by devoted followers of all ages and both sexes. That alone is enough to safely say that it has a wide and broad appeal. It should also appeal greatly to people who are deeply put off by the idea that they can "never" eat a certain kind of food again, or, if they do, that they would be abandoning their program. There are a lot of real-world concessions in this plan that make it very appealing.

I very much doubt there are vegetarians who would have an easy time of this plan, and I know for a fact it would be impossible for vegans. If you have a problem eating a fair amount of protein—nothing dangerous, mind you, just more than you might be used to eating now—you should probably look elsewhere, especially since "all protein" one day a week is a lifelong feature of the Dukan Diet.

Those with real food addiction problems may want to look elsewhere as well. Though the concept of "celebration" meals sounds like an awfully good, reasonable real-world idea, fact is, if you're an addict, it's going to be a problem, akin to telling an alcoholic he can have one "celebration" glass of wine.

JONNY'S LOWDOWN ★★★★½

I have a couple of reservations about this program, but for the most part, I think it's very smart and very original. Let's start with the reservations. Though Dukan seems incredibly savvy when it comes to nutrition and health, it is remarkable to me that he still completely buys into the low-fat thing, recommending nothing but nonfat dairy products, and non- or low-fat versions of any other protein foods. This is all the more puzzling as he seems to have a pretty good grasp of the hormonal impact of food yet disregards the fact that fat has exactly zero effect on insulin (the fat-storing hormone) and that a good deal of research in the past decade has questioned the long-held assumption that saturated fat intake is linked to higher death rates (it's not).

The second reservation I have concerns the 3rd and 4th phases of the program. I completely understand the concept of adding things back in gradually, but the recommendation to include two slices of whole wheat bread daily at the start of the Consolidation phase seems to me to be counterproductive. First of all, there's the issue of gluten/grain-sensitivity, which affects many people and which would make this a bad idea. Second of all, there's the blood-sugar issue, as nearly all breads are high glycemic. I would have much preferred a more gradual approach and the ability to customize (i.e., dump the bread if it's a problem for you).

Related to that concern is my issue with the "celebration" meal. In theory, it's a great idea. In practice, no one who is food-addicted or carb-addicted will have an easy time of it. One person I spoke to said that if she were allowed this "celebration" meal, it would be the beginning of a binge for sure—I'm not sure she's not unique in this respect.

The good news is that except for those issues—the nonfat thing, the reintroduction schedule, and the celebration meals—this is a really, really smart program. I'm especially fond of the "Protein Thursdays" notion (one day a week of protein to stabilize), and I particularly like the idea that the diet is designed to be relatively easy to follow for the rest of your life.

In the "real" world, most dieters will eventually have their own "celebration" meals where they throw caution to the wind and eat what they like. Problem is, when people do this, they feel they've "cheated," and tend to have some trouble getting back on track. One of the real selling points of Dukan is that he makes it possible to do what people are going to do anyway (occasionally wander off the reservation, that is) without actually going off the program.

I'd give this program five stars, but I had to take a half point off because he's so wrong on fat. Other than that, this is a terrific program and should work well for an awful lot of people.

7. The Fat Flush Plan

Ann Louise Gittleman, PhD, CNS

WHAT IT IS IN A NUTSHELL

A 3-phase eating plan designed for both fat loss and detoxification. The idea is both to lose fat and to make your body more efficient at processing it effectively, largely by targeting a sluggish liver, the main organ for detoxification and fat metabolism in the body. The first phase is fairly (though not completely) carbohydrate-restrictive—you can still have two portions of fruit a day and a ton of vegetables—with each subsequent phase adding back more carbohydrates until you reach maintenance.

About the Fat Flush Plan

The Fat Flush Plan started life as a 2-week eating program that was originally chapter 16 in Ann Louise Gittleman's pioneering book, *Beyond Pritikin*. Developed and expanded over the years, it eventually became the fully realized diet and lifestyle plan that is the cornerstone of this book.

Fat Flush brings a different spin to low-carb dieting by concentrating on what Gittleman calls the "five hidden weight gain factors": an overworked liver, lack of fat-burning fats, too much insulin, stress, and something that Dr. Elson Haas has called "false fat."

The Liver

In addition to being the main organ for detoxification in the body, the liver is also responsible for fat metabolism. Bile, for example, is made in the liver (and stored in the gallbladder) and is responsible for helping the liver break down fats. But bile can't work efficiently if it doesn't have the proper nutrients that make up the bile salts, or if it is congested or thickened with toxins, pollutants, hormones, drugs, and other nasty stuff. Hence, inefficient bile production can slow weight loss.

Another example of how impaired liver function can slow weight loss is "fatty liver," a condition that many overweight people develop. It's not life-threatening, but it's also not something you want to put on your holiday wish list. A very early symptom of possible liver disease frequently seen in alcoholics, it basically means that fat is backed up in the liver like cars on a multilane freeway trying to get through a single toll booth.

Modern life puts a lot of stress on the poor overworked liver. The number of commonly used substances (including medications and even some herbs) that can harm the liver is enormous, and includes Tylenol, some cholesterol-lowering medications, some estrogens used in hormone-replacement therapy and in birth-control pills, alcohol, and a host of other stuff.

Getting the liver in tip-top shape is one goal of the Fat Flush Plan, and that's something that virtually no other diet program addresses. Fat Flush does it by including well-known bile thinners like eggs (high in an amazing liver-supportive substance known as phosphatidylcholine, which also has the ability to break up fats in the bargain) and hot water with lemon juice.

Fat-Burning Fats

Gittleman was a pioneer in debunking the popular '80s notion that a no-fat diet was a good thing (*Eat Fat, Lose Weight*), and she was especially credible because she had been chief nutritionist at the Pritikin Center, which was (and still is) Command Central for the low-fat contingent. She specifically recommends supplementation with GLA (gamma-linolenic acid, a fatty acid found in evening primrose oil, borage oil, and black-currant oil) because it stimulates a special kind of fat in the body called *brown adipose tissue*, or BAT. BAT is metabolically active fat that surrounds vital organs and can actually help *burn off* calories.

Excess Insulin

Virtually every low-carb diet plan exists precisely because of the theory that too much insulin is the culprit behind weight gain for a huge number of people. *The Fat Flush Plan* addresses this with the now-familiar prescription of healthful fats, lean proteins, and low-glycemic carbohydrates.

Stress

The connection between stress and fat gain is mediated by excess production of the stress hormone cortisol, is firmly established by research, and is now making its way into the popular consciousness (which you know is happening once it hits the women's magazines), largely due to the pioneering work of Dr. Pamela Peeke. The connection is too lengthy to go into in detail here—those interested should check out Dr. Peeke's excellent book, *Fight Fat After Forty*, or read the very good explanation of the stress–fat connection in *The Fat Flush Plan*. Here's the condensed version: *stress makes you fat.* The Fat Flush Plan addresses stress by offering suggestions on improving sleep, getting moderate exercise, and removing dietary cortisol boosters such as caffeine and sugar.

"False Fat"

People love this term. When I wrote about it for iVillage.com, my article got more hits than almost anything else I had ever written and was featured on the America Online home page. People are fascinated by the notion that they could actually be carrying around something that *feels* like fat, *looks* like fat, but maybe, just *maybe*, isn't *actually* fat at all! The term is the invention of the wonderful integrative physician and author Dr. Elson Haas, who wrote a book about it (*The False Fat Diet*), and Gittleman honorably credits him with the concept, which is central to her discussion of the five hidden weight-gain factors.

Here's the deal: Food sensitivities can trigger hormonal reactions in the body that lead to both water retention and cravings. Water retention happens because incompletely digested molecules or peptides from the food you're sensitive to enter the bloodstream and are perceived as invaders by the immune system, which then mounts a full-fledged Pac-Man–like attack, releasing histamine and flooding the area with extra fluid. (This extra fluid can be up to 10 or 15 pounds in some people—it's not really fat, but it sure feels like it, and it can easily make the difference between you being able to wear your "skinny clothes" and having to wear your "fat jeans.")

During this immune-system response, the body also overproduces the hormones cortisol and aldosterone, which in turn increase sodium retention, attracting even more water to the cells and tissues. This whole immune cascade will cause you to release endorphins (natural "feel-good" opiates), which can, over time, easily give rise to a feeling that you're addicted to the very foods you're sensitive to. (Think of sugar, wheat, flour, and the like. Ever notice how no one ever says they're addicted to Brussels sprouts?) Finally, your levels of serotonin—the feel-good neurotransmitter—drop when the immune system goes into full alert, because the same white blood cells that carry serotonin are now too busy fighting off the invaders to bother with serotonin. Lower levels of serotonin almost always lead to increased cravings for high-carbohydrate foods, which in turn spikes your blood sugar, leading to a vicious circle of higher levels of insulin and more fat storage. Get it?

The Fat Flush Plan relies heavily on daily intakes of "cran-water," a mixture of unsweetened cranberry juice (not the "cocktail" stuff commonly found in supermarkets) and water. The juice contains arbutin, an active ingredient in cranberries that is a natural diuretic (as is the lemon in the hot-water-and-lemon-juice mix). The Fat Flush Plan also deals with the "false fat" issue by restricting the "usual suspect" foods that are likely to trigger food sensitivities: wheat, dairy, and sugar.

Phase 1 of the plan is about 1,100 to 1,200 calories (this is one of the few low-carb plans in which the author actually mentions the caloric intake) and is designed to jump-start weight loss. It's also meant to be a good cleansing program that supports the liver. You stay on it for 2 weeks; if you've got more than 25 pounds to lose, you can stick with it for a month, though it might get pretty boring.

In phase 1, you avoid:

- hot spices (because of possible water retention)
- oils and fats (other than daily flaxseed oil and GLA supplementation)
- all grains
- all starchy vegetables (potatoes, corn, peas, carrots, beans, etc.)
- all dairy
- alcohol and coffee (you are allowed one cup of organic coffee in the morning)

Other than that, the diet is flexible. No counting carb grams, figuring out protein minimums, or counting calories. You eat:

- up to 8 ounces a day of almost any kind of protein
- *in addition*, up to two eggs a day

- one serving of whey protein powder (not in the book, but later added to the phase 1 food list on the website)
- unlimited amounts of almost any vegetable but the starchy ones (which get put back in during the next phase)
- up to two portions of fruit per day

You can sweeten with stevia (xylitol wasn't widely available when Fat Flush first came out, but I'm willing to bet that xylitol would be acceptable). Each day, you have a fiber supplement, a GLA supplement, flaxseed oil, and the cran-water mixture.

Phase 2 is for ongoing weight loss, and it ups the calories to between 1,200 and 1,500. You stay on phase 2 until you're at or near your goal weight. The main difference between phase 1 and phase 2 is that during phase 2, you slowly add back some carbohydrates from the "friendly carb" list—one serving per day for the first week and two servings per day for the second week and beyond. The cran-water drink gets replaced with pure water, and most everything else stays the same.

Phase 3 is 1,500 (or more) calories per day and is designed for ongoing maintenance. There are more liberal choices in the oil and fruit categories, and you can now add dairy products as well as choose from a bigger list of "friendly carbs," working up to four servings a day. Most everything else remains the same—there are some minor changes in supplementation that are discussed.

The book also has sections on exercise (greatly expanded in *The Fat Flush Fitness Plan*), journaling, stress reduction, recipes, resources, and great FAQ.

The Fat Flush Plan as a Lifestyle: Who It Works for, Who Should Look Elsewhere

This is such an all-around sensible plan that it's hard to see how anyone wouldn't benefit from it. Within certain parameters (like the carb restriction and the prohibition on sugar), it's very flexible, and it's one of the few lower-carb plans where you can eat fruit right from the beginning. Gittleman seems to have a particular gift for writing for women, who appear to constitute the majority of her audience. Men do well on this plan, too, but need to make some adjustments. According to Gittleman, they should do phase 1 as is, but can usually jump to phase 3 so they can take in more carbohydrates right away. They also generally should increase the portion sizes of their protein and can double up on the whey protein powder.

People who need a lot of structure might find this plan too freewheeling for their tastes, and the maintenance plan allows more carbs than some people might feel comfortable with. In addition, if you suspect you have a carbohydrate addiction, the amount of carbs allowed on the maintenance phase could conceivably trigger binges.

JONNY'S LOWDOWN ★★★★★

This is one of the half-dozen best low-carb approaches to health around. I have minor quibbles, with the emphasis on "minor": there is a lot of talk about cellulite and how the plan can reduce it, which I think is highly speculative, as is the section on food combining. I'd like to have seen alpha-lipoic acid mentioned as an important supplement for liver health. In my opinion, there is disproportionate emphasis on flaxseed oil and not enough on fish oil, which provides equally important omega-3s that are harder for the body to make on its own. But with that said, the basic template—limited starch, some fruit, unlimited vegetables, lean protein, and high-quality fats—is a great program and would benefit anyone. The phenomenal success and public acceptance of this program is well deserved.

8. THE FAT RESISTANCE DIET

LEO GALLAND, MD

WHAT IT IS IN A NUTSHELL

An absolutely first-rate program with an original point of view and novel information that is not found in other diet books. Written by one of the great icons in integrative medicine.

About the Fat Resistance Diet

The Fat Resistance Diet is a rarity in diet books—it actually offers an original and unique perspective on the whole issue of weight gain and health.

This is all the more worthy of mention because the author—Leo Galland, MD—is literally one of the giants in the field of integrative medicine. Most of what Galland has written has been for other professionals—he's been one of the main educators in holistic medicine, and has written extensively about such issues as digestive health, leaky gut, inflammation, and immunity. Once every so often, he writes for the general public. When he does, pay attention. Galland believes that being unable to lose weight is a sign that some basic metabolic mechanisms are not working properly, generally due to choices we make. "The whole premise of the Fat Resistance Diet is that we have inborn, natural regulatory systems that support a healthy weight, but our food choices and our lifestyle interfere with their functioning," he told me when I interviewed him.

One of these inborn regulatory systems that seems to go awry in obesity is a hormone called *leptin*. Leptin is a hormone that was first discovered in 1994 by researchers at Rockefeller University who were studying obese mice. It's a protein hormone that lets your brain and body know how much fat you are storing. When leptin levels goes up, your appetite goes down. Leptin also speeds up your metabolism. So, for proper weight management, we want the leptin circuits working well. "The problem is that overweight people have developed resistance to leptin," Dr. Galland explained. "Their leptin levels are high but it's not depressing their appetite and it's not stimulating their metabolism."

So why doesn't leptin work so well in overweight people?

According to Galland, one reason is inflammation. "Inflammation disables the leptin signal," he told me. "It also contributes to insulin resistance, a central feature of obesity and diabetes."

Everyone has had a personal experience with inflammation. If you stub your toe—if you get a sore throat, if you have a mild asthma attack or stuffed-up sinuses, if you've been stung by a bee or bitten by an ant at a picnic—you've seen firsthand what mild inflammation can look and feel like. And it's not always bad—in fact, it's part of the body's healing process. Fluid flows to the area, white blood cells surround the injury in an attempt to isolate and remove any foreign pathogens. It's all your body's response to an injury or insult and as such, some inflammatory processes can be important parts of the immune response. Your body makes inflammatory biochemicals and anti-inflammatory biochemicals, and they need to be in balance in order for you to be healthy.

But here's the problem: when your body's inflammation factories are on overdrive, it's not a good thing. We're constantly exposed to toxins, irritants, medicines, and foods that cause or aggravate mild inflammation, inflammation that flies under our pain radar but is nonetheless causing damage, especially to our vascular system. This is why Time magazine did a cover story on inflammation some years ago, in which they called it "The Silent Killer." Inflammation is now recognized to be a component of every degenerative disease, from Alzheimer's to cancer to obesity to diabetes to heart disease.

Galland's program is all about controlling inflammation. In the Fat Resistance Diet, you do it with the natural anti-inflammatories that are found in herbs, spices, and a multitude of fresh whole foods like vegetables. According to Galland, if you control inflammation, you're on the way to controlling fat. "Inflammation is the critical link between obesity and chronic illness," Dr. Galland told me. In the presence of inflammation, the "fat control mechanisms" simply don't work.

Another aspect of the inflammation equation has to do with what's called *nutrient density*. You can help control inflammation with nutrients (for example, omega-3 fats, which are among the most anti-inflammatory compounds on the planet). "What matters most about the calories in any food are the nutrients that accompany them," says Galland. "The most critical nutrients are those needed to stop the slow-moving avalanche of obesity/inflammation."

Calories are important, but not nearly as important as what else is in the food that contains those calories. "A weight-reduction program that only looks at calories completely misses the boat," he says. "A 'calorie-controlled' diet consisting of 12 packs a day of 100-calorie Oreo snack packs might have the 'right' number of calories, but you'd be completely screwed up by the lack of fiber, the lack of protein, and the resulting blood-sugar roller coaster."

Some of the best anti-inflammatory spices and herbs include cloves, ginger, parsley, tumeric, cinnamon, and basil, all spices I wrote about at length in my book, The 150 Healthiest Foods on Earth. In fact, many of the foods and spices that made the list of the healthiest foods on earth were included precisely *because* they were so rich in natural anti-inflammatories (not to mention vitamins, minerals, protein, fiber, and omegas). "We need to re-educate our palate to learn to appreciate the wonders of these foods," Dr. Galland told me.

The Fat Resistance Diet is a lifestyle based around great food rather than the calorie restriction that is usually accompanied by the use of artificial sweeteners, sugar substitutes, and fake fats. The book contains incredibly valuable information about the role of these chemicals in inflammation and the inflammation–obesity connection. You can get a good idea of what's in store for you by reading the basic 12 principles of the Fat Resistance Diet in the accompanying sidebar.

THE 12 PRINCIPLES OF THE FAT RESISTANCE DIET*

1. Choose foods that are loaded with nutrients.

2. Avoid trans-fats.

3. Consume foods with plenty of omega-3 content.

4. Eat fish 3 times a week or more.

5. Eat at least 25 grams of fiber per day.

6. Eat at least 9 servings of vegetables and fruits daily.

7. Average one serving a day of alliums (onions, scallions, garlic) and crucifers (broccoli, cabbage, kale, cauliflower).

8. Get no more than 10% of total calories from saturated fat.

9. Use only unbroken egg yolks.

10. Don't follow a "low-fat" diet.

11. Eat two healthful snacks a day.

12. Use fruits for sweets.

*Used with permission.

The Fat Resistance Diet as a Lifestyle: Who it Works for, Who Should Look Elsewhere

I think the principles of this program would actually benefit everyone. People looking for an extremely structured program might not find it to their liking, but if you like understanding the principles behind why you're eating what you're eating, this is a great book for you. Weight loss in this book does not seem to be the main goal—rather, it's a natural by-product of the kind of healthy eating Galland recommends.*

JONNY'S LOWDOWN ★★★★★

A really original contribution to the weight-loss literature with some important information about influences on weight that don't ordinarily get addressed in

---

*Shortly after *The Fat Resistance Diet* was published, Dr. Galland and his son Jonathan Galland published an excellent accompanying cookbook—*The Fat Resistance Diet Cookbook.*

most diet books. If you've been frustrated with the usual calorie-based meal plans and standard exercise programs and want a different take on some of the metabolic obstacles to weight loss (as well as some solid information about what to do about those obstacles), this book is highly recommended. It's worth it just for the information on artificial sweeteners, chemicals, inflammation, and leptin control. Highly recommended.

9. The Hamptons Diet

Fred Pescatore, MD

WHAT IT IS IN A NUTSHELL

A lower-carb plan that's a twist on the Mediterranean diet: high in vegetables, fish, nuts, and omega-3 fats, but favoring macadamia-nut oil instead of olive oil. You choose from three plans—A, B, or C—depending on how much weight you would like to lose. Each plan has slightly different amounts of carbohydrate. All plans stress lean protein, nuts, vegetables, fish, and—you guessed it— macadamia-nut oil.

About the Hamptons Diet

The Hamptons Diet starts with the premise that the low-fat, low-cholesterol message of the past couple of decades was—if not wholly wrong—terribly miscommunicated. No disagreement there: fat phobia gave rise to the ridiculous notion that we could consume as many fat-free foods as we wanted. By now practically everyone realizes that this silly philosophy led us into our current predicament: near-epidemic levels of obesity and diabetes. The low-fat, high-carb diet, particularly as practiced by people using tons of processed high-glycemic foods, produces increased levels of triglycerides, which increase the risk for coronary heart disease. And high-glycemic diets have been linked with diabetes and with several kinds of cancers.

So far, so good. Dr. Pescatore points to the fact that the American Heart Association diet—which recommends limiting total dietary fat to less than 30% of the diet and saturated fat to less than 10%—fails to lower triglycerides and actually lowers HDL (good cholesterol). In addition, the AHA diet has never consistently shown long-term improvement in any heart-disease outcome. The original low-fat advice was also predicated on the simplistic idea that blood cholesterol was the whole picture when it came to cardiac risk. We now know that there are a host of measures that are far better predictors of heart disease than total cholesterol. These include triglycerides, HDL (good) cholesterol, LDL particle size, inflammatory markers like C-reactive protein, homocysteine, blood pressure, lipoprotein(a), and others, many of which respond quite poorly to a high-carb diet, particularly one high in sugars. And, as Dr. Walter Willett recently proclaimed, research has shown that the percentage of fat in the diet—contrary to the advice of the last two decades—has shown absolutely no relationship to any major health outcome.

So why worry about fat at all? Having been the associate medical director of the Atkins Center for many years, Dr. Pescatore understands well that the demonization of all fat was a ridiculous idea. But rather than taking a stand for the wholehearted repeal of fat-phobia, the Hamptons Diet takes a more cautious approach. The author points to the benefits of the Mediterranean diet, an eating regimen that has long been touted as healthy by many nutritionists. This diet is high in fish, nuts, lean proteins, vegetables, and especially monounsaturated fat. The classic Mediterranean diet "does not regard all fat as bad," and, in fact, doesn't limit fat consumption at all. It does, however, specify which fats to eat and which to avoid (more on this in a moment). The primary monounsaturated fat in the Mediterranean diet is olive oil, which even fat phobics have conceded is a "heart-healthy" fat.

Dr. Pescatore has found an oil he feels is even better for you than olive oil, and this is the gimmick of the Hamptons Diet. Dr. Pescatore replaces olive oil with macadamia-nut oil, an oil he claims has miraculous benefits for several reasons. First, you can use it in both hot and cold recipes. Second, it has a perfect ratio of omega-6 to omega-3 fatty acids (1:1). Third, it has a higher concentration of the healthy monounsaturates (omega-9 fats) than olive oil. And fourth, it has a high smoke point, which decreases the risk of trans-fatty acid formation. Dr. Pescatore's company, MacNut Oil, imports the macadamia-nut oil he recommends in his resource section. That's not necessarily a bad thing—macadamia-nut oil is a good food, and many of us sell products that we truly believe in and use ourselves—but it's worth disclosing.

There are six basic tenets of the Hamptons Diet:

1. Eat fish that is rich in omega-3 fats (for example, sardines, mackerel, salmon).
2. Eat nuts.
3. Do not eat trans-fats.
4. Do eat "healthful" fats (stay tuned). The author states: "In the

Hamptons Diet, we use the most healthful oil—macadamia nut—
and in the pure Mediterranean diet, olive oil is used.")
5. Consume ample quantities of vegetables and some fruits.
6. Consume moderate amounts of alcohol.

There are also three levels, or programs, somewhat cutely labeled the
"A List," the "B List," and the "C List" in an amusing takeoff on the social
stratification that is de rigeur in the diet's namesake hometown. The "A"
program is for people who have more than 10 pounds to lose, and limits
carb intake to 30 grams a day. There is also a long, detailed suggested list of
A List–appropriate proteins, vegetables, fruits, spices, nuts, and nut butters.
The B List is a transitional program for people who have fewer than 10
pounds to lose and are on their way to maintenance (the C List). On the B
program, you consume between 40 and 60 grams of carbs (less for women),
and can choose from another 8 protein sources and an additional 3 dozen
veggies. You can also now add some whole grains and fruits. And on the C
program, which is for maintenance, you have an even wider range of grains
and fruits to choose from, as the daily carb content goes up to 55 to 65
grams for women and 65 to 85 grams for men.

So why all the fuss about macadamia-nut oil? Well, like olive oil, it contains an omega-9 fatty acid called oleic acid. Oleic acid, according to Dr.
Pescatore, increases the incorporation of omega-3 fatty acids into the cell
membrane, which is a good thing. He postulates that this might decrease
the incidence of breast cancer, though he doesn't tell us how. We do know,
however, that oleic acid has been shown to decrease total and LDL (bad)
cholesterol, but, perhaps more important, it also lowers triglycerides and
raises HDL (good) cholesterol. Dr. Pescatore takes the position that since
we know that olive oil does these things, and since macadamia-nut oil has
even more of the active ingredient (omega-9 oleic acid) than olive oil does,
it stands to reason that the cardiac and perhaps anticancer benefits might
be even more pronounced in the Hamptons Diet than in the classic Mediterranean diet.

The Hamptons Diet, to its credit, does say that "some saturated fats are
OK" and recommends, for example, eggs as a good source of "lean protein."
Also to its credit, it makes the point that we need to eat much less of those
omega-6 fats we were told were healthy in the days when low-fat was king—
the polyunsaturated oils like grapeseed, corn, safflower, sunflower, soybean,
and cottonseed. Kudos to Pescatore for making this point, often missed in
other programs. I couldn't agree more.

The Hamptons Diet as a Lifestyle: Who It Works for, Who Should Look Elsewhere

This is a perfectly fine program for most people, though I suspect it's going to appeal more to people who have fewer than 20 pounds to lose. Its recipes and food lists are not for those on a strict budget—reading the menus makes me think of four-star restaurants and red velvet ropes. And it is clearly meant to be marketed to those who see themselves as part of the glamorous set, though that's more a statement about the marketing and the title. If you can afford the food and the exotic recipes appeal to you, and if you don't have a ton of weight to lose, go for it. Those who prefer a little more basic stuff or a little more structure might be put off.

JONNY'S LOWDOWN ★★★★★

Full disclosure: I like Fred Pescatore. He's a good guy. He means very well, he's knowledgeable, and, as medical director of the Atkins Center, he did a great deal of good by showing how to apply the principles of the Atkins approach to the treatment of children (his Feed Your Kids Well *remains my favorite book on children and diet). And it's hard to fault this program. The book has a definitive section on oils, is on the money on the issue of trans-fats, urges organic foods, and limits processed junk. What's not to like?*

The Hamptons Diet is clearly Dr. Pescatore's attempt to brand himself as an entity separate from his mentor Robert Atkins. I can understand this. My only real criticism of the Hamptons Diet is a personal one—I wish he had taken a stronger stand against those who deem all saturated fats the enemy. I guess I hold him to a higher standard than say, Dr. Agatston of South Beach fame. Unlike Agatston, Dr. Pescatore is a nutritionist, and a very good one at that; he has to know that if you followed all the principles in his book and still consumed saturated fats from healthy sources (à la Atkins for Life), you would be just fine. My guess is that he opted for a program that is more acceptable to the masses, who still believe that saturated fat is the worst thing you can eat.

The book is chock-full of great recipes, the information is on track, the information on oils is outstanding, and the supplement program is well thought-out.

10. The Low GI Diet Revolution

Jenny Brand-Miller, PhD, et al.

WHAT IT IS IN A NUTSHELL

A diet program based entirely around the concept of glycemic index.

About the Low GI Diet Revolution

The Low GI Diet Revolution is based on the concept of glycemic index, which has revolutionized the way we think about carbohydrates.

Briefly, here's how it works. In 1981, David Jenkins and Thomas Wolever of the University of Toronto came up with a system for classifying carbohydrates according to how fast they raise blood-sugar levels. At the time, people were still talking about carbohydrates in terms of "simple" and "complex," an outdated system which still, sadly, persists to this day and is utterly irrelevant (more on that in a moment). The glycemic index was a far more useful way to classify carbohydrate foods.

In the "olden" days—when I first studied nutrition—we classified carbohydrates into two groups—simple and complex. Remember, all carbohydrates are made up of units of sugar (called "saccharides"). The *simple* carbohydrates contain either one unit of sugar (a *monosaccharide*—like glucose and fructose*) or two units (a *disaccharide*—like sucrose, which is simply one molecule of glucose plus one molecule of fructose). The "complex" carbs are even longer chains, known as *polysaccharides* (poly meaning "many").

We used to believe that the "simple" carbs were bad because they were so quickly digested and absorbed and the "complex" ones (like, for example, pasta and bread and bagels) were "good" because they took longer to break down.

Unfortunately, that turned out to be wholly false.

Many "complex" carbs (such as bread) break down so quickly in the bloodstream that you might as well be swallowing table sugar. And conversely, many "simple" carbs (such as an apple) break down much more slowly and are loaded with nutrients and phytochemicals to boot. So the old

---

*Fructose is a "simple" sugar that doesn't raise blood sugar very much at all; but when it's isolated from fruit and made into a liquid sweetener, it does a lot of damage in other ways.

saw about "simple" carbs being ones to avoid and "complex" carbs being ones to consume turned out to be nonsense.

Much more useful is to think about carbs in terms of whether they are "slow-burning" or "fast-burning"—in other words, how quickly do they raise your blood sugar, and how long do they keep it elevated?

Enter the glycemic index.

When scientists test a carbohydrate food to determine its glycemic index, they pick a fixed amount of carbohydrate—50 grams—and then feed it to people and measure what happens to their blood sugar. They rate the results on a scale of 1 to 100, with 100 being the score for pure glucose (or white bread). Foods tested this way that score 70 or over are considered "high-GI foods," foods that score between 56 and 69 are considered "medium-GI foods," and foods that score 55 or under are considered "low-GI foods."

Since the whole principle of low- (or controlled-) carb eating is based on the idea that you want to control your blood sugar, eating "low glycemic" makes a whole lot of sense. High blood sugar leads to high levels of the fat-storing hormone, insulin, and low-glycemic (or low-carb) diets prevent that from happening.

Furthermore, a lot of research has shown that low-GI diets are really healthful. They help improve your body's sensitivity to insulin (since your body produces less of it, the cells "listen" to it better); they improve diabetes control; they reduce the risk of heart disease; and they can also help people lose weight. What's more, low-glycemic diets keep you full longer and help stave off hunger and cravings. And recent research has linked high-glycemic diets to some forms of cancer. So, all in all, eating "low" on the glycemic scale makes a lot of sense.

But the glycemic index has some problems. For one thing, the "rating" only applies to a food eaten alone. (Once you group foods together, the impact on your blood sugar is very different.) Second of all—and maybe most important—the glycemic index number only tells you the effect of 50 grams of carbohydrates, which doesn't reflect real-world portions. For example, carrots got a bad rap for being so high on the glycemic index, but there's only 3 grams of carbohydrate in a carrot, not 50. You'd have to eat a bushel of them to really raise your blood sugar significantly. And conversely, pasta—which has a "moderate" glycemic index—is rarely eaten in 50-gram portions. You're more likely to consume about 200 grams, which will send your blood sugar off the charts.

To compensate for this, scientists invented the "glycemic load," which is a far more accurate measure of a food's "real-life" effect on your blood sugar because it takes portion size into account. For example, carrots have a glycemic index of 92 (high!), but once you take into account the typical portion size and figure out their glycemic load, it's very low (under 10). Foods which are between 0 and 10 on the glycemic load are considered low, 10–20 medium, and over 20 high.

Jennie Brand-Miller, the author of *The Low GI Diet Revolution*, is the research scientist who's done the most to popularize the glycemic index and to bring it into the popular lexicon. She's published a ton of research on glycemic index, and her tables of glycemic index (and glycemic load) for hundreds upon hundreds of carbohydrate foods are widely considered the industry standard. (You can find the glycemic index and glycemic load for just about any food that has been tested at http://www.mendosa.com/ gilists.htm.)

The Low GI Diet Revolution is Brand-Miller's entry into the diet book world, and it's her attempt to bring low-GI eating to the masses. Except for a few missteps, it's a pretty good program.

First the missteps. She repeats a number of myths about low-carb diets (much of the weight loss is muscle mass, not body fat; saturated fat causes heart disease; the brain can only use glucose as a source of fuel). She also doesn't do much to address the fact that the *glycemic load* is a much better indicator than the glycemic index. But given the enormousness of her contribution to the conversation about carbs, insulin, and health, let's overlook those mistakes for the moment and focus on what's good about this program.

The Low GI Diet Revolution uses a novel approach to determining what you should eat. First you look at a table for your weight and determine what your "energy level" is. (By "energy," the authors are not talking about "get up and go"; they're talking about "calories," which is the technically correct use of "energy" in nutrition.) So, for example, women who weigh less than 154 have an "energy" level of "1," those who weigh 155 to 176 are "2," 177 to 198 are "3," and so forth. (There is a similar table for men.)

Once you know your "energy" number, you simply go down to the graph and look at the number of servings of protein, carbs, and fat you should consume. Each "energy level" (from 1 to 10) has a recommended number of servings from each of these three groups. For example, if you're a woman who weighs 175, you look on the chart and see that your "energy rating" is 2; for an energy rating of 2, your recommended daily intake would be 4 servings of carbohydrate-rich foods, 4 servings of protein-rich foods, and 2 servings of fat-rich foods.

A carbohydrate-rich serving is one that contains 20 to 30 grams of carbs (like grains and starches). A protein-rich serving contains 10 to 15 grams of protein, and a fat-rich food contains 10 grams of fat. In addition, everyone eats at least 5 servings of vegetables (which tend to be very low in actual grams of carbs) and 2 servings of fruit each day. The authors consider this program to be a very good "compromise" between a low-carb and a low-fat program.

Once you know the carb, protein and fat content of food—not hard to learn from reading labels, using calorie books, or checking online—it's pretty easy to follow.

The Low GI Diet Revolution as a Lifestyle: Who It Works for, Who Should Look Elsewhere

Overall this is a good program. By limiting your "carb-rich" foods, you will automatically be reducing the high-ticket items like starches but will still be able to eat some of them, a big plus for people who don't do well on—or don't need—a very carb-restricted diet. The 5 servings of vegetables and 2 of fruit will make sure you get all the valuable nutrients and phytochemicals contained in the plant kingdom (though I'd argue you could eat even more vegetables than that), and if you pretty much stick to the recommendations, your calories will be moderately—but not painfully—low.

However, if you are insulin-resistant, very carb-sensitive, or very overweight, you may need much more carb restriction than this program provides, and you may want or need more protein or fat in your diet than the amount recommended by the authors.

It's also worth noting that this isn't so much a weight-loss program as it is a general guide to eating. Those who have a lot of weight to lose may need a bit more fine-tuning than the general guidelines of this program provide and may want to look elsewhere.

JONNY'S LOWDOWN ★ ★ ★ ½

The Low GI Diet Revolution is not really a weight-loss program per se—it's much more of a general eating plan based on the principles of low-glycemic eating. For the average person willing to make the effort to learn the protein, carb, and fat content of their food, it's a good program from which you will undoubtedly see some health benefits like appetite control and better energy. It's a very good starting place for weight loss, but be prepared to fine-tune the program a lot if your main goal is to lose weight.

Three and a half stars simply because the general idea of low-GI eating is such a good one.

---

11. The Paleo Diet

Loren Cordain, PhD

WHAT IT IS IN A NUTSHELL

All the lean meat, poultry, fish, and seafood you want, plus unlimited fruits and nonstarchy vegetables. No dairy, cereals, legumes, or processed foods.

About the Paleo Diet

The Paleo Diet is perhaps the most sophisticated example of the "Stone-Age" or "caveman" type of diet book, and Dr. Loren Cordain is one of the best-known researchers in the field of what might be called "nutritional anthropology" or "Paleolithic nutrition." The general theory behind the Paleo Diet—and others like it—is this:

- Being fat comes primarily from eating a diet that is *completely unsuited* to our ancient genes and digestive system.
- The human genus spent a couple of million years adapting to and functioning on a diet *entirely* different than the one we eat today.
- Our digestive systems—identical to those of our caveman ancestors— are simply unsuited for the staples of today's diet: dairy, refined sugar, fatty meat, and processed food.
- By returning to the diet that humans lived on for the vast majority of their time on earth, we can correct a great many of the problems in human health, including but not limited to obesity.

The argument for this position is pretty strong. DNA evidence shows that genetically, humans have hardly changed in the 2.5 million years the genus has been on the planet. The human genome has changed less than 0.02% (one fiftieth of 1%) in forty thousand years. Most of the diseases of modern civilization—cancer, obesity, diabetes, and heart disease—have happened at the same time that we've experienced a sea change in our diet, and the modern diet is completely different from the one humans have lived on for the overwhelming bulk of our time on the planet.

Through fossil records and research on contemporary hunter–gatherer societies, we have a pretty good idea of what Paleolithic peoples ate—and it didn't look like anything you'd find at Burger King.

Consider the diet of our Paleo ancestors, before the invention of modern foods: they ate no dairy (how easy would it be to milk a wild animal?) and no cereal grains; they didn't salt their food; the only sweetener they used was honey, which they ate rarely (when they could find it); wild-animal foods dominated their diet (so protein intake was high and carb intake was low); and since all carbs came from wild fruits and nonstarchy vegetables, fiber was very high.

Beginning to get the picture?

On the other hand, the average American diet contains:

- 31% calories from cereals
- 14% calories from dairy
- 8% calories from beverages, especially sodas and fruit juices
- 4% calories from oils and dressings, especially processed oils and omega-6's
- 4% calories from sweets like candy, cookies, and cake

That means 61% of calories in a modern diet come from foods that were largely unknown before the adoption of agriculture (a drop in the time bucket as far as evolution is concerned), and *most* of them weren't even available until a couple of hundred years ago, when food processing became the norm. The remaining 39% of our calories come from animal foods, but ones that are very different from those of our cavemen ancestors. The animal foods the average American is likely to consume are mostly hot dogs, fatty ground beef, bacon, and highly processed deli meats. (When looked at in this way, is it any wonder there are studies linking "meat" consumption in industrial societies to a number of health issues? Maybe meat as a category has gotten a bum rap, and it's the kind of meat we eat that's the problem!)

Cordain claims that a return to a diet of our ancestors—what has been described elsewhere as eating what you could hunt, fish, gather, grow, or pluck—is the answer not only to obesity and overweight, but to a multitude of other health problems. Though it seems like he stresses protein as the most important component in the diet, in actuality he makes it clear that protein *alone*—without fat or the alkalizing influence of tons of vegetables and fruits—is a big problem. Add those and the problem disappears: "There is no such thing as too much protein as long as you are eating plenty of fresh fruits and vegetables," Cordain says. And he is pretty flexible about the possible balance among them, pointing out that some hunter–gatherer societies that survived into the twentieth century lived healthy lives free of chronic disease while getting 97% of their calories from animal foods (the Inuit of Alaska), while others got the majority of their calories (65%) from plant foods (the !Kung of Africa). Most Paleo societies fall somewhere between these two extremes. No Paleo peoples, however, ate refined sugar.

On the Paleo Diet, fully 50% to 55% of your calories come from lean meats, organ meats, poultry, fish, and seafood. The rest come from vegetables (except for starchy ones like potatoes and yams) and "healthful" fats (more about these in Jonny's Lowdown). It's simple and easy. There is no calorie-counting, no protein-gram counting, no fat-gram counting, and no carb-gram counting. By staying within these guidelines, Cordain claims you will:

- have built-in protection against overeating because protein (and fiber) naturally feels more satiating
- enjoy the increased metabolic activity (and increased calorie-burning) that protein provides (see chapter 3 for studies that show this)
- control insulin and reduce insulin resistance, making weight loss a breeze

The Paleo Diet itself allows "cheating." There are 3 levels of commitment, with level 1 allowing you three "open" (read: cheat) meals a week, level 2 permitting two such meals, and level 3 only one.

Many people not previously familiar with the material in chapter 3 of this book will find Cordain's passionate argument against grains surprising, as we have been so conditioned to think of grains, especially whole grains, as wonderful foods. Cordain is particularly expert on this subject, having written the seminal paper "Cereal Grains: Humanity's Double-Edged Sword,"[6] and what he has to say on the subject is worth considering even if you don't adopt this particular dietary program.

The Problem with Grains

Here's the synopsis: the agricultural revolution began about ten thousand years ago in the Middle East. Dwindling food resources—especially wild game—and rising populations gave birth to the need for smarter, more efficient ways for people to support themselves and their families. Some enterprising people figured out how to sow and harvest wild wheat seeds. Then they tried barley. Then legumes. Livestock—sheep, goats, and pigs—wasn't far behind. Later, cattle. Domesticated farm animals were milkable. Over time, there was a complete change in the diet of most of humanity.

Without the agricultural revolution, we would not have civilization as we know it. Our ability to farm—to domesticate animals for dairy products, to raise cattle, and especially to grow and cultivate grains—was responsible for allowing us to live in denser conditions and encouraged towns and cities to develop. It allowed us to become independent from our original food source—hunted game.

But this new lifestyle came with a price. Early farmers were shorter in stature than their forebears had been. Examination of their bones and teeth showed more infectious diseases and shorter life spans. Egyptian mummies frequently reveal obese bodies. There were more cases of osteoporosis, rickets, and vitamin- and mineral-deficiency diseases, in large measure because of cereal-based diets (whole grains and legumes contain "antinutrients," pyridoxine glucosides and phytates, that respectively block absorption of B vitamins in the intestines and chemically bind iron, zinc, copper, and calcium and block their absorption). And the skulls of those living on modern foods revealed teeth filled with cavities and jaws that were misshapen and too small for the teeth (Dr. Weston Price's seminal 1939 book, *Nutrition and Physical Degeneration*, contains many pictures that dramatically illustrate this phenomenon).

Then came fermentation and salting. Grains were fed to livestock, making them fatter but also changing the quality of their meat and their fat. (Interesting, isn't it, that grains are the food of choice for fattening livestock and yet are still recommended by the dietary establishment as the foundation food of a weight-loss program!) Meat was preserved by pickling, salting, and smoking. Two hundred years ago, things got even worse. We now had ways to refine sugar and flour and to can foods, almost always with the addition or creation of trans-fats, sugar, refined oils high in omega-6s, and high-fructose corn syrup, not to mention additives, preservatives, emulsifiers, and other toxins.

As Cordain says, imagine Paleo man with a Twinkie or a pizza. He wouldn't even recognize them as food.

Cordain is one of the few writers to talk about something called the acid–base balance, a very hot subject in nutrition these days. Briefly, it goes like this: everything reports to the kidneys as either an acid or an alkaline (base). When there is too much acid, the body needs to neutralize it with alkaline substances like calcium. Meats are one of the top five acid-producing foods; but the other four—grains, legumes, cheese, and salt—were rarely or never eaten by our Paleo ancestors, who buffered the acid load of their meat with plenty of fruits and vegetables. The main "buffering" compound in the body is calcium, and the main storehouse for calcium is the bones; this is how high-protein diets got their (false) reputation for causing bone loss. Cordain correctly points out that loss of calcium does not happen when there are plenty of fruits and vegetables in the diet, and especially when other acid-producing foods (like cereal grains and dairy) are absent.

The Paleo Diet as a Lifestyle: Who It Works for, Who Should Look Elsewhere

The straightforward simplicity of the Paleo Diet—all you want of *these* foods, none at all of *those*—makes it pretty easy to follow and a good choice for those who are put off by counting grams, calories, and carbohydrates, figuring out protein allowances, or computing food blocks. But that same lack of rigidity makes it a poor choice for those who need more structure. And although it restricts nearly all of the usual problem foods for carbohydrate addicts, the unlimited fruit could easily be a problem for those who are insulin-resistant. In addition, since it is not primarily a weight-loss diet, it may be frustrating for those whose main focus for the immediate future is on losing fat.

JONNY'S LOWDOWN ★ ★ ★ ½

The Paleo Diet is a frustrating program to rate. On one hand, you have to give tremendous credit to a no-grain diet that eliminates sugar, dairy, and trans-fats and recommends tons of vegetables. How bad can that be? Most people— especially those who eat the typical American diet—are going to reap such enormous benefits from this program that I want to give it five stars just for that alone.

On the other hand, there are some major problems. For one thing, Cordain completely buys into the cholesterol–heart disease hypothesis; I believe that this hypothesis, in its current form, is less than a decade away from being dumped on the pile of scientific flotsam and jetsam. He also accepts the dogma that all saturated fats are bad, largely because they raise cholesterol (some do; many don't; and ultimately it may not matter much). Cordain puts eggs on the "avoid" list for their cholesterol content (something we now know is completely irrelevant, since dietary cholesterol has virtually no impact on serum cholesterol) and warns against such natural traditional fats as butter and cream, which he puts in the same category as such trans-fat nightmares as nonfat dairy creamer and frozen yogurt. He recommends canola oil (I don't agree; see chapter 5). He puts sweet potatoes—a "good" starch by almost anyone's standards—in the same class as french fries and tapioca pudding. He makes the somewhat problematic statement that "fruit won't make you fat on this diet even in unlimited amounts." And he completely misrepresents other low-carb diets, saying that they call for complete restriction of all carbohydrates to "between 30 and 100 grams a day," which, though basically true, does not mean—as Cordain says it does—that "fruits and vegetables are largely off-limits." In fact, this statement is not only demonstrably false but inconsistent; 100 grams of usable carbs a day buys you an awful lot of broccoli!

That said, he's a good guy and a sincere and responsible scholar, and his overall recommendations will propel a person eating the average American diet light-years ahead in his quest for good health. Done with care, Cordain's diet may also make you lose weight.

12. The Paleo Solution

Robb Wolf

WHAT IT IS IN A NUTSHELL:

The Paleo Solution is a program based on our ancestral diet of protein, vegetables, and fat. It is accompanied by one of the best and most complete descriptions of how the modern high-carb diet works to promote obesity, diabetes, and virtually every other disease of civilization.

About the Paleo Solution

Desperate times call for desperate measures.

I imagine that's what Robb Wolf—the author of this first-rate book—might have been thinking when he first started his journey back to health. He had been a strapping 180 pounds, a teenage state champion in power lifting with an amateur kickboxing record of 6–0. Then, in an attempt to get "healthy," he went on a vegetarian diet for several years. Many giant plates of steamed rice, tofu, and veggies later, he found himself a sickly and emaciated 140 pounds with sky-high triglycerides (over 300), hypertension, and an A–Z catalogue of digestive disturbances including constant gas and bloat—all this at the ripe old age of 26.

Long story short: this young man—armed with a degree in biochemistry and gifted with both a passion for learning and an excellent built-in BS detector—went on a mission to figure out what went wrong. He found the solution, regained his health, and this book is the result.

"You can walk into your doctor's office with horrible blood work, all the while eating a low-fat, high-carb diet of whole grains," he writes. "You can then shift to an ancestral way of eating that involves lean meats, seafood, seasonal vegetables, and fruit. Walk back into your doctor's office with perfect blood work, yet he will not believe that eating more protein and fat is what fixed your broken blood work."

The "ancestral way of eating" to which Wolf refers is the core of the Paleo Solution Diet. It worked for Wolf, and it may well work for you. "We are not genetically wired for a 50 percent carbohydrate, bran muffin diet, despite what the USDA, AMA, and FDA have to say on the topic," says Wolf. "*Capisce?*"

Yes, Robb. We capisce.

For the purposes of this review, I'll concentrate on the fat-loss résumé of The Paleo Solution, but you should know that there's a lot more in this book than just a prescription for weight loss. This book could easily be used as a modern-day primer on basic endocrinology for the intelligent reader who is not a professional nutritionist. It's very strong on subjects like grains and fat, offers some excellent information on cardiovascular disease, and contains a terrific discussion of cholesterol. Wolf is excellent at describing exactly what all the hormones do, how they "talk" to each other, and how their messages are jumbled by the modern high-carb diet. This is great information, and he presents it with a rare combination of accuracy and humor.

Now let's get to the fat-loss part.

The Hormonal Effect of Food (Redux)

Virtually every diet discussed in this book—including my own—talks about the hormonal effect of a diet too high in sugar or carbs. If you've sampled any of the diet reviews—or read my own explanation of what happens when you eat excess carbs—you already know all about insulin and its fat-storing action. But Wolf brings up some other, lesser-known hormonal effect of excess carbs, one of which is of great importance in the weight-loss equation. Here's how it works.

You may recall from high school biology that glycogen is the storage form of glucose. When glycogen stores in the liver are filled up, the excess glucose (sugar) is converted to fat, specifically a short-chain saturated fat called *palmitic acid*. The palmitic acid (PA) is combined with a glycerol molecule and made into triglycerides, which are packaged together with proteins and cholesterol into a molecule called a VLDL (very low-density lipoprotein). These VLDLs, with their rich PA content, move all around the body, but they *really* come alive once they are in the brain. And guess what PA does in the brain? It decreases our sensitivity to *leptin*, the hormone that tells us we're full.

When there's too much PA in the brain, we literally become "leptin-resistant." Leptin is a hormone that sends a "satiety" signal to the brain, essentially saying, "Hey guys, we're full, no more food needed, stop scarfing it down." When the brain stops "listening" to leptin, appetite no longer works correctly. Your body produces more and more leptin in a futile attempt to get the brain to "know" that you're full, but the brain isn't paying attention. You remain hungry despite the fact that your blood sugar is high, your belly is full, and leptin is shouting at you to stop eating. It's like one of those horror movies where someone is screaming a warning at you that the monster is right behind you, but the train is roaring into the station and you can't hear them! Leptin is screaming "stop," but your brain can't hear it 'cause it's so full of carb-created VLDLs!

There's more. Your liver is converting sugar into fats and VLDLs at such a high rate that some of this fat begins to accumulate in the liver itself, leading to non-alcoholic fatty liver disease (NAFLD). (NAFLD is the main focus of one of the other excellent diets discussed in this book, the Eadeses' *6-Week Cure for the Middle-Aged Middle*.)

If this weren't bad enough, consider that the pace at which all this happens is sped up considerably by fructose, a known driver of NAFLD. Fructose turns up the glucose-transport molecules in the liver, making the liver, in Wolf's words, "hungry for sugar." This in turn leads to increased PA production, which leads to—you guessed it—even greater leptin resistance.

As Wolf puts it, "The wheels are seriously falling off the wagon by this point."

So now we've seen at least two ways in which a high-carb diet makes you sick and fat. First, the high carb intake is driving your blood sugar through the roof, which in turns drives your insulin levels through the roof. Unless you're very, very lucky, this scenario turns into full-blown insulin resistance, which makes it fiendishly difficult to lose weight and sets you up for metabolic syndrome, diabetes, obesity, and heart disease. And second, the high level of carb intake puts a huge burden on the liver, leads to an overproduction of triglycerides and VLDL, and ultimately leads to leptin resistance, meaning the brain no longer listens to the hormone signal that tells you to stop eating. You keep eating, you get fatter, insulin and leptin resistance get worse, and—from a health perspective—you're pretty much out of luck.

Wolf also brings something we've discussed earlier in this book into the picture: the nasty little molecules appropriately nicknamed "AGEs."AGEs (advanced glycation end-products) are the products of a reaction between proteins in our body and sugars. The sugar gloms onto some normally slippery, healthy proteins and makes them sticky and less able to travel through the bloodstream. AGEs damage proteins, DNA, enzymes, and even receptors for both insulin and leptin, which is the very last thing you need. They "age" the body and are implicated in many degenerative diseases. (Our old friend fructose is seven times more effective at forming AGEs than glucose. Just sayin'.)

The point is that all this damage—and the weight gain that goes along with it—comes from the ridiculously high amount of carbohydrate in our diet, which we are in no way genetically prepared for.

According to Wolf, this loss of hormonal sensitivity—particularly for insulin and leptin—leads to a host of health problems, of which overweight is just one. Controlling these hormones is the key to losing fat, but—as he himself found out—it's also the key to healing.

So What Can I Eat?

The ancestral diet that Wolf advocates is really very simple: meat, poultry, seafood, vegetables, and fat (and a little fruit). No dairy, no grains, and no legumes. This prescription shares a lot with the original Paleo Diet, written by Wolf's acknowledged mentor, Professor Loren Cordain. But there are a few differences, one of which has to do with fat.

Wolf takes a much more reasonable position on saturated fat than his mentor, Cordain, took in *The Paleo Diet*. (One of the only things I strongly disagreed with in Cordain's book was his agreement with the position that "saturated fat is the devil." Wolf's is much closer to my own position, so, naturally, I like his view more. "Saturated fat has historically been implicated as a causative factor in everything from CVD to cancer," he writes. "*However, closer analysis has shown this assumption to be largely inaccurate.*") He also points out that the ratio of omega-6 to omega-3 fats is of far more importance in disease progression than saturated fat. This, too, is a position I wholeheartedly agree with. No wonder I'm such a fan of this book!

Wolf's "day job" is that he owns one of the best gyms in the country (voted in the top 100 by *Men'sHealth*), so it's no surprise that his section on exercise is the best I've ever seen in a low-carb diet book. It's thorough, intelligent, and nothing like the cursory, boilerplate stuff that often gets tagged on as an afterthought in so many diet programs. There are programs for different levels of fitness, and they are well-designed and intelligent. Of course, you could choose to follow the diet and do your own thing in the exercise department, but you can't go wrong following any of the exercise programs carefully described (and illustrated with photos) in this book.

This is not a "diet" book in the conventional sense. The program is more like a philosophy of eating and health, and rather than give you a specific menu to follow, Wolf gives you a shopping list. He does give you a 30-day meal plan, but that's more like training wheels, providing a suggested guide for meal planning based on the ingredients he's included. What you learn from this book is what to put on your shopping list and what to leave off. He himself has a list of fifteen meats, fifteen veggies, five fats, and twenty herbs and spices, all easily available from your grocery store, which you can combine in thousands of ways. He suggests you pick five meats, five veggies, five fats, and as many herbs and spices as you can carry. "If you take one item from each of these columns and consider that a meal, you have 22,500 meal options," he says. The eating prescription is simplicity itself:

"Put some oil in a pan, start browning meat, add herb or spice, and then add a vegetable. Cook for five to ten minutes. Eat." Try for 30 days.

The Paleo Solution as a Lifestyle: Who It Works for, Who Should Look Elsewhere

Let's be honest: this is a pretty drastic departure from the way many people have eaten all their lives. In Paleo world, dairy, grains, and legumes are definitely off the menu, and even some foods considered acceptable on most low-carb plans have cautions attached, especially for people with autoimmune or inflammatory issues. Even fruit is minimized, especially at first, thought it's not totally banned. "There is no nutrient in fruit that is not available in veggies, and fruit may have too many carbs for you," he says. But Wolf is not a zealot, and even has some suggestions for "easing into" the Paleo lifestyle, one meal at a time.

Still, this is also not the kind of program where you're taken by the hand and treated like a baby. This is like the Marine Corps of diet books— it's not for the faint hearted, and you better be ready to say good-bye to a lot of familiar foods (or, more accurately, "food products"). It seems to me to be particularly suited to those rugged, individualistic types of both sexes who don't need to have everything spelled out for them and are perfectly capable of constructing their own meals from a clear, basic shopping list. If that's you, you should give this program a go. It's particularly suited for those with multiple health issues that haven't gotten a lot of help from the conventional medical system and are ready to take an *un*conventional—if historically sensible—approach. According to Wolf, the ancestral diet solves a lot of problems, and weight is only one of them.

The program is definitely not vegetarian-friendly, though if you're really committed, you might be able to make a go of it. Vegans, don't even bother.

JONNY'S LOWDOWN ★★★★★

This is one of the best low-carb diet books I've ever read, and it's hard to think of a situation in which it wouldn't produce a huge benefit in your overall health. You can keep this book on your shelf as a reference on digestion, hormones, and the effects of carbohydrates on your health. It has the best and most thorough exercise program of any diet book I've ever seen. He's got some excellent, albeit technical, information in here, but it's presented in a highly readable and often very funny manner, and he never talks down to the reader.

I recommend this book wholeheartedly.

13. THE PRIMAL BLUEPRINT

MARK SISSON

WHAT IT IS IN A NUTSHELL:

The Primal Blueprint is a high-fat, moderate-protein, low-carb, Paleo-type diet that is smart and sensible and incredibly effective. It's a bit more flexible than some of the other Paleo-oriented diets, especially when it comes to dairy, but it shares a lack of love for grains and legumes. The emphasis is on lifestyle, not diet, and it's very user-friendly. The author holds that if you follow the basic template 80% of the time, you will get the results you want.

About the Primal Blueprint

There's a lot to like about the Primal Blueprint—for example, everything.

The basic premise is similar to other "Paleo-centric" programs: *We are genetically adapted to a diet of foods we could hunt or gather.* For Sisson, like the other "Paleo-ists," being overweight and sick is a direct consequence of our reliance on foods and "food products" that are processed, man-made, and introduced relatively recently into the human diet. To Sisson, a return to the caveman way of eating—or a reasonable facsimile of it—will restore us to health (and to leanness).

What's not to like?

On the Primal Blueprint, you'll eat meat and other protein sources, as many vegetables as you can possibly consume, and all the fat you like. For those who like visuals, there's a terrific "Primal Blueprint Food Pyramid," at the base of which is *meat, fish, fowl,* and *eggs.* These foods constitute the bulk of your dietary calories. Next up on the pyramid is *vegetables,* with an emphasis on locally grown and/or organic. The next level consists of *healthy fats,* which includes saturated fat. Butter, coconut oil, avocados, coconut products, olive oil, and macadamias are all mentioned as good fats. (In my view, the fact that saturated fat is *not* demonized—as it is in the original Paleo Diet—gives this program additional credibility.)

Moderation foods are the next level of the pyramid. These include locally grown, in-season, high-antioxidant fruits like berries, high-fat dairy (preferably raw, fermented, and unpasteurized), starchy tubers, quinoa, wild rice (for athletes), nuts, and seeds. The small triangular peak of the pyramid contains herbs and spices, *sensible indulgences* (such as red wine and dark chocolate), and supplements.

For anyone who might be skeptical that such a simple program can work, I suggest looking at the before-and-after pictures of some of the Primal Blueprint success stories. They're nothing short of stunning. I was particularly impressed with the women in this section, since "meat-centric" programs so often appeal to men. The pictures of the women who have followed the Primal Blueprint should forever put to rest the idea that Paleo diets are just for men. Both sexes seem to do equally well on this program, and the photographic proof is right there.

Sisson is very clear from the beginning that this is not a "diet" program in any conventional sense. "The Primal Blueprint is a lifestyle with some important but extremely flexible eating guidelines," he writes. He starts the book with the "Ten Primal Blueprint Laws," of which only two have anything to do with food:

1. Eat plants and animals.
2. Avoid poisonous things.
3. Move frequently at a slow pace.
4. Lift heavy things.
5. Sprint once in a while.
6. Get adequate sleep.
7. Play.
8. Get adequate sunlight.
9. Avoid stupid mistakes.
10. Use your brain.

Sounds simple, but it's about as smart a set of guidelines as you could come up with if you want to be lean and healthy.

A Word about Exercise

Sisson is no fan of long, drawn-out, strenuous aerobic sessions for either weight loss or health. Law number three (above) is to move frequently at a slow pace, law number four is to lift heavy things, and law number five is to sprint from time to time. Taken together, this means an exercise program that's a blend of frequent low-intensity energizing movement (e.g., walking, hiking, easy cardio), regular, brief strength-training sessions, and occasional all-out sprints. He explains why and how in detail in the book. Did I mention that he's on-the-money on this one? No? Well, he is.

He's also on-the-money about a whole lot more. The section on heart disease ("How to Sneeze at Heart Disease") is superb. He dismisses the cholesterol hypothesis and advances the position that heart disease is caused by oxidation and inflammation (a view cardiologist Stephen Sinatra, MD, and I also take in our book, *The Great Cholesterol Myth*). His discussion of fat is excellent, clear, and accurate. So is his discussion of sleep and play.

In fact, there's hard to find much in this book that *isn't* terrific.

The temptation—for me—is to tell you about *all* of the positive aspects of this book, but I'm going to resist that temptation and just give you one example: what Sisson calls "The Carbohydrate Curve." He writes, "Your body composition success is overwhelmingly dependent on controlling your carbohydrate intake and hence, your insulin output." A graph in the book plots "grams of carbohydrate per day" against outcomes like *burn more fat, maintain body comp, store more fat,* and *obesity and illness.* Eat in the 100 to 150 gram "maintenance zone" and you won't gain fat. Eat in the 40 to 100 gram "sweet spot" zone and you'll lose body fat. It's simple, easy-to-follow, and—best of all—it works.

Conventional Wisdom versus Primal Blueprint

Even if you don't want to read this book in full, I suggest you pick it up and at least study the chart in the very beginning of the book, comparing "conventional wisdom" to "Primal Blueprint." Sisson details the conventional wisdom on a variety of categories, including cholesterol, eggs, fiber, meal habits, strength training, cardio, weight loss, sun exposure, footwear, prescription drugs, and goals, accurately summarizing the "wisdom" of the authorities and then contrasting it with the principles of the Primal Blueprint. As you would expect, the two columns present very different points of view. If the surprising contrasts on these pages speak to you as much as they did to me, you'll understand what's in store for you if you go "primal."

The Primal Blueprint as a Lifestyle: Who It Works for, Who Should Look Elsewhere

It's hard to think of someone for whom this program would not work. It's also very hard to take issue with the principles on which it's based, principles that are rock-solid and very smart indeed. The only question is whether you'll be able to follow the program, since—like all Paleo-centric eating plans—it pretty much eliminates most of the "comfort" foods we consume daily, and many of the foods we've been taught are universally healthy (like grains).

This is definitely not a "quick-fix" diet. The author is scrupulous about stressing the lifestyle aspects of the program, and only one (possibly two) of the "Ten Primal Blueprint Laws" has anything to do with food. That said, weight management is an almost-guaranteed "side effect" of living Primal (or Paleo, take your pick). But it's not for those looking for instant gratification. Following this excellent program is going to take some readjustment and some rethinking of your beliefs about what's healthy and "necessary" in the human diet and about what's causing all the problems (hint: it's not fat!).

If you're willing to do this kind of fundamental reassessment and you're prepared to give this plan a trial for the recommended 21 days, you will undoubtedly become a convert to this way of life.

Since the program is pretty heavy on protein and fat, vegetarians will have a problem with it. If you're a vegetarian for health reasons, you owe it to yourself to read the book. If you're a vegetarian for ethical or moral reasons, the book is probably not going to change your way of thinking, and you'll be happier elsewhere. Vegans, don't even bother.

JONNY'S LOWDOWN ★★★★★

The story of how The Primal Blueprint *came to be published and went on to become an Amazon bestseller and an Internet sensation is an interesting one. Mark Sisson is a former world-class marathoner and Ironman triathelete with a bachelor's degree in biology who describes himself as "an athlete, a coach, and a student, on a lifelong quest for exceptional health, happiness and peak performance." He's the founder and publisher of MarksDailyApple.com, the leading "Paleo" blog on the Internet. But when he tried to get his book published, door after door slammed in his face. "Mark, you're not a doctor," he was told. "You have no credibility. You need a celebrity attached or it won't go anywhere. Ditching grains? Eating more fat? Making workouts slower or shorter? It just won't fly with today's reader."*

Except it did. Sisson published the first edition himself, and it sold over 130,000 copies in six printings and climbed to the top of the charts on Amazon. Deservedly, I might add.

When I first I combed through this book trying to find something to disagree with, I came up empty-handed. It's pitch-perfect on just about everything. I particularly like the way Sisson presents the material—even if you've seen this stuff before, you'll love the way he lays it out. At the beginning of each chapter he tells you what the chapter is going to cover, and at the end he summarizes the important points. There's a ton of tips sprinkled throughout the book, and a wonderful "Primal Approved: At A Glance" section that summarizes what foods you should eat, what foods you should avoid, what exercises work, and what lifestyle changes matter.

All in all, this is one of the best of the new crop of diet/exercise/weight-loss books, and I recommend it without reservation.

14. PROTEIN POWER

MICHAEL EADES, MD AND MARY DAN EADES, MD

WHAT IT IS IN A NUTSHELL

A three-phase plan in which you do the following:
  •Eat no less than a minimum calculated amount of protein per day (you are free to eat more but not less)

  • Eat no more than a maximum amount of carbohydrates per day (you are free to eat less but not more)

  The maximum amount of carbohydrates depends on which phase of the diet you are in. Phase 1 is intervention and allows up to 30 grams of carbohydrate a day; phase 2 is transition and allows up to 55 grams; phase 3 is the maintenance phase, and the amount of carbs will vary according to the individual.

About Protein Power

In the Eadeses' plan, you first determine your protein needs through an easy-to-follow series of steps:

1. Measure your wrist, then your waist.
2. Refer to a chart to estimate your body fat from these measurements.
3. Now you calculate your total number of fat pounds. For example, if you're 200 pounds with 20% body fat, you would have 40 fat pounds.
4. Subtract the number of fat pounds from your total weight to get the number of lean body-weight pounds (muscle, bone, and the like). Using the above example, you would subtract 40 pounds from 200 and wind up with a lean body weight of 160 pounds.
5. Multiply your lean body weight by an "activity factor" to get your minimum daily protein needs (in grams). The activity factor ranges from 0.5 for someone who is completely sedentary to 0.9 for a competitive athlete. For example, if the 200-pound guy with 40 fat pounds and 160 lean pounds were sedentary, he'd multiply 160 by 0.5 for a total of 80 grams of protein per day minimum.

Knowing your lean body weight also allows you to calculate a realistic weight goal, which is done using the worksheets and very easy formulas.

Note: In *The Protein Power Lifeplan*, the authors have simplified the process even more. You don't even have to take your wrist or waist measurements, compute your lean body mass, or multiply by an activity factor. There's a simple table in which you look for your height and weight, and the table tells you immediately what your minimum protein requirement is. It couldn't be easier. It's not as refined and accurate as the method in the original *Protein Power*, but it will give you a decent estimate of your minimum requirement and is good for people who just don't want to do the calculations. (My personal opinion: the calculations are easy.)

Once you know your minimum daily protein needs, you simply decide what phase of the diet you're going to be on. Phase 1, intervention, is for those who have a lot of fat to lose and/or who want to correct a health problem. In phase 1, you take in 30 grams or less of carbohydrate a day (in *The Protein Power Lifeplan*, this number is amended to 40) plus, of course, *at least* your minimum protein requirement. Phase 2 is the one to go with if you want to lose a little fat, recompose your body (i.e., change the ratio of fat to muscle or, as people often say, "tone up"), or improve your general health. In phase 2, the maximum carb allowance is upped to 55 grams a day, in addition, of course, to the protein allowance determined above. You can eat *more* than your minimum protein requirement but not less, and you can eat *less* than your maximum carb allotment but not more. The rest of the diet comes from fat.

Nearly everyone will fall into one of four categories of minimum protein requirement—less than 60 grams a day, between 60 and 80 grams a day, between 80 and 100 grams a day, or between 100 and 120 grams a day. You find the category you belong to and then refer to the corresponding chart. The chart will tell you exactly what protein foods in what amounts you can have *per meal and snack*. For example, if you're in the 80-to-100-gram category, you should be getting about 34 grams of protein per meal. The chart shows you exactly how to make any combination you can think of from meat, fish, poultry, eggs, hard cheeses, soft cheeses, curd cheeses, or tofu to get the right amount of protein per meal.

Like nearly all the diet or lifestyle plans discussed in this book, Protein Power is all about controlling and balancing insulin. The Eadeses have a clever way of determining the actual insulin-raising (or active) carbohydrate content of foods. Even though fiber is not metabolically active, it's technically counted as a carbohydrate on food labels and the like. But it doesn't raise insulin at all, since it's not even digested. So the Eadeses have come up with a formula in which you subtract the fiber from the total carb content of a food to get what they call the "effective carbohydrate content," or ECC.

That's the only number you have to pay attention to when counting your carbohydrate grams. For example, 1 cup of fresh raspberries has 14 grams of carbohydrate but 6 grams of fiber, so you'd subtract the 6 grams of fiber from the 14 grams of total carbohydrate to get a mere 8 grams of ECC, and only those 8 grams would count toward your carbohydrate allowance for the day. (This is now standard operating procedure for most low-carb diets, some of which call the number "effective carbs," some "net carbs.")

The book has charts of the ECC for a huge number of foods, so you don't have to figure them out for yourself. You use these charts to put together your daily carbohydrate allowance (or, if a food is not listed in the chart, you can easily compute it yourself from the label's listing of total carbs and total fiber). Counting only effective carbs, you could easily have 1 cup of broccoli, 1 cup of cabbage, 3 celery ribs, 1 cup of green beans, 1 cup of lettuce, ½ cup of mushrooms, 1 cup of zucchini, 1 cup of spinach, and 1 cup of raspberries in one day on phase 1. Even though the total carb content of these foods is about 44 grams, 16 of them are fiber; subtracting the 16 from the 44 (all done for you in the charts) leaves you with only 28 grams of usable (effective) carbohydrate, well under the cutoff for phase 1 and not even close to the cutoff for phase 2.

Calories are barely mentioned in *Protein Power.* The idea is that calories are self-regulating if you are eating the foods that put you in correct metabolic balance (an idea that runs throughout many low-carb diet plans). The Eadeses do warn you that since you may not be as hungry on a low-carb plan as you were before, you can easily *under*eat, so it's important to be sure that your calories don't fall below 850 to 1,000 a day. (The 850 figure seems really, *really* low—nearly every other weight-loss expert, including myself, uses 1,000 to 1,250 as the bare minimum, and some even suggest not dropping below 1,250. If the food eaten produces a hormonally balanced state and the calories are coming from good stuff, most women will drop weight on 1,250 calories and most men on 1,500.)

On the other hand, especially in *The Protein Power Lifeplan,* the authors explain that if you're doing everything right (i.e., eating the minimum protein requirement and not exceeding the maximum carb allotment) and you're *still* not losing weight, you might be consuming too many calories, especially calories from fat. Nuts seem to be a frequent culprit: since nuts are only fat and protein, many low-carbers munch on these with abandon because they have very little effect on insulin. But while a 1-ounce portion (which is pretty small!) may have only 160 calories and a few grams of carbs at most, three to four portions can add an awful lot of calories (and carb grams) to a diet plan and could effectively slow down or stop weight loss altogether. As with most low-carb plans, the message here is this: though calories are not the whole story by a long shot, they still matter, so don't ignore them.

Phase 3 is the maintenance phase, which is what you stay on once you've reached your goal. To get there, you add 10 grams of carbohydrate to your daily allotment in phase 2, and stay there and stabilize for about 5 to 7 days. Then you add another 10 grams. You continue in this way until you find the amount of carbs you can take in and still keep your weight stable. The Eadeses have found that *most* people will stabilize when they've reached the point at which the number of carb grams equals the number of protein grams, but they discuss the exceptions to this general rule and tell you what to do if you don't fit the template.

The maintenance phase is pretty cool. There is really no food you can't have "in some quantity at some time." The trick is knowing what you're doing. As the authors put it, there are foods that are "so rich in sugars and starches, such potent unbalancers of your metabolic hormones, that you cannot have unlimited amounts of them anytime you want unless you are willing to accept the consequences of that action." They even have recovery guidelines for those times when you throw caution to the wind and have a "nutritional vacation," such as on birthdays, holidays, and the like. You simply return to phase 1 for 3 days (or until you have lost any of the weight you might have gained), move to phase 2 for the rest of the week, and then return to your maintenance level of carb consumption.

The thing about *The Protein Power Lifeplan*, and to a lesser extent the original book, is that it is about so much more than just a diet. There is absolutely first-rate information about cholesterol and the "cholesterol hoax," plus wonderful explanations of how insulin works in the body and its relationship to heart disease, high blood pressure, diabetes, and obesity. There is a terrific exposition on the Paleolithic Diet. And in *Lifeplan*, the authors go into even more detail on all of these topics, plus they include discussions of antioxidants, leaky gut syndrome and autoimmune responses, sugar, iron overload, magnesium, brain health, and a further expansion of the nutritional plan.

Lifeplan also has a cool concept. It suggests three levels of "commitment" to health: the purist, the dilettante, and the hedonist. All of these approaches share the same requirements for protein, the same need for high-quality fat, the same prohibition on trans-fatty acids, and the same limitations of carbohydrate grams (depending on what phase you're in). (Even at the lowest level of commitment, the hedonist, you're still way better off than you would be following the standard American diet or, for that matter, the standard high-carb, low-fat diet.) All of the levels should theoretically give the same weight-loss results. The difference is in overall health benefits.

The purist regimen is really restrictive. Purists eat *no* cereal grains or products made from them (à la *The No-Grain Diet* of Joseph Mercola). They eat *no* dairy or legumes (such as beans). They eat *only* organic fruits and vegetables and *only* natural meat and poultry—no processed foods, no sugars (except occasionally honey), no artificial sweeteners, no caffeine, and no alcohol. It's probably the most healthful diet in the world to follow, but also next to impossible for most folks. However, for people with serious health issues, it may mean the difference between life and death.

Next up is the dilettante. You aim for organic foods whenever possible but are not obsessive about it. You still avoid some grains (wheat, for example) but can eat others (like oats and rice). You eliminate high-fructose corn syrup but can have some other sweeteners, even table sugar (in very limited amounts), and the prohibition against alcohol and caffeine is lifted. This is the program the Eadeses themselves follow.

Finally, there is the hedonist, where everything goes, within the limits of your carbohydrate allowance. You still have to keep to the basic parameters of the program, but you can fulfill those requirements with just about any foods you wish. Obviously, the high-carb content of some foods, such as potatoes, may make it impossible to fit portions of those foods into the phase 1 plan, when carbs are limited to 7 to 10 grams per meal and snack. But once you're on phase 2 or 3, you can eat anything you want as long as you don't exceed the maximum number of carbs for the day.

Protein Power as a Lifestyle: Who It Works for, Who Should Look Elsewhere

This is a great plan if you have a lot of weight to lose or if you have any of the health conditions discussed in the book. In its maintenance phase, it's a great plan to follow, period. But you've got to be willing to do a little figuring. You can't eyeball portions on the first two phases (which you can do on the Zone or even on phase 3 of this plan). You've got to be exact about carb-gram content and about meeting your minimum protein needs. The calculations to figure out your protein needs could put some folks off (although it's a nonissue in *Lifeplan*). Having to check ECC for every food might be a pain and could be a real problem if you eat out often, unless you get really familiar with the carb content of a lot of foods. If you're willing to put in the effort, it's totally worth it. If you're not into counting, measuring, and keeping really clear records (in your mind, if not on paper), this is going to be a hard plan for you, and you might be better off with a simpler formula.

JONNY'S LOWDOWN ★ ★ ★ ★ ★

It's hard to find anything wrong with this plan and the concepts and theories behind it. In some ways it's like the Zone with an induction phase, which may be why Barry Sears, whose Zone diet is way higher in carbs and lower in fat, is still able to endorse it (phase 3, the maintenance phase of Protein Power, is not far from Zone-like eating). The only credible argument I've heard against this type of plan is from endocrinologist Dr. Diana Schwarzbein, whose dietary regimen is not considered high-protein but is definitely still on the lower-carb side of the fence (see The Schwarzbein Principle *on page 239). Her concern is that too much protein without enough carbohydrate will raise the hormone cortisol, which has a whole other set of problems attached to it. It's a fair objection, and only time and additional research will clarify these hazy areas. In the meantime, I'm continuing to recommend* The Protein Power Lifeplan *as a basic textbook to all my clients who just want to live a healthy lifestyle and manage their weight. It's hard to find anything commercially available that's more comprehensive.*

15. THE ROSEDALE DIET

RON ROSEDALE, MD

WHAT IT IS IN A NUTSHELL

A novel higher-fat approach to low-carb that focuses on leptin, a hormone involved in the regulation of appetite.

About the Rosedale Diet

How can you fault any diet book that clearly states the following: "The high carbohydrate–low fat diet being prescribed to diabetic patients is precisely the wrong approach"? Answer: You can't.

The Rosedale Diet is a gem. It's is the creation of Ron Rosedale, MD, the doctor who, when Mike and Mary Dan Eades (of "Protein Power" fame) left Colorado to move on to other projects, took over the directorship of their clinic for metabolic medicine. Rosedale has long been one of the most sought after educators in nutritional and metabolic medicine, and this book is his first entry into the popular diet world. And it's a winner on every count.

While the Rosedale Diet is clearly a "low-carb" plan, it takes a somewhat different approach to weight loss, one that is focused on a hormone called *leptin*.

Here's the deal with leptin. Back in the '90s, researchers were excited to discover this protein hormone which seemed to regulate appetite. Leptin signals the brain that it's time to stop eating. Rats that were leptin-deficient ate a ton of food and, when injected with leptin, lost weight easily. The excitement in the research community was palpable. Researchers at Rockefeller Institute believed they just might have found the holy grail of weight loss. They reasoned that obese people must be leptin-deficient, and that if leptin (or a drug that mimicked it) could be given to obese individuals, their appetite would be regulated automatically and the pounds would drop off.

No such luck. Turns out that what worked in rats didn't work at all in humans. Obese people, as it happens, have plenty of leptin.

The problem is, their bodies don't "listen" to it.

They are, to use the term Rosedale uses, *leptin-resistant.* "Leptin is produced by your fat cells," Rosedale explains. "It tells your brain when to eat, how much to eat and most important, when to *stop* eating." Just as type 2 diabetics have plenty of insulin (but their cells don't respond effectively to it), obese people have plenty of leptin, but all that leptin falls on deaf cellular ears. In obese or overweight people, leptin does not seem to be able to effectively communicate its message to "stop eating."

Rosedale explains it elegantly: *"When leptin levels can be properly 'heard,' it alerts your brain and other body tissues that you have eaten enough and stored away enough fat, and it's now time to burn off some excess fat. This feedback system is designed to prevent you from getting fat. In order for leptin to be heard clearly, however, leptin levels must remain stable and low. When leptin levels spike too high, too often, your cells stop listening to leptin. In medical terms, they become 'resistant' to leptin."* In other words, your brain continues to tell you "be hungry, eat, and store more fat!"

The Rosedale Diet is all about getting rid of "leptin resistance."

Interestingly, the same foods that aggravate insulin resistance—the central factor in obesity, diabetes, and metabolic syndrome—also promote *leptin resistance*: sugar and high-carb diets. The Rosedale Diet abandons the outdated classification of carbohydrates into "simple" and "complex" and instead classes them into "fiber" versus "nonfiber" (or what some people would call "slow-burning" versus "fast-burning"). Fiber, good; nonfiber, not so good. Not surprising, and totally accurate. On the Rosedale Diet, most grains are avoided (especially for the first 3 weeks), but nonstarchy vegetables are plentiful.

Rosedale isn't of the opinion that protein should be unlimited, and I think he may be right on this. He recommends limiting protein to 50 to 75 grams a day. Remember, protein doesn't have a neutral effect on insulin (the way fat does). "Extra protein can be converted into glucose and burned as sugar, which causes spikes in leptin and insulin levels, which in turn cause sugar cravings," he points out.

Rosedale's variation on the low-carb theme is lower in protein than, for example, the Eadeses' program, and—perhaps counterintuitively—concentrates on fat. (Remember, fat is the one macronutrient that has virtually no effect on insulin!)

Rosedale's take on fat is some of the sharpest and most accurate writing I've yet seen, and should be read by everyone. For openers, he distinguishes between "good" and "bad" fat, but he actually knows what he's talking about. Don't expect the usual "saturated fat is bad, unsaturated fat is good" platitudes. "Some types of fat are bad for you all the time," he says, "and some types of fat are bad for you only some of the time. The health effects of fat often depend on what you eat with it."

Amen.

He warns against too much omega-6 (found in vegetable oils that the conventional establishment thinks are healthy all the time), completely forbids trans-fats, and even points out the fact that saturated fat sometimes has an *advantage* in the diet. But he doesn't recommend eating a huge amount of saturated fat since, in general, "it is the toughest fat to burn." "If you are looking to shed pounds, it is best to limit (not eliminate) your intake of saturated fat."

I have to give Rosedale credit also for being just about the only nutrition doctor I've ever read who actually questions the universal mandate that omega-9s (monounsaturated fat such as that found in olive oil) is great. "I'm not convinced that monounsaturated or omega-9 fat has any special health properties, yet people who eat monounsaturated fats seem to be protected against certain common diseases." He suggest that the health benefits seen by people consuming the Mediterranean diet (which is famously high in olive oil) get those health benefits more because of the amazing beneficial phenols and antioxidants in olive oil and nuts rather than the omega-9 fat itself. "I believe that the major benefit of monounsaturated fat is what it is *not*," he says. "It is *not* bad for you and doesn't have any of the negative effects of other oils."

Clearly, Rosedale is a guy who thinks for himself.

The Rosedale Diet is divided into 2 levels: Level 1 and Level 2. "I consider Level 1 to be the healthiest possible diet," Rosedale says, "and one that will not only help you lose weight quickly, but will give you the best shot at longevity." On the diet program, you stay on Level 1 for at least 3 weeks, though you can opt to stay on it forever. "It is basically the diet that I follow most of the time," Rosedale says. Level 2 contains a wider variety of foods (a few more servings of fruits and starches) but is still a hugely healthful diet.

On the first 3 weeks of the Rosedale Diet (Level 1), you'll eat nuts, nut butters, avocado, olives, all kinds of fish, poultry, game, veggie burgers, and even some selected dairy. Protein powders are OK, as is plain tofu, and there's the usual list of "free" vegetables, from asparagus to zucchini. A few high-fiber starches, limited legumes, tea, and just about any spice you can name round off the list. You don't count calories, but eat until you're full, which winds up being less than "usual" because you don't crave sweets and your body is becoming less leptin-resistant.

After the first 3 weeks, you can opt to move to Level 2 and begin to add a wider variety of foods, including fruit and legumes, coffee and wine. Off the menu—pretty much permanently—are milk, most full-fat hard cheeses, processed meats, certain legumes (including peanut butter, which I'm not sure I agree with), very starchy vegetables, sugar, commercial fruit juices, soda, and all fried foods. (I have a few minor disagreements with some of the foods on the "banned" list, but for the most part I think he's nailed it!)

How long can you stay on the diet? The short answer is forever, if you want to. "I consider the Rosedale Diet the optimal diet for life and I urge patients to stay on it forever," he says. "If you keep your leptin levels down, you will not experience the constant hunger or food cravings that helped make you overweight and sick in the first place, and that makes diets difficult or impossible to maintain."

The Rosedale Diet as a Lifestyle: Who It Works for, Who Should Look Elsewhere

For those who are metabolically suited to a hunter–gatherer diet of protein, vegetables, and fat (with a few judiciously chosen extras thrown in for good measure), this is a terrific weight-loss plan that you can actually stay on for life.

If you're OK bucking the conventional establishment "wisdom" on fat, this is a program definitely worth looking at. Your friends may think you're nuts for eating so much fat, but if you can ignore them, you'll be glad you did. The only danger here is the same danger that exists with Atkins—assuming that once you lose the weight, you can continue eating this way plus add back all the junky carbs you used to eat. This program works, but not when you add a bunch of useless carbs to it.

JONNY'S LOWDOWN ★★★★★

One thing you can say about the Rosedale Diet that you can say about few other diet books on the market is this: you will actually learn something from it. The information on leptin alone—and its relationship to insulin, stress, and aging—is worth the price of the book. The diet is designed to "turn off your hunger switch," which certainly makes sticking to a plan a lot easier than gritting your teeth and relying on willpower all the time. Well worth reading and well worth following.

16. THE 6-WEEK CURE FOR THE MIDDLE-AGED MIDDLE

MICHAEL EADES, MD AND MARY DAN EADES, MD

WHAT IT IS IN A NUTSHELL

The authors of Protein Power turn their attention to the problem of visceral abdominal fat (VAT)—also known as the "spare tire." VAT is an important factor in diabetes, obesity, and "middle-aged spread," and it's one that has enormous health consequences. Particularly suitable for those over 40.

About the 6-Week Cure for the Middle-Aged Middle

Without question, two of the smartest advocates of low-carb dieting in the world are the husband-and-wife team of Mary Dan Eades, MD and Michael Eades, MD. (Their best-selling books *Protein Power* and *The Protein Power Lifeplan* are discussed on pages 226–231.) In their latest, *The 6-Week Cure for the Middle-Aged Middle,* they focus their sights specifically on the problem of middle-aged girth.

Though most people aren't aware of it, fat really comes in two "flavors"—visceral and subcutaneous. The later is more unsightly—it's the stuff that makes your thighs push against each other in your jeans, the stuff that causes you to ask "Does my butt look big in this?" But the former—visceral fat—is far more dangerous.

"Typically, in middle age, people are afflicted with visceral fat," explain the Eadeses. While subcutaneous fat is basically contained within a non-rigid, rubbery wall (the skin) and tends to puddle when going from vertical to horizontal, visceral fat is typically contained within the abdominal wall. It's visceral (abdominal) fat that correlates the most with bad health outcomes and conditions like insulin resistance and diabetes. That's the reason you've heard (correctly) that "apples" (people who store their fat around the middle) are at more risk for health problems than "pears" (people who store it in the thighs and butt). While both can be "unsightly," it's the abdominal fat that is a real health concern. Getting rid of visceral fat—or what is properly known as VAT (for visceral adipose tissue)—is the focus of The 6-Week Cure.

This program couldn't have arrived at a more opportune time. Just as I was originally writing this review, the November 12, 2008 issue of the *New England Journal of Medicine* was published, featuring a widely reported study showing that belly fat was linked to early death. In the study, which followed 360,000 Europeans for over 10 years, those who had the most belly fat had double the risk of dying compared to people with the least amount of belly fat. That's pretty striking. And that's on top of previous research showing an association between VAT (belly fat) and a host of other diseases including some cancers, diabetes, and even dementia.

VAT also correlates with something that's becoming endemic in this country, although at the moment it's flying under the radar—non-alcoholic fatty liver disease (NAFLD). "A recent study on middle aged people in the Dallas area who had no known health problems showed that 34 percent of this population had liver fat accumulation," Michael Eades told me. "And a recent autopsy study from San Diego found that 12 percent of adolescents who died from accidents *already* had fat accumulations in their livers. Those who were overweight had a much greater accumulation."

"Clearing fat from the liver is essential to getting rid of VAT," explain the Eadeses. They give techniques to do this in the book. Surprisingly, consumption of saturated fat helps *rid* the liver of fat, at least in animal studies. Here's how we know: Researchers give animals alcohol to get them to develop fatty livers quickly. If they add vegetable oil and/or fructose to the mix, the livers fatten more quickly. If they add saturated fat, it's difficult to get the animals to develop fatty livers even in the face of continued alcohol consumption. "If you look at the epidemic of NAFLD in this country, it pretty much correlates in time with the advice to reduce saturated fat and replace it with vegetable fat," says Mike Eades, "not to mention the increase in the consumption of fructose." While the Eadeses are quick to point out that correlation doesn't mean causation, it's certainly easy to make that leap, especially in the light of the animal research.

Early in this book, I discussed the work of an old-time GP in New York named Blake Donaldson, MD (see page 23). Donaldson was a mainstream physician who experimented with all-meat diets for his patients, largely as an attempt to treat allergies. The Eadeses discuss Donaldson, as well as another old-timer named Walter L. Voegtlin who, quite independently, experimented with the same all-meat diet as a way of treating ulcerative colitis and Crohn's disease. Both serendipitously discovered an interesting "side effect": all their patients lost weight!

In *The 6-Week Cure for the Middle-Aged Middle*, the Eadeses "deconstruct" the principles behind the all-meat diet and put it back together in the form of a protein shake. You start on three shakes a day plus a protein meal, then move to what is basically an all-meat diet. In the last 2 weeks of the 6-week diet, you progress to a more typical low-carb diet. "Results have been pretty spectacular in the patients we've worked with, many of whose histories are described in the book," Mike Eades told me.

In virtually every book on low-carb eating, the focus is on the oversecretion of insulin. The mechanism is now familiar to anyone reading this book—blood sugar rises, insulin is secreted, the cells eventually become resistant to its actions, and the body secretes more and more insulin in an (often futile) attempt to get blood sugar back down. But insulin can build up in the bloodstream in two ways, not one. The first is oversecretion; the other is undermetabolism. And undermetabolism is a unique focus of the Eadeses' program.

Here's how it works. One of the many jobs of the liver is to metabolize proteins (one of which is insulin). But when fat builds up in the liver, the liver slows down and doesn't work as well. It becomes sluggish, much like a bloated computer loaded down with unwanted programs. Ridding the liver of fat allows it to work better and to more rapidly break down and metabolize circulating insulin. If the insulin that's hanging around is metabolized more efficiently, by definition there will be less of it hanging around. Less insulin hanging around has the effect of making the cells more sensitive to the insulin that's left. (This is, after all, one of the major goals of a sugar-and-insulin-lowering low-carb diet.) And more sensitivity to insulin means that we can make less of it to get the job done.

So by focusing on lowering fat buildup in the liver, the Eadeses have taken on an often-neglected piece of the metabolic puzzle. Their low-carb diet attacks high blood sugar and insulin from both the "manufacturing" side and from the "metabolizing" side. "Everyone in the low-carb field focuses on the oversecretion brought on by carb intake, but the other side of the equation is just as important," Mike Eades told me. And since elevated insulin not only increases fat buildup in the liver but also makes us store visceral fat in the first place, lowering insulin helps interrupt the vicious circle. Less insulin, less visceral fat and reduced fatty liver. It's a double whammy.

The book has some really interesting stuff on the evolutionary psychological basis for our attraction to a slim waistline. If you know the Eadeses as I do (or if you read Michael's always-fascinating blog at http://www.protein power.com/drmike), you know that their interests are wide-ranging (as in opera, cooking, travel, and philosophy). So it's no surprise that the book contains some really interesting stuff on the evolutionary basis for our attraction to a slim waistline and draws on material from anthropology to a kind of Literary Darwinism. That part of the book won't help (or hurt) you in your weight-loss efforts, but readers like me find that stuff utterly fascinating. Maybe you will too.

Besides the diet itself, the book is filled with helpful hints for supporting your liver (always a good idea) and helping rid itself of unwanted (and metabolism-slowing) fat buildup.

The 6-Week Cure for the Middle-Aged Middle as a Lifestyle: Who It Works for, Who Should Look Elsewhere

The Eadeses have treated probably several thousand people in their long career, and they've had pretty spectacular results. They're two of the smartest and sharpest people I know, and it's rare that I find anything significant that we disagree on (OK, sometimes politics and music, but that's another story). That said, I would simply caution that in my opinion not everyone is metabolically suited to a very high-protein diet. I don't think there's anything "bad" or "dangerous" about it; I just think people respond differently to dietary strategies, and some people just may not like such a high-protein intake, especially when meat is involved. If you're one of them, this might not be for you. But if you're willing to give this a try, it might produce some very dramatic results. Remember, Vilhjalmur Stefansson went on just such a diet for a year while being supervised and monitored at Bellvue (see page 17), and by every single measure his health was robust and he had no problems.

JONNY'S LOWDOWN ★★★★★

With detailed, weekly guidelines for diet and nutrition—including 80 recipes that make following the plan simplicity itself—the 6-Week Cure for the Middle-Aged Middle is a terrific program for blasting fat, particularly the dangerous kind of belly fat known as VAT (visceral abdominal fat).

Visceral fat and fatty liver are both big problems to people wanting to stay healthy and lean. This program is a revolutionary approach to both. All in all—if you're not opposed to the idea of eating meat—this is a terrific program that should find a lot of advocates.

17. THE SCHWARZBEIN PRINCIPLE

DIANA SCHWARZBEIN, MD AND NANCY DEVILLE

WHAT IT IS IN A NUTSHELL

A program designed not specifically for weight loss but for metabolic healing, which, when successful, results in weight loss. Schwarzbein says, "You need to get healthy to lose weight, not lose weight to get healthy." In her second book in the series, The Schwarzbein Principle II, you compute your protein requirement and your maximum carbohydrate allowance for each meal and snack, then construct your menu accordingly.

About the Schwarzbein Principle

Let me start by saying this: if you are a dedicated low-carber, the original *Schwarzbein Principle* should be in your library, regardless of whether you choose to follow the program. It's as good a basic reference book on hormonal health, the need for good fats, the arguments against a low-fat diet, and the relationship of hormones to health and aging as we're likely to see. If you're not yet familiar with the case against the low-fat diet and the concept of eating plenty of good fats (which include saturates!) and protein, this is a great place to start. If these concepts are old-hat to you and you want to actually try the program, the second book, *The Schwarzbein Principle II*, is the place to begin. The original is the overview and will give you the basics; *Schwarzbein II* is a more fully realized eating plan.

The Schwarzbein Principle can be summed up as follows:

- All systems of the human body are connected.
- One imbalance creates another imbalance.
- Eating too many man-made carbohydrates is the number one reason for hormonal imbalances.
- Poor eating and lifestyle habits—not genetics—cause diseases of aging.

The actual eating plan depends on where you fit in a matrix of four metabolic types. What type you are depends on the operating health of two of the major hormonal systems in your body: your *insulin metabolism* and your *adrenal metabolism*. Most people reading *Living Low Carb* understand by now the concept of insulin resistance and the role elevated insulin levels play in weight gain. We saw in chapter 3 just how this mechanism operates, and it is the underlying concept in almost every one of the diet plans discussed in this book. What has *not* been emphasized in any of the plans so far is adrenal health.

The adrenal glands are responsible for the secretion of two critical hormones: *cortisol* and *adrenaline*. These are also known as *stress hormones*—they are involved in the "fight or flight" response. Cortisol is a major hormone. It keeps your blood pressure from dropping too low, and you need it in every cell of your body—without it, you would die. Adrenaline is another major hormone; it keeps your heart beating. Adrenaline is the primitive hormone that saved our butts from being eaten when confronted with a saber-toothed tiger on the savanna. That's why cortisol and adrenaline are called the "fight or flight" hormones—in response to stress (like a life-threatening emergency), they prepare you for either picking up a club to fight off a bear or running like hell for the nearest tree.

These hormones served our Paleolithic ancestors well as a kind of "turbo" system for emergency response. The problem is that our current lifestyle causes them to charge around our systems far more than is strictly necessary. They are our constant companions. Our poor overworked adrenals respond to daily stresses and secrete them when we're stuck in traffic, when we have a report due, when we get into a fight with the hotel clerk, when the telemarketer interrupts our dinner, and when we have a fight with our boyfriend/girlfriend/husband/wife/son/daughter/boss. And just like our poor pancreas can eventually "burn out" from the constant demand put on it to produce enough insulin to deal with a chronically high-carbohydrate diet, so can our poor adrenals eventually reach a similarly exhausted state. This is what Schwarzbein and others call *adrenal burnout*. It is hardly uncommon.

So if we're interested only in weight loss, why should we care about our adrenals?

Well, first off, the adrenal hormone cortisol, like all hormones in the body, sends a message. Several, actually. One is to break down muscle for fuel. If you break down muscle, you do two things: you lower your metabolic rate (since muscle is where the fat and calories are burned), and you reduce the number of muscle cells that are able to accept sugar, leading to more sugar being stored as fat and eventually more insulin resistance. Cortisol also sends a message to the brain to "refuel" for emergency, leading almost inevitably to stress eating.

Since cortisol is involved in breaking down the bodily proteins—both functional and structural—eventually, if levels of cortisol remain high, the body will do something to protect itself against breaking down too much. Can you guess what hormone it sends in as reinforcement? Insulin. Too much cortisol eventually triggers insulin, the storage hormone, to counter the catabolic (breaking-down) processes in an attempt to rebuild the ship. If this happens frequently enough, you will eventually have high levels of insulin and will become insulin-resistant. Remember that adrenaline helps your body *use up* your biochemicals; insulin helps your body *rebuild them*— including the fat stores! Hence, chronically high cortisol can wind up being a cause of insulin resistance.

It gets worse. Chronic oversecretion of the stress hormone cortisol will cause you to use up serotonin. Less serotonin almost always goes hand in hand with cravings, especially for sugar and carbohydrate. Those cravings, a kind of biochemical "mandate," can be irresistible even for people with amazing willpower. Give into the cravings—as most people will—and the cycle continues. You use up serotonin anytime your cortisol and adrenaline levels get too high—when you don't sleep, when you are stressed, and when you overuse stimulants (including refined sugar, nicotine, and caffeine). This is one reason why stress management figures so prominently in the Schwarzbein program.

In the Schwarzbein Principle, you first determine which of four metabolic categories you fit into:

1. insulin-sensitive with healthy adrenals
2. insulin-sensitive with burned-out adrenals
3. insulin-resistant with healthy adrenals
4. insulin-resistant with burned-out adrenals

These four categories represent varying degrees of metabolic damage and require very different eating plans for healing. The underlying thinking here is that you *must* heal your metabolism before you can begin to lose weight. The program consists of five elements:

1. nutrition
2. stress management
3. cross-training exercise (usually of a low-intensity level)
4. eliminating stimulants and drugs
5. hormone replacement therapy, if needed

All five elements don't have to be done at once. The transition into metabolic health is gradual and gentle and takes place in stages.

You first determine your protein needs using a very simple formula. Those with healthy adrenals do not have to monitor protein; they can "listen to their bodies," though guidelines are given for those who want them. The formula and guidelines give *minimum* protein needs and should be divided among the three meals (and usually two snacks) that you will eat every day. You can eat more protein if you want, but not less. Then you determine your carbohydrate allowance, which is also divided into three meals and two snacks. You do not count calories, and you do not measure or count fat.

Carbohydrate allowances range from a low of 15 grams per meal and 7½ grams per snack (60 grams per day) to a high of 45 grams per meal and 20 grams per snack (175 grams per day), though the high end of the range is only for the rare person who is insulin-sensitive with healthy adrenals and is very, very active. There are meal plans given for 15, 20, 25, 30, 35, and 40 grams of carbs per meal. There are vegetarian versions of all meal plans, and there are even low-saturated-fat versions of most of the meal plans for those very special cases where saturated fat has to be limited (Schwarzbein does not normally limit saturated fat).

Carbs—though much more limited than in standard diets—are not eliminated and, in Schwarzbein's view, are essential to the success of the program. The reason is this: if you eat too many carbs (and too much food), your insulin levels will rise too high and you will become insulin-resistant if you aren't already; if you already are, too many carbs will certainly make matters worse. But if you don't eat *enough* carbs, you will raise adrenaline and cortisol too high, using up your precious biochemicals and eventually becoming insulin-resistant anyway.

The Schwarzbein Principle as a Lifestyle: Who It Works for, Who Should Look Elsewhere

People who flock from all over the country to Diana Schwarzbein's practice in Santa Barbara, California, are frequently people at the end of their rope—they have tried every diet, damaged their metabolisms, and turned their hormonal balance on its ear. She has an amazing success rate, but you clearly have to be patient. This is not a diet for weight loss; it is a program for metabolic healing, and in many cases you have to be prepared to actually gain weight before you begin to lose. In addition, the careful computing of grams of carbohydrate per meal and snack doesn't appeal to everyone. If you're willing to be patient and are looking at the long-term picture, you've probably come to the right place. If you need more immediate results, if you're concerned only with weight loss, if you can't deal with counting carbs, or if you don't feel you've damaged your metabolism all that much, this might not be the best place to start.

JONNY'S LOWDOWN ★★★

You simply cannot say enough good things about Diana Schwarzbein. She truly is a giant in the field and one of the most knowledgeable, cutting-edge endocrinologists in the country. Interestingly, many of the people I interviewed for this book started with more basic plans like Atkins and then, when they got closer to maintenance, moved to the Schwarzbein Principle. As an overall plan for health, this is five-star material. But as a weight-loss diet—which it was never intended to be—it may not be the ideal entry-level plan, as it requires a good deal of patience and a lot of commitment.

18. The South Beach Diet

Arthur Agatston, MD

WHAT IT IS IN A NUTSHELL

A 3-phase diet plan. For the first 2 weeks, you cut out bread, rice, potatoes, pasta, baked goods, fruit, sugar, and alcohol. During the 2nd phase, you add back just enough carbs to let you continue to lose weight. In the 3rd phase, when you've reached your goal weight, you can add back still more carbs from any category of food you like.

About the South Beach Diet

The South Beach Diet is very . . . *friendly.* Written by a cardiologist, it has the benefit of a terrific marketing campaign, sports a great-looking cover, and borrows the cachet of a sleek, sexy, very "in" area of Miami known for its celebrities, models, and generally very good-looking people. That gets your attention. More important is the fact that the information deserves it.

According to the author, Arthur Agatston, the South Beach Diet was designed *not* with weight loss as its main goal, but to improve the heart health of his patients "by changing their blood chemistry." Agatston says his heart patients—and his diabetic ones—lost weight "like crazy" ("10, 20, 30, even 50 pounds within months"), much of it from their midsections. The diet caught on and wound up featured on the local ABC affiliate station in a segment in which Miami Beach residents who wanted to lose weight were put on the diet and then followed around for a month. The station, WPLG, scored big with the feature, and it became an annual "South Beach Diet challenge" for 3 years. Eventually, the South Beach Diet became known nationally, and it was enthusiastically endorsed by a wide range of people, including former president Bill Clinton.

Here's how it works: For the first 14 days, you are on a decidedly low-carb regimen in which you cut out all bread, rice, potatoes, pasta, baked goods, dairy, fruit, sugar, and alcohol. Eggs are unlimited. You can have most kinds of cheese (except for Brie, Edam, and full-fat cheese), certain sugar-free desserts, and a couple of kinds of nuts. You can also drink coffee. According to Agatston, you will lose between 8 and 13 pounds in the first 2 weeks, and most of that will come off your midsection.

In phase 2, you reintroduce fruit, certain cereals, bran muffins, pasta, whole-grain breads, and other starches, albeit in small amounts. On this phase, you continue to lose weight at the reasonable rate of 1 to 2 pounds a week. When you get to your goal, you go on phase 3, which is your lifetime-maintenance "forever" plan. At this point, you can eat anything—there are no restrictions on what kind of carbs you can take in, which, of course, makes it very attractive for some people. Regarding these "foods you love," the author says, "You won't be able to have all of them, all the time. You'll learn to enjoy them a little differently than before—maybe a little less enthusiastically. But you will enjoy them again."

Agatston starts with the same basic premise as the low-carb theorists: high amounts of insulin are responsible for weight gain, and limiting carbs stabilizes both blood sugar and insulin. He explains, "The equation behind most obesity is simple: the faster the sugar and starches you eat are processed and absorbed into your bloodstream, the fatter you get." He suggests eating foods and combinations of foods that cause *gradual* rather than *sharp* increases in blood sugar (i.e., proteins and fats with minimal carbs). He makes distinctions between good carbs (low-glycemic, whole-grain) and bad (processed, sugary, high in starch). So far, so good.

The author is a cardiologist and takes a traditional approach to "good fats" and "bad fats." Though one could dispute his wholesale damnation of saturated fats, one could also argue that his condemnation of them is likely to make him more acceptable to the medical establishment, which is a good thing, as his thinking on the subjects of carb consumption, blood sugar, insulin, and weight gain is right on the money. And while he and I might have a friendly disagreement over saturated fats, we concur that trans-fats are the worst, and Agatston hammers this important point home time and again. And no one is going to object to his inclusion of plenty of good marine fats like fish oils.

The popularity of the diet is probably due to how realistic it is. ("It's important for people to like the food they eat. Eating is meant to bring pleasure even when you're trying to lose weight. That's a sensible way to think about food and it's one of the basic principles of the South Beach Diet.") Agatston has some great recipes for desserts, like a tiramisu made from ricotta cheese and cocoa powder, as well as some good side dishes, "mashed potatoes" made from cauliflower. But the most appealing part of the diet may be the fact that after the initial Atkins-like spartan regimen, you can add back just about any carbs you want, as long as you keep the portions small and continue to lose weight; when you get to your goal, you can eat anything you want as long as you don't gain.

This could be a problem for some people. Such unstructured eating looks great on paper and works great for many, but it can be a slippery slope for others. Start by adding one slice of bread or one piece of chocolate cake, and for many people, the ballgame is over. It's like letting an alcoholic have one drink. But if you can follow his advice and stick to the moderate portion doctrine, you'll allow those "favorite foods" to become occasional treats rather than mainstays of your diet. In this scenario, you'll love the foods you're eating, you won't feel overly restricted, and the health benefits you receive are likely to be enormous. This is truly healthy, realistic, controlled-carb eating for the masses.

The South Beach Diet as a Lifestyle: Who It Works for, Who Should Look Elsewhere

People who want to have their cake and eat it too, *literally*, will love this plan. Because it makes a lot of concessions to "real-life" eating habits and, after the weight-loss period, does not restrict any food whatsoever, it's bound to have a ton of appeal. And if you are the kind of person who can do moderation, it's a great diet, providing plenty of protein, good fats, vegetables, and just enough carbohydrates to keep the demons at bay. However, this liberal way of doing things is potentially problematic for people who like specified amounts and clear instructions and want to know exactly what they can and can't eat. If you fall into this category, you might be better off either staying on the first phase a bit longer or starting with a more structured plan and graduating to South Beach later on.

JONNY'S LOWDOWN ★ ★ ★ ½

This is a decent program, although it shares many of conventional medicine's prejudices and misconceptions (including a phobia of saturated fat). Some of my colleagues have criticized it for "not being anything new" (one Internet pundit called it "Atkins for the first two weeks and then the Zone"), a criticism that's not entirely unjustified.

But the genius of Agatston is that he has taken this information and made it extremely user-friendly and accessible, and has done so while making sure not to alienate his more conservative colleagues in the medical profession. This makes it much more likely that his important message will actually be heard. The friendly tone, accessibility, and overall permissiveness of the plan practically guarantees that its intelligent, lower-carb message will reach thousands of people who might have ignored the more "militant" platforms. For that we owe Agatston a lot of thanks. Adopting some form of the South Beach Diet would represent a giant step forward for most Americans, and because it is presented in such an unintimidating way—and possibly even because it is not substantially outside the medical mainstream in its avoidance of saturated fat—it's more likely that people will adopt it.

---

19. South Beach Recharged

Arthur Agatston, MD and Joseph Signorile, PhD

WHAT IT IS IN A NUTSHELL

The South Beach Diet plus an exercise program.

About South Beach Recharged

Let me be honest: in the first two editions of the book you're reading right now (when it was titled *Living the Low Carb Life*), I rated the original South Beach Diet a little higher than it deserved (I gave it five stars).

Here's why. At the time, any deviation from the god-awful "wisdom" of conventional dietetics was a blessing, and South Beach was certainly a departure from the mainstream. I felt it deserved kudos for emphasis on protein and vegetables and for its movement away from processed carbs. It was also (still is) an extremely user-friendly diet, and one to which conventional docs would not raise major objections since it was so low in saturated fat.

But truth be told, the original South Beach Diet could easily (and not unfairly) be characterized as "Atkins for two weeks followed by the Zone." It wasn't original. It "bought into" the demonization of saturated fat, and it was downright uninformed about supplements.

But still. In that market—which, remember, worshipped the God-awful USDA Food Guide Pyramid—it was a breath of fresh air.

South Beach Recharged is quite a bit better than the original. It still suffers from conceptual incoherence (although it's in 3 "stages" the 3rd stage is virtually incoherent and impossible to explain), it's still very conventional on saturated fat; but overall the book has some really good things to recommend it, and I'd take this version over the original any day of the week.

The most obvious difference between the original South Beach and South Beach Recharged is the addition of an exercise program based on my favorite type of workout, interval training (more on that in a moment). It's also clearly meant for people who are fairly new to exercise, which is not necessarily a bad thing at all—the program is uncomplicated, doesn't require equipment and is easy to follow, thus removing some significant barriers to exercise for a lot of people.

The exercise portion is based on walking, but it's not just your usual exercise prescription (e.g., "30 minutes walk"). Instead, the program uses the principles of interval training. You walk at one of four intensities—easy pace, moderate pace, "revved up," and "supercharged." Like all interval-training programs, the idea is to alternate short bursts of high-intensity exercise with slightly longer and more laid-back periods of "active rest" (which means continuing to exercise, but at a much lower level of intensity while you catch your breath). In the case of South Beach Recharged, you alternate fast walking for between 15 and 60 seconds with longer "recovery periods." You can build up intensity and difficulty by making the "fast" periods longer and the "relaxed" periods shorter. Gym rats take note: you can also use aerobic equipment like an elliptical machine for the interval program if you want.

Agatston favors interval training because "it send[s] your metabolism soaring when you work your body at higher intensities, but you have to work hard for only a short time to achieve that result." He's right. I've written a lot about interval—or "burst"—training in my book *The Most Effective Natural Cures on Earth*, and I've been a big fan of this kind of workout for years.

To accompany the interval walking, Agatston has a strength-and-flexibility component called the "Total Body Workout." (You do the interval walking and the Total Body Workout on alternate days.) The Total Body Workout is comprised of basic exercises all of which can be done at home with minimal equipment (a chair, a step, a towel, and so forth). They're well described and well illustrated. Both the interval walking and the Total Body Workout program have a Phase 1, a Phase 2, and a Phase 3, presumably to accompany the diet portion of the program. Everything you're supposed to do is laid out for you with elegant clarity—Phase 1: week 1, week 2; Phase 2: week 1, week 2, and so on.

There's also a welcome section on belly fat and inflammation and a discussion of the different metabolic risks for "apples" (who store their fat around the middle), and "pears" (who store it around the thighs, hips and butt). And he's bullish on fish oil, which is always a plus. Plus there's an excellent recipe section—always a selling point of the South Beach franchise—which is terrific as usual.

South Beach Recharged as a Lifestyle: Who It Works for, Who Should Look Elsewhere

This is a perfectly acceptable program that will work for most people, especially those who find very low-carb programs to be unmanageable. It's also perfectly suitable for those who just have an extra 10 or 20 pounds to lose. Those who have a lot more than 10 or 20 pounds to lose and those who are insulin-resistant might find a better fit with another program. The diet is often frustrating to people who prefer a lot more specific instruction about what they can and can't eat. If you're OK with more general guidelines, you might like this program a lot.

JONNY'S LOWDOWN ★ ★ ★ ½

The dietary program is pretty much the same as the original South Beach Diet. He's still anti-saturated fat, he's still pretty liberal on bread, he's still just a tad short of "cutting-edge" on the latest research on low-carb diets, and I still can't figure out for the life of me what "Phase 3" is. But all in all this is a very user-friendly program made a whole lot better by the addition of a very "doable" exercise program.

It will appeal to a lot of people, deservedly.

20. THE ULTRASIMPLE DIET

MARK HYMAN, MD

WHAT IT IS IN A NUTSHELL

Exactly as advertised: a very simple basic program that's relatively low-carb, easy to follow, and nutritionally sound. It's packed with great information about two factors too infrequently covered in other weight-loss books: toxicity and inflammation.

About the UltraSimple Diet

The UltraSimple Diet is one of a new generation of weight-loss books—others include *The Fat Resistance Diet* and *The Rosedale Diet*—that focus on lesser-known but incredibly important factors in the weight-loss equation.

In the case of The UltraSimple Diet, the culprits are twofold: toxicity and inflammation.

"For many of you," writes the author, Mark Hyman, MD, "toxicity in particular may be frustrating your weight-loss attempts. You may be carrying around a truckload of toxins that are disrupting your body's natural mechanisms for health." And getting healthy, as Hyman explains, is the key to losing weight.

I've long been a fan of Mark Hyman. A former yoga teacher and "country doctor" who continues to practice in New England, he's someone with impeccable credentials who is actively affiliated with the Institute for Functional Medicine, one of the premiere organizations bringing nutrition, medicine, and holistic healing together under one conceptual roof. His previous book—UltraMetabolism—was a best seller, (deservedly so) and The UltraSimple Diet is a distillation of the principles of that book, applied to the task at hand—weight loss.

"Just restricting calories is a recipe for disaster and inevitably leads to failure," Hyman says. According to Hyman, toxicity can frequently explain why people seem to reach a plateau or "hit the wall" when attempting to lose weight, where, after an initial drop in weight, further weight loss proves next to impossible. "Unless you get rid of this toxic load," he writes, "you might find yourself continually hitting this wall."

The UltraSimple Diet is subtitled Kick-Start Your Metabolism and Safely Lose up to 10 Pounds in 7 Days. The usual objection to this kind of promise is that when you lose weight this quickly, it's "just water weight." "The truth is that you want to lose water weight," he says. "Inflammation and toxicity cause fluid retention." By cleaning up your system with this type of detoxifying and anti-inflammatory diet, you will drop both fluid (and toxins) quickly. You'll be on your way to a healthful weight and—even more important—better health. After losing the initial toxic fluid and inflammation, you can continue to drop fat at the reasonable rate of about ½ pound to 2 pounds per week.

So how do you do it? Simple. You take away the things that make you toxic and inflamed.

The "major toxins," according to Hyman, are not much of a surprise: coffee, sugar, alcohol, processed food, fast food, junk food, trans-fats, and high-fructose corn syrup top the list. "By eliminating [these] major sources of inflammation in your diet—food allergens, sugar and flour products, and bad fats—your body can heal," he promises.

This book lives up to the promise of its title: it's really "UltraSimple." Here are the six basic steps in a nutshell:

1. Get rid of bad foods (i.e., those that create toxicity and inflammation).
2. Add good foods (foods that are both detoxifying and anti-inflammatory).
3. Detoxify (Hyman teaches you how to make a special cleansing and detoxifying "UltraBroth").
4. Reduce inflammation (here you use his recipe for "UltraShakes").
5. Relax ("Take a fabulously relaxing and detoxifying 'UltraBath' every night before bed").
6. Reflect ("Read and write in your journal about what you're doing and how you're feeling during the program").

That's it. There's a special recipe for a "liver-detoxification" cocktail to promote bile flow, some simple stress-reduction techniques, a very easy exercise prescription (30 minutes a day of walking), and a few recommended nutritional supplements. Couldn't be easier.

Before starting, you take a Toxicity and Inflammation Quiz, designed to help you determine just how toxic and inflamed you really are. You'll answer questions about common symptoms ranging from nausea, constipation, and bloating to mood swings, energy, and headaches. The quiz takes only about 10 minutes to complete and should give you a good idea of what you need to work on. Best of all, you can monitor your progress by seeing how you score after a week on the program. Most people score significantly better!

According to Hyman, the toxic load you're carrying—mostly, by the way, in your fat cells, where toxins tend to get stored—can undermine weight loss in a variety of ways:

- By impairing two key metabolic organs—the thyroid and the liver
- By damaging energy-producing cellular structures called *mitochondria*
- By harming brain neurotransmitter and hormone signaling that affects your appetite
- By increasing inflammation and oxidative stress, both of which promote weight gain

A central part of the program is identifying food sensitivities, which Hyman (and others, including me!) believe are a huge part of the chronic health and weight problems many people suffer with. "Though they are real and well-documented in medical literature, they are generally ignored by conventional medicine," Hyman states. Part of the benefits you'll see from following this plan undoubtedly has to do with giving your body a break from "the usual suspects" for food sensitivities (and allergens)—gluten, dairy, yeast, eggs, corn, and peanuts. Hyman gives an excellent and very easy to understand explanation of the difference between classic "allergies" and the far more common (and frequently undiagnosed) food sensitivities or delayed food reactions that can easily sabotage weight loss.

Like many of the plans in *Living Low Carb*, you're a little stricter during the 1st "phase," which in this case lasts just 7 (relatively easy) days. After that, you go into "Reintroduction" mode. There's a list of foods to "reintroduce" during Phase 1 Reintroduction (which continues over 2 weeks). After that, you're in Phase 2 Reintroduction and you can begin to test your reaction to some of those "usual suspect" foods that for many people (but not all) are triggers for delayed food sensitivities. Hyman smartly suggests adding those foods one at a time so that you can really monitor your body's reaction to them.

Some "foods" are permanently banned—high-fructose corn syrup, trans-fats, artificial sweeteners, and the like. Good riddance.

The UltraSimple Diet as a Lifestyle: Who It Works for, Who Should Look Elsewhere

This is a book that lives up to its name—it's truly UltraSimple, especially if you don't mind making a nice homemade soup/broth and whipping up a couple of rice protein shakes. Be aware that with the UltraSimple Diet—like with most "detox" plans—there's always the possibility of a short (but possibly uncomfortable) "healing crisis" where you feel a little crummy at first as your body gets rid of the stuff it shouldn't be holding on to in the first place. So if you're about to tackle a huge project or give an important presentation, this might not be the week to try this program—you'd be better off waiting for a less stressful week.

"Though most people can safely do the program, there are a few people who should not do it or should do it only under a doctor's supervision," Hyman cautions. Among those for whom it's not recommended are anyone with cancer or a terminal illness, anyone with kidney failure or borderline kidney function, anyone who is underweight or malnourished, children under the age of 18, and pregnant or nursing women.

That said, virtually everyone could benefit from a program that stresses a reduction in toxic load and inflammation, and the book is worth reading just for what you'll learn about the impact of those two variables on weight and overall health.

Hyman was co-medical director for Canyon Ranch, one of the premier health spas in the United States, and the program reflects that sensibility. It's a program that easily could serve as the basis for a week at a spa: easy exercise, whole foods, nutrient-dense broths and shakes, and a healthy dollop of relaxation and reflection. What's not to like?

21. UNLEASH YOUR THIN

JONNY BOWDEN, PhD, CNS

WHAT IT IS IN A NUTSHELL

Unleash Your Thin is a complete program in a box, consisting of 2 hours of DVDs, 6 CDs, a full 166-page manual, a 300-plus-page workbook, plus a full 6-week menu plan and recipes. The plan is unique in that it attacks the psychological underpinnings of cravings, binges, failures, and plateaus and gives you real-world tools for dealing with them in a positive way.

About Unleash Your Thin

Unleash Your Thin is an updated, expanded, and improved version of the highly successful "Diet Boot Camp" program. UYT is a two-pronged approach to weight loss, and in this regard, different from virtually every other program I've reviewed. According to the authors, two major issues derail most weight-loss efforts, and the Unleash Your Thin program addresses both equally.

The first cause of weight gain is hormonal. It works like this: foods you eat trigger specific hormones and enzymes in the body, which are either favorable to fat loss or favorable to fat gain. Although calories do matter, they are not the whole picture, as calories from sugar, for example, affect the hormonal environment very differently than, say, calories from fat.

The main player in this hormonal environment—at least from a weight-loss point of view—is insulin. Insulin, also known as "the hunger hormone," and, more insidiously, as "the fat-storing" hormone—is released by the body as soon as your blood sugar goes up, which it does every time you eat. Insulin's purpose is to escort that excess sugar into the muscle cells where it can be "burned" for energy. Unfortunately, for many people—(anywhere from

25% of the population to 75%)—the system doesn't work very well. For these folks, blood sugar goes up, insulin goes up, but the muscle cells aren't having any of it. They basically shut their doors (a condition known as "insulin resistance"), which results in a number of things happening, none of them good (at least not if you're trying to stay trim).

See, not only does insulin help store fat, it also *prevents* fat burning. High levels of insulin literally "lock the doors" to the fat cells, keeping everything inside. Insulin's "sister" hormone, glucagon, does pretty much the opposite of what insulin does, opening the doors to the fat cells and allowing fat to be "burned" for energy. Unfortunately, when insulin is high, glucagon can't do its job. Creating a hormonal environment where insulin never gets high enough to create this ideal environment for fat storage is the first goal of the Unleash Your Thin program.

If you've read this far in the book, you undoubtedly now understand that the type of food that raises insulin the most is carbohydrates. Unleash Your Thin wisely keeps carbohydrates at a fairly low level for 2 weeks, allowing your "fat-burning switch" to stay permanently in the "on" position.

But that's just the *first* promise of the program.

According to the manual, the major obstacle to weight loss isn't just the hormonal environment, which, after all, is pretty easy to correct with a low-carb diet. No, the major obstacle to weight loss is *poor mental conditioning*— our inability to resist addictive foods that make us fat, sick, tired, and depressed.

The manual and DVD goes into great detail about exactly why this is so, and much of the information contained within will make you piping hot mad. Food companies scientifically engineer their "food products" with just the right combinations of tastes that light up our craving buttons. Sugar, salt, and fat are added and layered in precise proportions to create a massive, toxic food environment that literally taunts us with the mocking slogan, "Betcha can't eat just one!" The Unleash Your Thin program is predicated on the idea that unless you can master these cravings and your behavior around these foods, the best information about what to eat won't help you.

If the first premise of the program is to eat in a way that turns "on" your fat-burning switch, the second, equally important premise is that you have to reprogram your "behavioral control switch," the one that gets literally disabled in the presence of craving-producing foods.

The 4 Phases

Phase 1 of the UYT program is unique in that it is focused on preparation and habits rather than on specific changes in what you eat. "You don't go into battle without a battle plan," writes the author. This week of preparation is focused on buying the right food, "bulletproofing your kitchen," eating meals with specific beginnings and endings, answering lots of questions in the workbook that will help clarify your goals, clearly identifying your own trigger foods and toxic-eating situations, and doing a number of other things to increase mindfulness around eating. You can think of Phase 1 as the psychological equivalent of a physical conditioning and warm-up program that an athlete might do prior to getting on the field.

If Phase 1 is like conditioning prior to the big game, Phase 2 is when the big game starts. During this 2-week phase, you eat only protein and vegetables with one piece of low-sugar fruit a day (apples are recommended). There is also one optional portion of either avocado or nuts. You can cook your veggies in any fat you like (butter, coconut oil, olive oil, etc.), you don't have to count calories or grams, and you can eat until you're full. It's actually a very easy program to stay on, and weight loss is noticeable.

In Phase 3, which lasts 2 weeks, you reintroduce foods like dairy, grains, and starches, but in a very controlled way. The first week of Phase 3 is all about dairy; the second week is all about grains and starches. The purpose of each week is to gently reintroduce foods in these respective groups and notice your reactions. You make notes in your food diary, which helps you decide exactly how much (if any) dairy, grain, and starch foods you can keep in your diet after the program is over.

Phase 4 is only 1 week, and it looks pretty much like what you're "permanent" eating plan will look like. This final week allows you to assemble meal plans with just the right amount of those reintroduced foods to keep your fat burning switch in the "on" position, minimize symptoms, and keep food triggers at bay.

Throughout the program there are incredibly sophisticated exercises that allow you to literally recondition your brain so that your "behavioral control circuits" aren't disabled every time you smell a Cinnabon in the food court! The program gives you lots of "real-world" exercises—like pairing a really disgusting image with a food that makes you fat—helping to break the link between that food and unmitigated "pleasure."

A unique feature of the program is detailed menu plans (found in a separate book) plus original recipes especially created by chef Jeannette Bessinger, coauthor of *The Healthiest Meals on Earth* and several other books. However, since the authors recognize that it's unlikely that anyone will follow exact menu plans for 6 weeks, there is a very clear "roll your own" section that shows you how to effortlessly assemble your own Unleash Your Thin–friendly meal from a list of acceptable foods.

The authors are very clear that exercise is vital for health and for weight maintenance but they do not emphasize it too much in this program. Why? Because they (correctly) believe in the maxim from 12-step groups everywhere: Keep It Simple, Stupid. They believe that focusing on one thing at a time improves the odds of both compliance and success (not to mention mastery!). If you're not exercising when you start the program, you can certainly begin with one of the beginner's workouts, but you can also put it off until you're more comfortable with the eating plan. (Spoiler alert: when you do begin exercising, the authors recommend high-intensity burst training or circuit training as the best way to burn fat efficiently and effectively. That seems to be in accord with most state-of-the-art recommendations on exercise and fat loss.)

Unleash Your Thin as a Lifestyle: Who It Works for, Who Should Look Elsewhere

It's hard to imagine any demographic for whom the Unleash Your Thin program wouldn't be suited. It's probably especially good for those who have issues with motivation and willpower and who are continually derailed in their weight-loss efforts by cravings, binges, frustration, and stress.

This program would definitely be better suited to nonvegetarians; protein figures prominently in this plan, and vegetarians by definition will have a more limited number of protein choices. However, vegetarians who eat eggs and/or fish, and those who can tolerate whey protein powder should have a fairly easy time of it. Vegans should probably look elsewhere.

JONNY'S LOWDOWN: ★★★★★ (WITH DISCLAIMER)

Full disclosure: As primary author, I can't be wholly unbiased about this program. But I can honestly say that Unleash Your Thin is the most complete system I've ever seen for losing weight and, especially, for maintaining that weight loss in the real world. In its previous incarnation as Diet Boot Camp, it has earned thousands of endorsements from real people getting real results. The Unleash Your Thin program is like a turbocharged Diet Boot Camp with greater depth, scope, and reach. I can honestly say that even if I had not had a thing to do with this program, I would still consider it a solidly five-star affair! Highly recommended.

(Unleash Your Thin is available on http://www.jonnybowden.com).

22. Women'sHealth Perfect Body Diet

Cassandra Forsythe, MS

WHAT IT IS IN A NUTSHELL

An excellent plan for women that allows you to tailor the dietary component depending on your level of carb sensitivity, which you determine from some very smart questionnaires included in the book. Strong on both dietary information and exercise, and highly recommended.

About Women'sHealth Perfect Body Diet

Without a doubt, this is one of the best diet and exercise books ever.

It's smart, well informed, practical, and contains incredibly useful information that reflects a great deal of what we've learned about low-carb eating these past years.

It's easy to see why this book will appeal to women and why it deserves a wide audience. It begins with a foreword from the editor of *Women'sHealth*, Kristina M. Johnson, in which she states clearly the goals they had in mind when deciding to publish a *Women'sHealth* official diet and exercise guide, goals that are likely to appeal to a lot of women:

- The *Women'sHealth* Perfect Body Diet should be custom-fit for every woman. ("After all," she adds, "hormonally speaking, our bodies vary tremendously. I want the best plan for *me*.")
- The *Women'sHealth* Perfect Body Diet should make me feel strong. Not weak. Not starving.
- The *Women'sHealth* Perfect Body Diet should be easy to maintain as a permanent lifestyle change. ("Studies show that 95 percent of dieters gain back the weight they lose within 1–5 years," she adds. "Give me something I can stick to for life.")

If these goals interest you, read on, because Cassandra Forsythe's book delivers on its promise.

The "diet" is actually *two* distinct dietary plans. Forsythe recognizes that we're hormonally and metabolically different, and that some people are good at metabolizing sugar (carbohydrates) and some aren't. Carbohydrates are particularly detrimental for women who don't metabolize them well, Forsythe correctly explains. "Too many carbs actually slow down your fat-burning furnace so that your metabolism is not running as hot as possible," she says.

A clue to which group you're in (and which diet plan to follow) is found by looking at your body shape. You've probably heard about "apples" and "pears," a common way of describing body types that focuses on where your fat is stored. "Apples" are rounder and tend to store their fat around the middle. "Pears" are bottom-heavy and tend to store their weight around the butt and thighs. To this well-known dyad, Forsythe offers a third body type—"avocados." These are folks who could go either way (more on this in a moment).

It's pretty well known at this point that there are some people who absolutely thrive on a vegetarian diet while others drag around all day feeling tired all the time; and some people absolutely thrive on a high-protein diet while others feel bloated and heavy. Clearly there are huge individual and metabolic differences in how we respond and adapt to different diet strategies. Your body type—apple or pear—actually says a lot about your metabolism and suggests what kind of dietary program you'll respond best to.

To decide which of the two dietary plans to follow, you take an ingenious test for "Carbohydrate Intolerance." The test is simple. There are two breakfasts—a high-carb breakfast and a low-carb breakfast. On the first day (say, Monday) you eat the high-carb breakfast; on the second (Tuesday), you eat the low-carb one. At 6 timed intervals after eating breakfast, you simply answer a series of easy questions relating to how you feel—your energy, your mood, your hunger, and so forth. (The whole process of answering the 10 questions probably takes less than 2 minutes, so even filling out the quiz six times is a time commitment of less than 15 minutes!). On Wednesday, you eat your regular breakfast and go about your business. You repeat the process on Thursday (high-carb breakfast) and Friday (low-carb breakfast) just to confirm the results, and you take an average of your scores for high-carb and low-carb days. (Incidentally, though the process may sound involved as you read this, trust me, it's simplicity itself and takes very little time.)

Once you discover your level of carb intolerance, you're ready to begin the program. (Incidentally, there's nothing like actually experiencing the comparison between how you *feel* with a high-carb breakfast versus how you feel with a low-carb one. Experiencing it for yourself is better than any theoretical explanation and will help motivate you to stick with the plan that's best for your metabolism.)

Apples are also more likely to score higher on the "carb-intolerant" scale and should start on the Greens and Berries Plan (see the following page). Pears, on the other hand, can usually tolerate relatively higher levels of carbs, and should begin on the Grains and Fruit Plan (see below). Those avocados among you who could go either way will learn a lot from doing the 5-day breakfast test, and it will be pretty clear which plan to start on. The good news is you really can't go wrong on either plan; and if one doesn't quite work, you can adjust it toward the other.

The Greens and Berries Diet (best for apples) is the one that's lowest in carbs, most of which come from—as you might expect—green vegetables and berries.

Here are the specifics:

The Greens and Berries Diet (for Apple Shapes)

20–30% carbohydrates	90–125 grams
35–45% fat	60–70 grams
30–35% protein	120–140 grams

The Grains and Fruits Diet is similar to the Zone in its distribution of protein, fat, and carbohydrates, and it allows for some grains and a wider variety of fruit.

Here are the specifics:

The Grains and Fruit Diet (For Pear Shapes)

35–45% carbohydrates	150–180 grams
25–35% fat	50–55 grams
25–35% protein	100–120 grams

Two things become immediately apparent, both of them good. One, there's a *range* of recommended percentages, allowing for some flexibility within the plans and discouraging too obsessive an approach to meal planning. Two, both plans have considerably fewer carbohydrates than the average American diet, and considerably fewer than the usual amount recommended across the board by organizations like the American Dietetic Association.

And that's good news.

There's one more secret ingredient in the Women'sHealth Perfect Body Diet: glucomannan. Never heard of it? Read on.

If there's one supplement that I'd recommend for weight loss it would be this: fiber. And that's exactly what glucomannan is. "It makes your stomach full without adding any extra calories to your diet, and it's an indispensable tool for helping you stick to the Perfect Body Diet," Forsythe says.

Using glucomannan is a terrific idea. It's the most soluble fiber found in nature: it can expand to 100 times its own water weight, helping you to eat fewer calories and feel full longer. The book tells you exactly how to add this super fiber to your diet easily. Come to think of it, supplementation with fiber from glucomannan isn't a bad idea for people on *any* diet.

The book also contains an excellent exercise section for strength-building and toning that is well photographed and described well.

Women'sHealth Perfect Body Diet as a Lifestyle: Who It Works for, Who Should Look Elsewhere

This is an all-around excellent fitness-and-diet book for women, probably one of the best I've ever seen. While there are very good exercise-and-fitness books around, many of them are lacking in the kind of thorough, well-thought-out and scientifically accurate nutrition program that *Women's-Health Perfect Body Diet* offers. Similarly, many good nutrition books are a little light on the exercise component. This one has both, and as such, it's hard to think of a woman who wouldn't benefit.

JONNY'S LOWDOWN ★ ★ ★ ★ ★

A smart, well-written, scientifically accurate program that takes into account individual differences and offers two distinct plans, depending on your level of carb intolerance. Both plans are excellent, with one plan being a little higher in carbs than the other. Both plans permit some flexibility within the ranges of the recommended amounts of protein, carbs, and fat, and should appeal to people wanting to individualize their programs.

The exercise program is terrific, the explanations are clear, and the information about both nutrition and exercise is first-rate. I especially like the way they make use of the fiber supplement glucomannan and integrate it into the program. Bonus points for an excellent recipe section.

23. THE ZONE

BARRY SEARS, PhD

WHAT IT IS IN A NUTSHELL

An eating plan consisting of 40% carbohydrates, 30% protein, and 30% fat. Zone orthodoxy calls for eating five times a day—three meals and two snacks, each of which should contain the 40/30/30 distribution.

About the Zone

Tell Barry Sears, creator of the Zone, that his eating plan is a high-protein diet, and you're likely to be met with either an icy stare or a frustrated sigh, depending on his mood. Most often, you'll get a resigned explanation that you sense (correctly) he's given a thousand times. "The Zone," he says patiently, "is *not* a high-protein diet: it is a protein-*adequate* diet. The amount of protein recommended on the Zone is very similar to what Americans are currently consuming. The amount of fruits and vegetables that are recommended on the Zone diet is nearly three times the amounts recommended by the U.S. government, even though the amount of total carbohydrates is lower."

He's got a point. This just might be the most misunderstood and falsely maligned popular dietary approach of all time, considering the fact that it has probably had the most influence on changing the dietary tenor of the times, especially in altering the prevailing attitude about fat as the demon behind obesity and disease. Let's go over just what the Zone is and what it isn't.

The Zone is not a high-protein diet, despite the fact that critics—who seem never to have read the book—continue to refer to it as such, especially in popular magazines. The amount of protein on the Zone diet could hardly be considered high (except by the intransigent right-wing of the dietary establishment, the American Dietetic Association). On a 1,500-calorie diet, 30% protein—the amount recommended by Sears—works out to 112 grams of protein (roughly 16 ounces) a day. That's about 4 ounces per meal and 2 ounces per snack for the average man, nowhere near an excessive amount.

The Zone is also not a low-carb diet. Do the math—you're always eating slightly more carbohydrates at every meal than you are eating protein or fat. In fact, 40% of your meal is carbohydrates, yielding, with the same

1,500-calorie intake, 150 grams of carbs a day. Just for comparison, Atkins allows 20 grams per day on the induction phase of his program. The Zone allows more than seven times that amount. The Zone diet gets most of its carbohydrates from fruits and vegetables and uses the starchy carbohydrates—breads, pastas, rice, cereal, and the like—sparingly, almost, says Sears, "as condiments."

The Zone was never meant solely as a weight-loss diet. It was designed to reduce heart disease through the control of inflammation, and its success and popularity surprised Sears as much as anyone. The fact that so many people lose weight and feel terrific on it—and that it has been adopted by a number of celebrities—put it in the public arena and made Sears either a hero or a monster, depending on what academic pundit you listen to.

The Theory Behind the Zone: A Short Lesson in Nutritional Endocrinology

Think of your body and its organs, glands, hormones, and other chemical compounds as one huge biological Internet, where messages (sometimes conflicting ones) are constantly being sent out, received, interpreted, misinterpreted, and acted upon. Hormones are particularly potent messengers; when you receive a message from a hormone in your biological e-mailbox, you pay attention. Insulin is a hormone—a major one. It's secreted by the pancreas in response to the increased blood sugar that you get after you ingest food (particularly carbohydrates). Insulin is intimately tied to levels of blood sugar. If you eat a Snickers bar, your blood sugar rises and the pancreas says, *"Uh-oh, dude ate a Snickers; let's get to work."* It secretes some insulin. The job of that insulin is to bring the blood sugar back down into the normal range. It does this by "escorting" the sugar out of the bloodstream and into the cells. According to Sears, excess insulin is the culprit behind skyrocketing rates of obesity, a premise he shares with all low-carb diet writers.

There are two basic ways to raise insulin levels. One is to eat too many carbohydrates. The other is to eat too much food. Americans do both.

The word "zone" in the title actually refers to an *optimal range* of insulin levels. The diet claims to keep insulin levels from rising too high by replacing some of the carbs in the typical American diet with fat (which has no effect on insulin) and protein (which has some effect, but not as much as carbs). The balance among carbs, protein, and fat at each meal and snack is designed to prevent blood-sugar levels (or insulin levels) from going too high (or too low). This, combined with the fact that the diet is not too high in calories, is responsible for the weight-loss effects on the diet.

The *health* effects of the diet are caused by a different, though related, pathway. Remember that the Zone diet was birthed in the midst of a high-carb, low-fat diet mania. All of us in the field of nutrition were seeing clients who had virtually cut fat out of their diets (and almost always replaced it with carbohydrates). They thought they were eating healthfully. It was not unusual in those days (and even now, for that matter) to see a woman eating a bagel and orange juice for breakfast, a salad for lunch, a nonfat frozen yogurt for an afternoon snack, and pasta for dinner, then wondering why she wasn't losing weight. The Zone almost single-handedly put the argument for inclusion of good fats in the diet back "on the table." And it is through the inclusion of this fat that the Zone diet is thought to have one of its most significant health effects.

Here's how it works: The body makes an entire class of "superhormones" called eicosanoids out of the "raw materials" of essential fats. Eicosanoids are made by every one of the 60 trillion cells in your body. They don't circulate in the body—they're made in a cell, they do their action in the nearby vicinity, and then they self-destruct, all within a matter of seconds, like those little tapes they used to give Peter Graves on *Mission: Impossible*—so they are virtually undetectable in the bloodstream. But their importance on human health is incalculable. The 1982 Nobel Prize in Medicine was awarded for eicosanoid research. Your doctor may not know much about eicosanoids, but he or she has undoubtedly heard of prostaglandins. Prostaglandins are eicosanoids made by the prostate gland and were one of the first groups of eicosanoids to be studied.

The type of fat you eat influences the kinds of eicosanoids you make. Eicosanoids come in many "flavors" and types, but for our purposes we'll identify two major classes: the "good" and the "bad." The good are responsible for preventing blood clots, reducing pain, and causing dilation (opening) of the blood vessels, among other things. The bad are responsible for promoting blood clots, promoting pain, and causing constriction (closing) of the blood vessels. The point is not to get rid of *all* the bad ones, but to have a balance between the good and the bad. (For example, if you didn't have eicosanoids that promoted blood clots, you would bleed to death from a minor wound.) Aspirin works by knocking out *all* eicosanoid production for a while, which is a little like killing a fly with a sledgehammer. Corticosteroids do the same thing. The fat included in the Zone diet specifically fosters the creation of good eicosanoids and an optimum balance between the good and the bad.

The insulin connection is this: insulin stimulates the key enzyme involved in producing *arachidonic acid*, which is the "building material" of the bad eicosanoids. So by controlling insulin levels with the Zone diet, you not only lose weight, you also reduce many of the symptoms and health risks that come from an imbalance of good and bad eicosanoids. The promise of the Zone is that controlling insulin will result in increased fat loss, decreased likelihood of cardiovascular disease, and greater physical and mental performance. By controlling eicosanoids, you will have decreased inflammation and increased blood flow, which will help improve virtually every chronic disease condition and improve physical performance.

So, What Can You Eat?

A lot. The best protein choices on the plan are skinless chicken, turkey, all kinds of fish, very lean cuts of meat, low-fat dairy products, egg whites, tofu, and soy meat substitutes. For carbohydrates, Sears likes all vegetables except corn and carrots and all fruits except bananas and raisins. The heavy starches like pasta, bread, cereals, rice, and the like are used very, very sparingly. For fats, use olive oil, almonds, avocados, and fish oil.

It's really simple to make a Zone meal, actually, and doesn't require a lot of complicated calculations. All you have to do is divide your plate into thirds. On one third of the plate, put some low-fat protein—a typical portion would fit in the palm of your hand and be about the thickness of a deck of cards. Then fill the other two thirds of the plate with vegetables and fruits. Once in a great while, part of that two thirds can consist of pasta or rice, but again more as a condiment than a main dish. Add a dash of fat, and you have the basic Zone meal.

The Zone as a Lifestyle: Who It Works for, Who Should Look Elsewhere

The one criticism you hear about the Zone from the average person is that it is difficult to follow. Technically, if you're trying for the exact proportions of 40/30/30, that's correct. The fact is that you really *don't* have to achieve Zone-perfect proportions to get the beneficial effects—an approximation works perfectly well—but the lack of precision may be a problem for people who like their diets very exact and specific. Some people find that thinking about food in terms of Zone "blocks" is cumbersome. If you happen to love doing the math, and the computations of grams, calories, and so on is something you eat for breakfast, this is the perfect diet for you.

This is a great program if you are not overweight but just want a healthful way of eating that will in all likelihood reduce your risk for a number of unpleasant diseases and conditions. If you are only moderately overweight and believe you are not insulin-resistant (i.e., do not have a particular problem with carbohydrates), it's a great way to eat, but you will have to watch calories. If you are very overweight or very sedentary—or both—this program is probably too high in carbohydrates for you, and you might be better off using one of the more carb-limited programs (such as Protein Power or Atkins), at least to begin with.

The other thing to consider in choosing this program as a lifestyle is whether you can tolerate this level of carbohydrate. If you are carb-addicted, getting 40% of your calories from carbs may seem outrageously high. The program *does* allow things that trigger carb cravings—like bread and even pasta, albeit in small amounts—but for some people, small amounts are too much. Remember, it *is* entirely possible to create Zone-perfect meals using only vegetables and fruits as carbohydrate sources, and if you're able to live with that, you will do fine.

JONNY'S LOWDOWN ★ ★ ★ ★ ★

It's hard to underestimate Dr. Sears's contribution to the current nutritional zeitgeist. He almost single-handedly forced the dietary establishment to reevaluate the prohibition on fats. I have a few minor disagreements—I don't believe saturated fats from natural sources like butter and eggs are a problem, and I also don't agree with his position that supplements aren't necessary if you are eating correctly (a position, to be fair, that he has modified considerably in recent years). That said, the Zone template of 40% carbs, 30% protein, and 30% fat is darn close to ideal as a starting point for a healthful diet. I'm a huge believer in biochemical individuality and not in the "one size fits all" diet mentality, but we still need a basic template from which to individualize our diets; the Zone is as good a basic template as exists anywhere. Some people may need fewer carbohydrates; some may even need more. But the 40/30/30 plan beats the USDA Food Guide Pyramid (or its updated version, My Plate) as a place from which to begin constructing an individual diet plan.

CHAPTER 10

Frequently Asked Questions

*I*n this chapter, I've posed and then answered the questions that I see most often on my website, as well as those I'm asked most frequently in seminars and workshops around the country. I've also incorporated the questions that I've seen come up time and time again on Internet sites dealing with low-carbohydrate diets. The questions are organized into categories, such as Losing Weight on Low-Carb, Food and Water, and Exercise.

Losing Weight on Low-Carb

How Long Will It Take Me to Lose 10 (or 100) Pounds?

There is absolutely no way to know the answer to this question. A lot depends on how much you have to lose and how you respond to your program. Everyone is fundamentally different on a metabolic, genetic, and biochemical level, and each body responds differently. Even people on identical programs are likely to experience different amounts of weight loss on different timetables. Rule of thumb: in the first week or so of a low-carb diet, you may lose a bunch of weight—maybe even 7 to 10 pounds if you are considerably overweight—but eventually you should settle in to an *average* of 2 pounds of weight loss per week, more or less. Don't be discouraged if your weight loss is less—many other things could be going on. And even at the rate of 1 pound a week, you'll still lose 50 pounds a year.

Is a Low-Carb Diet for Everyone?

Memorize this and tattoo it behind your eyelids: no single diet is for everyone. The Bantu of South Africa thrived on a diet of 80% carbs, and some groups of Eskimos thrived on a diet of nearly zero carbs. However, here in America and in most of the industrialized nations, it's fairly safe to say that nearly everyone would benefit from a *lower*-carb diet than is currently the norm. And *everyone* would benefit from changing their carbs from the highly processed, sugar-laden, fiberless fare of convenience, fast, and packaged foods to what we might call "real" carbohydrates—things you could pluck, gather, or grow.

How low in carbohydrates you personally need to go must be determined by trial and error. If you are a basically healthy person looking to stay that way and weight loss is not a real issue for you, the best template to start with is the one advocated by Barry Sears, which is approximately 40% of your food as carbohydrates, 30% as protein, and 30% as fat. Interestingly, this is very close to what many of the plans discussed in this book—among them the Atkins diet, Protein Power, and the Fat Flush Plan—recommend for maintenance after your weight target has been achieved. And no less a luminary than the renowned Harvard epidemiologist Dr. Walter Willett has said, without actually mentioning the Zone diet, that a diet containing 40% carbs, 30% protein, and 30% fat may well be the healthiest alternative to the moribund USDA Food Guide Pyramid's (or its updated version, My Plate's) recommendations.

Once I Reach My Goal Weight, Can I Add Carbs Without Gaining Weight?

Posts on Internet bulletin boards respond to this type of question with the acronym YMMV, which means "your mileage may vary." Translation: everyone responds differently, so try it out. All of the classic programs basically suggest adding carbs back in a controlled and measured way until you discover for yourself the "magic" amount that allows *you* to maintain your goal weight. Be aware, though, that some of the foods you cut out—for example, wheat—may have been causing other problems in addition to weight gain (see chapter 4), so monitor your reactions carefully if you start adding those back.

Should I Weigh Myself Regularly?

Yes. The scale is a great way for you to check in with reality, as long as you know how to use it right. You need to learn *not* to beat yourself up about the number. You need to understand that water retention can mask fat loss. You need to understand that body composition can change with weight-training exercise, and that you could be losing fat while gaining muscle (which would not necessarily show up right away on the scale). And you need to understand that everyone loses at a different rate. You may go for a period of time with no change whatsoever and then all of a sudden have a "whoosh" of weight loss. That said, the scale *will* keep you honest. *Eventually*, the scale will reflect fat loss. It will tell you—in combination with other cues, like how you're feeling and what your measurements are—whether what you're doing is working. If you want to figure out your critical carb level, you'll have to use the scale at some point to find out whether additional carbs are slowing you down. Many people have been delighted to find out that they actually could have a few more carbohydrates than they previously thought, and that it didn't slow down their weight loss appreciably or, if they were already at their goal weight, it didn't cause them to gain. But you'll never know any of that if you don't watch the numbers.

What Are Net Carbs? What's the Difference between Net Carbs and Effective Carbs?

There is none. Net carbs and effective carbs are two different phrases for the same thing. The idea is that fiber, even though it's "counted" as a carbohydrate on food labels, isn't absorbed, so it shouldn't really be counted. To get the net, or effective, carbohydrate content of a food, simply go to the label and subtract the number of grams of *fiber* from the number of grams of *carbohydrate*. For example, 1 cup of raspberries has 14 grams of carbohydrate, but 8 of those are from fiber. Subtract the 8 grams of fiber from the 14 grams of *total* carbohydrate, and you get the number of net carbohydrate grams per cup: 6.

What Is the Minimum Daily Requirement for Carbohydrates?

Zero. There is no biological requirement for dietary carbohydrate in human beings. You would die without protein and you would die without fat, but you can live just fine without carbohydrates. I'm not suggesting that you should—just that you can.

Low-Carbing and the Body

Why Am I Getting Headaches during the Induction Phase of My Diet?

Headaches are a frequent side effect of switching abruptly from a high-carb to a low-carb diet. One of the reasons for this is that your body and your brain need to adapt to using fat and ketones as a primary fuel source after being accustomed to using sugar. Your brain can certainly use ketones, but it takes a few days to make the adjustment, during which you may get a headache. It usually goes away by itself, but one thing you can definitely do is drink more water. In fact, if you don't drink enough water, you may get a "ketone headache" even *after* your body has adapted to the diet. The other thing you can do is up your carbs by 5 to 10 grams a day until you're feeling better, then lower them gradually. Preventing some of the side effects is one reason for doing a 3-day transition from your previous way of eating into this new low-carb lifestyle.

Recent research indicates that it may not be just the "keto-adaptation" that's causing the headaches or lethargy. It might be withdrawal. Since both wheat and sugar are now known to act on the brain, it's not impossible that some of your temporary discomfort may be very similar to what people go through when they stop smoking. If you can somehow get yourself through it, it'll definitely be worth it.

I'm Getting Leg Cramps, Especially at Night. Why?

This is almost always due to a mineral deficiency, particularly potassium, calcium, and magnesium. Remember that insulin tells the body to hold on to salt and water. When your insulin levels fall, especially during the first week on your low-carb diet, the kidneys will release that excess sodium— and you will begin to lose a lot of water. This will usually result in a loss of potassium as well, and one of the symptoms of potassium loss is muscle cramping (as well as fatigue). Dr. Alan Schwartz, medical director of the Holistic Resource Center in Agoura Hills, California, recommends taking one to two potassium supplements (99 milligrams) with each meal, especially in the first week of your low-carb diet. Magnesium supplementation is also a good idea.

Note: nuts help prevent potassium and magnesium imbalances. While you have to watch your intake of nuts during the weight-loss phase of your program, they nonetheless are chock-full of these valuable minerals.

Does a Low-Carb Diet Cause Kidney Problems?

No. This is one of the great myths about low-carbing, but it is exactly that—a myth based on an incomplete understanding of the facts. It is true that people with preexisting kidney or liver problems should not go on very high-protein diets, but it is *not* true that either high-protein diets or low-carbohydrate diets in general *cause* kidney problems. If your doctor tells you otherwise, ask him or her to show you the research that confirms that finding. Your doc will not be able to, because there is none. There is not even a problem with protein in the diet of diabetics, who are frequently given to kidney problems. "There is no evidence that in an otherwise healthy person with diabetes eating protein causes kidney disease," says Frank Vinicor, director of diabetes research at the Centers for Disease Control and Prevention.[1] (For a more detailed explanation, see chapter 6).

Is Low-Carbing Good for Diabetes?

It is not only good; it is *essential.* "Diabetes is a disease of carbohydrate intolerance," says physician and diabetes specialist Lois Jovanovi , chief scientific officer of the Sansum Medical Research Institute in Santa Barbara, California. "Meal plans should minimize carbohydrates because *people with diabetes do not tolerate [them].*"[2] (Emphasis mine.) Dr. Richard Bernstein, author of *The Diabetes Solution* and a diabetic himself, has been fighting the medical establishment over this since the 1970s. "What is still considered sensible nutritional advice for diabetics can over the long run be fatal," Bernstein writes.[3]

The American Diabetes Association's high-starch diet is so behind the curve that it's ludicrous. Jovanovic sums up the conventional high-carb advice for diabetics in one word: "Malpractice!"

Can Stress Stall Weight Loss?

You bet. Not only can stress stall weight loss, it can *reverse* it. Stress—which can come from lack of sleep, extremely low-calorie dieting, and, of course, from life itself—causes the release of hormones such as cortisol and adrenaline. These stress hormones send messages to the body to break down muscle for fuel, resulting in a lower metabolic rate. They send compelling messages to the brain to eat (e.g., the well-known "stress eating" phenomenon). Cortisol also tells the body to store fat around the middle. Because cortisol basically breaks down biochemicals in the body, chronic elevated levels of cortisol can trigger a protective reaction from the body in the form of insulin secretion (since insulin builds up structures in the body, including, of course, the fat cells). This makes chronically high levels of cortisol one possible cause of insulin resistance.

Another way stress can screw up weight loss is by its effect on serotonin. Stress *eats up* serotonin. Less serotonin is produced because stress interferes with the good, deep, restful sleep needed by the body to replenish its serotonin stock.[4] The demand for serotonin becomes greater, while the production of it is lower. Serotonin depletion is never, *ever* conducive to weight loss, as it works against you in very powerful ways.

What Is Leptin?

Leptin is a hormone involved in appetite control. Early research at Rockefeller University showed that obese mice were very low in leptin, leading to a lot of excitement about the possibility that giving leptin to obese people would somehow result in weight loss. No such luck. It turned out that obese people have plenty of leptin. What seems to be happening is that they have what might be called leptin resistance—their cells don't respond to it, in a scenario not unlike that of insulin resistance.

Leptin is produced by fat cells—when the fat cells are full, they release leptin, which sends a signal to the brain to stop eating—but this mechanism doesn't seem to work in obese people. *Less* leptin means *more* appetite; as body fat is lost, leptin levels drop,[5] which in turn sends a message to the brain telling you to eat more. This mechanism may be one of the many that makes regaining weight after a diet so easy; it's as if this feedback mechanism is hard at work to preserve you at a set weight. Drugs to treat this "leptin resistance" are in development and, if they prove promising, may one day help to fight obesity.

This Is My First Week on a Low-Carb Diet. Why Do I Feel Lightheaded?

Loss of minerals could be the culprit. Remember that when you lower your insulin levels, you lose salt and water (but, in the process, lose potassium as well). This, plus the tons of water I hope you're drinking, could conceivably result in enough electrolyte loss to lower blood pressure to the point where you might feel lightheaded or even faint. Replace some of the lost salt with either salty foods or with some table salt. Try ¼ teaspoon of potassium chloride (Morton Lite Salt) and ¼ teaspoon of table salt to start, and see if that helps. Don't forget to take potassium supplements.

How Do I Know if I'm Insulin-Resistant?

The best way is with a fasting insulin test. This test tells you what your baseline level of insulin is when no food is around to spike it. If you're not insulin-resistant, you shouldn't have a lot in your bloodstream when you haven't eaten. Lab ranges will vary; you should not be above seventeen, and the optimal level is below ten. A blood sugar test won't tell you if you're insulin-resistant. You could have blood sugar in the normal range, but it could be taking an enormous amount of insulin to keep it there.

Without a fasting insulin test, the best "low-tech" way is to look at your body's "insulin meter"—your waistline. If you're storing a bunch of fat around your middle, chances are you're insulin-resistant. And though the argument about which comes first—obesity or insulin resistance—continues to rage, the fact is that they are so often found together that for all intents and purposes, if you're extremely overweight, you can assume you are also insulin-resistant. (There are exceptions; some heavy people are insulin-sensitive, and some thin people—who usually exercise a ton and never overeat—are insulin-resistant. These are not the typical cases.)

Does a High-Protein Diet Cause Bone Loss or Osteoporosis?

No. If anything, a diet high in protein does the opposite, particularly in the presence of adequate calcium intake and plenty of alkalinizing vegetables. There are a tremendous number of studies now showing that protein is essential for healthy bones and that, indeed, low protein intake can be an obstacle to bone-building. (For a more in-depth discussion of calcium, high protein, and bone loss, see chapter 6.) It's also worth remembering that the total amount of protein consumed on the typical low-carbohydrate diet of 2,000 calories (or fewer) is in no way excessive, even if it is a higher percentage of your diet than it had been before you revised your eating habits.

Can a Low-Carb Diet Cause Gallbladder Problems?

No, but if you have been overweight and have been on a very low-fat diet for a long time, a high-fat diet can make your gallbladder problems—like gallstones—apparent. Here's why. The gallbladder basically responds to fat in the diet with contractions that release the bile necessary to digest fat properly. When you've been on a very low-fat diet, there's not much for the gallbladder to do, so it gets lazy, and sometimes deposits accumulate and form stones, kind of like sediment forming in stagnant waters. When you suddenly go on a high-fat diet, the gallbladder now has work to do—it contracts in response to the fat, and it *may* pass these stones. The high-fat (low-carb) diet didn't *cause* the stones; they were already there and developed most likely in response to your very low-fat diet! But switching to a high-fat diet could trigger an attack. The solution: a moderate-fat version of the low-carb diet will trigger gallbladder contractions that are strong enough to release bile, but not vigorous enough to dislodge any stones.

What Can I Do about Constipation?

The two main causes of constipation on low-carb diets are not drinking enough water and not eating enough fiber, both of which you should be doing even if you're not constipated. Drink more water (see "How Much Water Should I Be Drinking?" on page 282), and make sure the vegetables and fruits you consume are high in fiber—spinach, broccoli, and raspberries are all good choices. Consider a fiber supplement (even sugar-free Metamucil, though I prefer Paleo Fiber or Cellulose Fiber, both available on my website, http://www.jonnybowden.com). Exercise almost always helps. And drinking hot water with a squeeze of fresh lemon juice first thing in the morning can help get things going as well.

A terrific "cure" for constipation is magnesium. Get the magnesium citrate form, start with 400 milligrams a day for a few days, and then, if needed, increase to 800. That almost always does it.

Cravings

Why Do I Get Cravings?

Cravings have many causes. Some are caused by nutrient deficiencies. In this case, what you crave is a clue to what's missing; for example, craving fatty foods could indicate that you're not getting enough essential fatty acids. Try adding omega-3 fats like fish oil; women can also try flaxseed oil. Many cravings are caused by blood-sugar imbalances. The common craving for carbohydrates in the evening can be caused by not having eaten enough protein and/or fat earlier in the day. Frequent small meals that contain protein and fat will help control the blood-sugar roller coaster that is often responsible for cravings. If a carb craving is absolutely irresistible, as a transition technique you should satisfy it with fruit (though you can blunt the insulin effect by adding some peanut butter or turkey).

A lot of cravings are caused by low serotonin states. Eating high-carbohydrate foods in this scenario is a kind of self-medication. The problem is that it creates a vicious cycle that results in weight gain and more cravings. Some supplements—for example, 5HTP—can help boost serotonin naturally, and there are a number of lifestyle ways to boost it as well, such as having a pet, being out in the sun, and making love! You also need to understand that some cravings are simply conditioned responses to stress and are more emotionally driven than anything else. That's why "comfort foods" are so named—we have been conditioned to eat them when things aren't going well and we need a little TLC. The more you work on developing alternative behavioral responses to these situations—like taking warm baths or going for a walk—the better off you'll be.

What Can I Do to Combat Sugar Cravings?

There are two supplements that are phenomenal for sugar cravings. One is glutamine—I recommend that you take a spoonful or two of the powder in water (available in health-food stores or through Internet sources). A spoonful of glutamine mixed with the sweetener xylitol and dissolved in a few tablespoons of half-and-half or heavy cream will knock the socks off even the worst sugar craving.

> *I don't care how much the experts say it's harmless, I know how sugar makes me feel: crazy. I start craving it like an addict, and once I start eating it I can't stop.*
> *—Jean N.*

You might also investigate a new product called Crave Arrest, a blend of ingredients such as tyrosine (a precursor to dopamine), 5-HTP (a precursor to serotonin), and B6, which is necessary for the conversion of tryptophan to serotonin. (Crave Arrest is made by Designs for Health and can be purchased through a link on my website, http://www/jonnybowden.com.)

Here are the top five techniques for busting cravings:

1. Control blood sugar by eating protein and fat every few hours, at every meal and snack.
2. Avoid *any* junk carbohydrates made of white stuff (rice, bread, pasta), as well as those that contain highly concentrated sweeteners, even if their carbohydrate content is permissible on your program.
3. Never let yourself become famished. Carry protein-based snacks like nuts, cheese, and hard-boiled eggs with you at all times.
4. Get enough sleep. Lack of sleep increases appetite and stimulates stress eating.
5. Learn to recognize the emotional triggers for cravings, such as fear,

tension, shame, anger, anxiety, depression, loneliness, resentment, or any unmet needs. Don't pretend they're not there—recognize them, accept them, embrace them, and own them. Then explore behavioral ways of dealing with them besides eating.

Supplements

Do I Need to Take Supplements?

The technology exists to give you health-protective and therapeutic amounts of vitamins, minerals, phytochemicals, antioxidants, and other compounds, many of which are simply not available from our food supply or, if they are, not in the amounts needed to make a difference to your health and well-being. You don't *need* to take vitamins, but then you don't need electricity either. The question is, why would you do without either of them if you didn't have to?

Doesn't Taking Vitamins Just Result in Expensive Urine?

If it does, then why bother to drink water? You just urinate it out at the end, right? Do you see how ridiculous this concept is? The expensive-urine comment, which is perpetuated by doctors who don't really understand nutrition and vitamins, implies that just because something eventually winds up in the urine, it didn't accomplish anything in the body. Why does a drug addict take drugs or an athlete take steroids? Drugs, both recreational and prescription, are detected in the urine, right? Does the fact that they're detectable in the urine mean that they didn't *work*? If that were the case, there's an awful lot of people wasting an awful lot of money on drugs and medications! It's funny how the same doctors who cry "expensive urine" in response to vitamin therapy never make the same remark about their prescription drugs that are just as detectable in the urine as vitamins are!

The fact that drugs—or vitamin residues—are detectable in the urine means absolutely nothing except that those substances went through the body and did their job. They didn't pass through and accomplish nothing, or else steroids wouldn't be banned by athletic organizations! The body takes what it needs, uses it, and excretes the rest. In addition, there's no way to know exactly how much of a given vitamin a specific individual actually needs. It's a lot better to take too much (with a few exceptions that might be toxic in very large amounts over an extended period of time, such as very high-dose vitamin A or selenium) and let the tissues decide how much they need and how much is excess. As nutritionist Robert Crayhon says in answer to this question, "Hey, I *want* expensive urine! In fact, I want the most expensive urine money can buy!"

What About Ephedra?

A recent post on an Internet diet board asked the following question: "Do people die from taking ephedra?" The question produced the single best response I've ever seen: "No, people die because they are *morons.*"

When ephedra has been used in supervised weight-loss research studies, it's been used in the dosage of 60 milligrams per day in three divided dosages (20 milligrams each) combined with 200 milligrams of caffeine per dose. In every supervised study using this dose, it has not shown itself to be dangerous, and the side effect of "jitters" was usually pretty well tolerated. It is *not*—I repeat, *not*—for people with high blood pressure; for people who are sensitive to ephedrine or caffeine; for people who have any kind of heart, kidney, or liver problems; or for people who are on *any* medication, including over-the-counter meds (unless cleared by a doctor). Ephedra works by stimulating brown-fat metabolism, thereby increasing the bodily production of heat (upping your metabolism *slightly*) and by suppressing your appetite. The possible side effects are very annoying and include nervousness, insomnia, and possibly dizziness. The benefits in the way of fat loss are very mild but probably do exist.

> I definitely noticed a difference in my skin when I began to supplement with fatty acids like fish oil. My hair and scalp weren't as dry and even my fingernails go stronger.
> —Bernice D.

But here's the thing. While I'm no great fan of ephedra, it has also been blamed for an awful lot of things it doesn't deserve. When a college athlete dies on the football field while practicing in 100° heat in full uniform, dehydrated, with a few hundred milligrams of ephedra plus who knows what else in his system, it's not exactly fair to blame ephedra. A recent field trip to my local vitamin shop uncovered ephedra pills with 250 milligrams *per pill*—more than ten times the recommended dose—and believe me, there are people who are taking several of these pills at a time. Let's also keep in mind that there are a couple of thousand deaths directly related to aspirin per year. Ephedra in small amounts, under controlled conditions, is not dangerous.

I'm more concerned about the adrenal burnout factor with ongoing ephedra use. This drug *is* a metabolic stimulant, and like any stimulant, it taxes the adrenal glands, which over the very long haul can not only hamper your weight-loss efforts but damage your health.

This discussion is probably moot, however. "Its time is over," says Dr. C. Leigh Broadhurst, who has herself used ephedra without incident. There's just too much bad publicity and public outcry about it." The FDA banned ephedra and ephedrine-based supplements as of April 12, 2004, a decision which was appealed and then later upheld in 2006 by the US Court of Appeals for the Tenth Circuit. The new "ephedra-free" diet pills have simply replaced ephedra with *Citrus aurantium* (bitter orange), which has many of the same fat-burning/appetite-suppressing effects but doesn't yet have the bad rap. (See next question.) If you *do* use ephedra, make sure you do not fit in any of the categories mentioned above, and never take more than the recommended dosage.

What about Over-the-Counter "Ephedra-Free" Diet Pills?

The new "ephedra-free" diet pills have simply replaced ephedra with bitter orange (*Citrus aurantium*), an herb that contains the active ingredient synephrine. Synephrine is chemically very similar to ephedrine and pseudoephedrine and has similar effects in terms of providing an energy boost, suppressing the appetite, and increasing metabolic rate and caloric expenditure. By stimulating specific adrenergic receptors, it is theorized that synephrine stimulates fat metabolism without the negative cardiovascular side effects experienced by some people with ephedra (also called "ma huang").

Bitter orange usually contains between 1% and 6% synephrine, but some manufacturers boost the content to as much as 30%.[6] It *does* have a thermogenic (fat-burning) effect.[7] In animal studies, synephrine caused weight loss, but it also increased cardiovascular problems.[8]

Bitter orange can also increase the side effects of many medications, including (but not limited to) Xanax, Zocor, Sudafed, Buspar, Celexa, Zoloft, Allegra, prednisone, Meridia, Viagra, and a number of blood pressure medications.[9] Do *not* take bitter orange if you have high blood pressure or are pregnant.

The bottom line is this: it *is* a stimulant, and the same cautions about other stimulants (like ephedra) apply. Just because the pill is "ephedra-free" does not mean that you should use unlimited amounts of it.

What's in Those "Fat-Burning" Formulas I See Everywhere, and Do They Help with Weight Loss?

A recent field trip to my local vitamin store to inspect a dozen of these formulas—labeled everything from "metabolism boosters" to "fat burners" to "lipotropics"—revealed a pretty standard revolving door of ingredients. Most used some combination of the following:

- bitter orange (*Citrus aurantium*), a stimulant that increases metabolism (thermogenesis) slightly and is discussed previously (see "What about Over-the-Counter 'Ephedra-Free' Diet Pills?")
- guarana, which is herbal caffeine
- white willow bark, which is basically aspirin and really doesn't add anything to the mix
- green tea extract, a.k.a. EGCG (epigallocatechin gallate), which *does* have thermogenic properties

Combinations of these ingredients can definitely suppress appetite, give you the jitters, and maybe, just maybe, burn a few extra calories.

Some "fat-burners" include a mix of carnitine and chromium. They almost never contain the best form of carnitine (tartrate) and rarely contain more than 500 milligrams (most nutritionists think the minimum amount necessary to impact fat-burning in an overweight person is 1,500 milligrams). As far as chromium is concerned, while I *have* seen formulas with 200 micrograms (the absolute minimum needed), I saw one that loudly proclaimed "contains chromium" and actually had a ridiculously low 13 micrograms. Understand that the amount most often given to people with blood-sugar problems is in the neighborhood of 600 to 1,000 micrograms; 13 micrograms would do absolutely nothing and is only there so that the manufacturer can say "contains chromium"—a complete rip-off.

Other ingredients that show up in the formulas, especially the ones labeled "lipotropics," are inositol, an essential nutrient and relative of the B family, and choline, another relative of the B family that mobilizes fat. Both choline and inositol (plus methionine) are involved in the liver's ability to process fats, so there's reason to think that these nutrients might help the liver move fat through it. If a sluggish liver is part of the reason you're holding on to fat, these nutrients could be helpful. As lipotropics go, I like the Fat Flush Weight Loss Formula from http://www.unikeyhealth.com, which contains reasonable amounts of choline, inositol, and methionine, plus the good form of carnitine, 400 micrograms of chromium, and an herbal mix that's good for the liver.

The other pair of ingredients often found in these formulas are tyrosine, an amino acid helpful for improving mood, and phenylalanine, an essential amino acid that can be converted into tyrosine. Both of these are precursors to dopamine, a neurotransmitter that makes you feel peppy and bright. Tyrosine is needed for the making of thyroid hormone, but it is highly unlikely that tyrosine will boost low thyroid, even though some supplement makers claim it does.

The important thing is to read the ingredients on the labels of the products you are considering. These formulas vary widely in their effects, depending on the amounts and quality of the ingredients included. At worst, they do nothing. At best, they'll give you a bit of a speedy feeling and maybe increase metabolic rate by a very small amount.

> *It was absolutely amazing to me when I really studied ketosis and found out that almost everything I had heard about how dangerous it was was utter hogwash.*
> *—Dana McG.*

Ketosis

What Is Ketosis?

Ketosis is a term used to describe what happens when the body switches to fat as its main source of fuel, which is exactly what you want to happen when you're using a low-carbohydrate diet to lose weight. When fat is the main source of fuel, there is an increase in the number of ketone bodies made as a by-product of fat metabolism. Ketones can be measured in the urine by means of ketone test strips.

Is Ketosis Dangerous?

Absolutely not. Ketones are a natural part of human metabolism—your body is always producing ketones. When you are in benign dietary ketosis, you are just making *more* of them, because fat, rather than sugar, has become the main source of fuel for your body. A strict ketogenic diet has been very successful in treating epilepsy in children and has been used for years at the Children's Hospital of New York-Presbyterian.[10] Children have been kept on it for years at a time. If there were dangers associated with ketosis, we would have heard about it by now. (For a full discussion, see chapter 6.)

Do I Need to Be in Ketosis in Order to Lose Weight?

No. First of all, ketosis doesn't *cause* weight loss. You can easily be in ketosis eating 10,000 calories of fat a day, but you'll never lose any weight that way. Ketosis is simply a by-product of fat burning. There have been many people who've lost weight on low-carb diets without being in ketosis, and there are many who have been in ketosis and not lost weight. Ketone loss, in the urine and the breath, accounts for only about 100 calories a day.[11] That said, there are some extremely metabolically resistant people who truly seem to do much better on Atkins-like induction plans in which they *are* in ketosis, carbohydrates are kept to very low levels (20 to 30 grams or so a day), and calories are moderately low.

You may want to go into ketosis just to get started, but the vast majority of people can lose weight over time on a low-carb diet by hovering around the border of ketosis. And as we saw in chapter 9, many of the programs don't emphasize ketosis at all—some programs deliberately keep you at a slightly higher carb level (50 to 90 grams a day) to prevent it. The point is this: if you keep your carbs low enough (and your calories reasonable), you will be lowering your insulin levels and breaking down fat. Exactly how low they have to be for you to continue to lose weight is something you will have to experiment with.

Why Don't My Ketone Test Strips Show a Positive Reading?

There are a number of reasons you may not get a positive reading, and you probably don't need to be too concerned about it. There are three ketone bodies—beta-hydroxybutyric acid, acetoacetic acid, and acetone—and the strips detect only the latter two, which are less than ⅕ of the total ketones produced. Beta-hydroxybutyric acid goes completely undetected. So it's entirely possible that you might not test positive on the ketone strips, yet if you performed a more sophisticated urinalysis, you'd find plenty of ketones floating around!

Other things can influence whether the strips change color, such as how much water you're drinking. If you're drinking a lot, which you should be, that'll very likely keep the strips from turning a deep color.

Of course, the possibility exists that they're not turning color because you're not in ketosis, probably because you are eating more carbs than you think or there are hidden carbs in your food choices.

Food and Water

How Many Calories a Day Should I Be Eating?

For weight loss, a good rule of thumb is to take your goal weight and multiply by 10. If you've got more than about 25 pounds to lose, multiply your *current* weight by 10 and then deduct 500 calories from that number. This formula doesn't work as well if you are at a relatively low weight—say 125 pounds—and are trying to drop only a few pounds. You should never, ever let your calories fall below 1,000 per day.

If you'd prefer not to do any calculations, you can remember it this way: the average weight-loss diet for men is about 1,500 to 1,800 calories and the average for women is about 1,200 to 1,400.

Remember that these formulas are only approximations. Every person's situation is going to be different based on one's own metabolic and historical factors, genetics, age, hormonal profiles, muscle mass, activity levels, and so on. The calorie calculators found on diet Internet sites woefully overestimate how many calories you "need," especially for weight loss. Ignore them. And remember that calories are important, but they're not the whole picture; the kinds of food you eat determine what messages are sent by your hormones, and the hormones are what control the whole shebang.

I'm a Vegetarian. Can I Low-Carb?

Yes, depending on the type of vegetarian diet you are following. If you're a vegan, it's going to be next to impossible, but if you can eat eggs and whey protein, it's definitely doable. If you can also eat fish, it's a snap. Check out *The Schwarzbein Principle Vegetarian Cookbook* (see "The Schwarzbein Principle," page 239) as well as the cookbooks in the Resources section.

It's worth noting that in 2009, researchers tested an all-vegan low-carb diet that later became known as "Eco-Atkins."[12] They kept carbs to 120 grams a day and all protein and fat came from nonanimal sources. People lost weight and saw their blood lipids improve considerably.

A note on vegetarianism: if you're avoiding eating animals for spiritual, ethical, or moral reasons, I am in great sympathy with you. I myself am a believer in animal rights, am a card-carrying member of PETA, and understand your feelings profoundly. But if you're doing it for health reasons, I urge you to rethink your position. Most people do better with some animal foods, and some people do a *lot* better on a *lot* of animal foods. Maybe one way to reconcile this for yourself is to patronize only those who sell meat from animals that have not been factory-farmed, have been *organically* raised, and have had a good and happy life. Just something to think about.

Why Is Water So Important for Fat Loss?

Drinking plenty of water is absolutely necessary for fat loss. When you're not drinking enough water, the kidneys can't work properly, so they start dumping part of their load onto the liver. The liver is the main fat-processing plant in the body, but if it has to take over some of the kidneys' work, it can't work at full operating capacity. It metabolizes less fat, so more fat remains in the body, and weight loss stalls.[13] Water is also necessary to get rid of the toxic wastes released from fat stores.

Water is also the absolute best treatment for water retention. The less water you drink, the more the body perceives this as a threat and sends signals that result in holding on to as much of that scarce water as possible. Sometimes this shows up as swollen hands, feet, and legs. When you're drinking enough water, this doesn't happen. There's no more "emergency," and the body releases stored water instead of retaining it.

How Much Water Should I Be Drinking?

More than you think. "Larger people have larger metabolic loads," says Dr. Donald Robertson. "Since we know that water is the key to fat metabolism, it follows that the overweight person needs more water." Robertson recommends 3 quarts a day. Many personal trainers recommend a gallon. I think the absolute minimum is 64 ounces plus an additional 8 ounces for every 25 pounds of excess weight you are carrying.

How Can I Get More Fiber in My Low-Carb Diet?

If your program permits it, include a serving of All-Bran or Fiber One cereal, which are the only commercial cereals that have a significant amount of fiber. Get some wheat or oat bran (not the cereals, the actual *bran*; you'll find it in the section of the health-food grocery that sells dry bulk items). You can mix the brans together in different proportions and cook it to make your own hot cereal mix, or you can use it as a breading or a filling. I also recommend adding fiber supplements (like psyllium husks or flaxseeds) to your program, but don't take them at the same time as other medications or supplements, because the fiber can inhibit absorption.

What Are Sugar Alcohols? Do They Count as Sugar?

Sugar alcohols—also called polyols—are sugar-free sweeteners that are carbohydrates but are not sugar. Common ones include maltitol, mannitol, sorbitol, and xylitol. They have fewer calories per gram than sugar: sugar has 3 calories per gram, while sorbitol has 2.6, xylitol has 2.4, and mannitol has 1.6. They don't cause sudden increases in blood sugar; instead, they are slowly and incompletely absorbed from the small intestine into the blood, and the portion that is absorbed requires little or no insulin. Since they aren't technically sugar, manufacturers are able to say "sugar-free" when they use sugar alcohols as sweeteners, but they're required to include these sweeteners in the carb count on the nutrition label (though not everybody does).

Scientists call them sugar alcohols because part of their structure chemically resembles sugar and part chemically resembles alcohol. They're certainly a lot better for you than pure sugar. Xylitol actually has health benefits. (I'm also a huge fan of the sugar alcohol *erythritol*, sold under the brand name of Truvia.) But some of them can cause slight gastric upset for some people, like a little gas or a mild laxative effect. And you have to be careful with portion sizes—even though the food may be technically sugar-free, the calories and grams of sugar alcohol can add up. And some folks—particularly carb addicts—say that products sweetened with sugar alcohols can trigger cravings just like products sweetened with sugar.

What Are the Best Oils?

There's a new star on the horizon: coconut oil. It can be used for anything and has amazing health benefits (see also next question).

For cooking, I recommend extra-virgin olive oil, virgin coconut oil (especially Barlean's 100% Organic Extra-Virgin Coconut Oil), grapeseed oil, or butter (I know it's not an oil, but it is fine for cooking and sautéing). Peanut oil is stable and can be used occasionally for stir-fries, but it is very high in omega-6, so don't overdo. You can use sesame oil, which is very good for frying, but remember that it contains a larger proportion of omega-6s, so don't use it exclusively. Almond oil is good for baking.

Flaxseed oil is terrific, of course, but *never* use it for cooking. It is a great source of alpha-linolenic acid (an omega-3 fat), but for that reason it can't be heated (though it can be poured or drizzled on hot foods such as vegetables). Omega-3 fats are very unstable and become extremely damaged when heated. Another terrific new oil that is a great source of the same omega-3 fat is perilla oil (a plant extract), but it should not be used for cooking.

For salads, try coconut oil, extra-virgin olive oil, any of the nut oils (macadamia, hazelnut, almond, walnut), avocado oil, or sesame oil. You can also use flaxseed oil or perilla oil. I don't recommend canola oil. To be used commercially, it has to be partially hydrogenated, refined, and deodorized, and in the process its omega-3s become a potent source of trans-fatty acids.[14] If you do use it, make sure to get organic, cold-pressed, or expeller-pressed canola oil (such as Spectrum), and only use it cold.

Oils you can say good-bye to permanently include safflower, sunflower, corn, soybean, and cottonseed. Buh-bye.

What's the Story with Coconut Oil? I Heard This Is a "Bad" Fat!

You heard wrong. Virgin coconut oil is a good, stable, healthful fat that actually has a number of healing properties, not the least of which is that it is anti-inflammatory.[15] The original bad rap for coconut oil came four decades ago, when researchers fed animals *hydrogenated* coconut oil that was purposely altered to render it devoid of essential fatty acids. The animals that were fed the hydrogenated coconut oil (as the only fat source) naturally became deficient in essential fatty acids, and their serum cholesterol increased.[16] Early commercial coconut oil was often hydrogenated (loaded with trans-fats), and all the good, healing stuff had been removed. That altered coconut oil *wasn't* very good for you. But *real* coconut oil is a health bonanza. The Pukapukans and the Tokelauans of Polynesia, for whom coconut is the chief source of energy, have virtually no heart disease, and research on these populations concluded that there was no evidence that their high saturated-fat intake (from coconut) had any harmful effects.[17] The saturated fat in coconut oil comes mainly from MCTs (medium-chain triglycerides), which are preferentially burned as energy and less likely to be stored as fat, making them a good choice for a weight-loss program. Coconut oil also contains a high proportion of the antiviral and antimicrobial lauric acid, as well as the antimicrobial capric acid and the potent "yeast fighter" caprylic acid.[18] Be sure to purchase the virgin or cold-pressed kind. In my opinion, there is none better than Barlean's 100% Organic Extra-Virgin Coconut Oil, which I use for almost everything.

MORE ON KETONES AND THE BRAIN

Dr. Mary Newport is the medical director of the newborn intensive-care unit at Spring Hill Regional Hospital in Florida. Her husband Steve had early-stage Alzheimer's. "I was watching my husband of 36 years fade away," said Dr. Newport.

Then she discovered coconut oil.

Dr. Newport began researching clinical trials and discovered a new medication that had shown unbelievable results in clinical trials. While generally, the best that can be hoped for with Alzheimer's is to slow the progression of the disease, this drug had produced actual memory *improvement*, something rarely seen in Alzheimer's patients. Unfortunately, her husband wasn't eligible for the trial—according to the results of a

MMSE test (a test commonly used to assess cognitive impairment), he scored too low and had too great a level of impairment.

But Dr. Newport didn't give up.

She researched the active ingredient in the new medication and found an in-depth discussion of its primary ingredient, a particular form of fat called MCTs—medium-chain triglyerides.

This is precisely the kind of fat found in coconut oil.

She decided to try it.

She purchased a jar of non-hydrogenated, extra-virgin coconut oil (one excellent brand is Barlean's Extra-Virgin Coconut Oil, available everywhere at health-food stores).

She started by adding a couple of tablespoons into her husband's oatmeal.

Almost immediately, her husband started showing improvements. He scored higher on the exam than he had scored in a year. More than 5 months afterwards, his tremors had subsided and he had become more social and interested in those around him.

The secret seems to be in ketones.

The body converts some of the MCTs into ketones, which are an additional source of fuel for starving brain cells. No one is claiming that ketones—or MCT oil, a purified form of the fat found in coconut—will cure Alzheimer's. But this inspiring story is yet another example of the way ketones can be helpful as an energy source for the brain.

"I started using 100% MCT oil for kids with brain problems about 25 years ago," says renowned neurosurgeon Larry McCleary, MD (author of *The Brain Trust Program*). "This generates more ketones and does it faster than coconut oil (and has fewer calories for the same amount of MCTs). It was part of a vigorous nutritional support program for kids with brain issues of many sorts—tumors, trauma, drowning, hemorrhage, etc. It produced dramatic results in them and it should help older people with disorders like Alzheimer's disease."

Ketones also appear to help children with epilepsy. Eric Kossoff, MD, is assistant professor of neurology and pediatrics at Johns Hopkins and the medical director of the Johns Hopkins ketogenic diet program. He's been using the ketogenic diet for years as a treatment option for epilepsy, and in 2003 developed a slightly gentler version of the diet called the MAP—Modified Atkins Program.

"In 2008, the ketogenic diet is not viewed as an alternative diet anymore," said Dr. Kossoff. "It's viewed as an option to meds, but most docs know it's an effective therapy for epilepsy."

What Are the Good Fats?

Good fats include all the oils mentioned previously as "good" *plus* natural, undamaged fats like butter, coconut, avocado, nuts, and the fat in fish.

The dietary establishment has long fostered the myth that fats are "good" or "bad" depending on whether or not they are saturated: saturated fats = bad, unsaturated fats = good. Not so. A much better way to categorize fats is by whether they are damaged or undamaged. You can damage fats in a number of ways. One way is by overheating any vegetable oil by frying at high temperatures—this creates toxic substances known as lipid peroxides. Another is through an industrial process known as partial hydrogenation, which creates something called trans-fats, by far the most dangerous of all fats. Trans-fats are found in almost all fast foods (french fries, for example, are doused in them), most margarines, virtually all commercially baked goods (including children's cookies), and movie popcorn, and in any products containing partially hydrogenated vegetable oils (look for these in the ingredients list on the package). Trans-fats are the true demons of the fat world, and the ones we want to avoid completely, as they are associated with all of the degenerative diseases common in the modern world.

> Every time I drink (alcohol), my diet goes out the window and I eat way more than I ever intended to. Cutting out alcohol—at least for now—has been the best thing I ever did for my waistline.
> —Kelley F.

Unfortunately, until recently, there has been no separation in the research between saturated fats and trans-fats, so saturated fats have been blamed for a great deal of the damage to the body that is actually the fault of trans-fats.[19] As of 2006, manufacturers are required to list trans-fats in the Nutrition Facts on food packaging, but the law allows manufacturers to say "zero trans-fats" provided there's less than half a gram per serving. This has led a lot of manufacturers to keep "suggested serving sizes" ridiculously low so that, in effect, you could easily be consuming a gram or two of trans-fats from "zero trans-fat" foods. The only surefire way to tell if a food has trans-fats is to read the ingredients. If it says "hydrogenated oil" or "partially hydrogenated oil," it's got trans-fats, no matter what the front label says.

What about Alcohol?

Here's the deal with alcohol: the body has no way to store the energy in it (7 calories per gram), so all "fat-burning" is put on hold while the body burns off the alcohol. Alcohol can also produce cravings, both for itself and for carbohydrates—Kathleen DesMaisons, PhD, an expert in addictive nutrition, considers alcohol dependence simply an extension of sugar sensitivity.[20] She also believes that although hard liquor is not technically a sugar, the beta-endorphin effect is a powerful trigger for cravings.[21]

That said, a lot of low-carb plans permit some alcohol, particularly red wine (in 4-ounce servings), which contains about 3 grams of net carbohydrate. Do the math and see if it works for you.

What Is the Glycemic Index?

The glycemic index is a numerical way of describing how carbohydrates in foods affect blood-sugar levels (an even more accurate measure is the glycemic *load*; see next question).[22] The index measures how quickly a 50-gram serving of a particular food converts to sugar. Foods with a high glycemic index cause a dramatic rise in blood sugar (and subsequent demand on insulin levels). That's why all low-carb diets suggest that you eat *low-glycemic* carbohydrates; these carbs (green vegetables, for example) have a much lower impact on your blood sugar and insulin.

What's the Difference between the Glycemic Index and the Glycemic Load?

The glycemic load is a more accurate predictor of what's going on with blood sugar and insulin than the glycemic index. Here's why. Suppose I put an empty bucket under a faucet and I want to know how much water is going to wind up in the bucket. You can see immediately that there are two variables I need to know: the water pressure (how high I turn on the faucet) and how *long* I'm going to leave it on. In the same way, if I want to know the impact of a particular food on blood sugar and insulin, I need to know two things: the glycemic index *and* how *much* of that food I'm going to eat!

The glycemic *index* tells you the impact that a 50-gram serving of a particular food will have on your blood sugar. The glycemic *load*, on the other hand, also takes into account the amount of carbs actually in the food. Remember that all the low-carb plans consider the number of net, or effective, carbohydrates in a serving, because we need to know that in order to determine the total impact the food is going to have on your blood sugar. Some foods have only a few grams of available carbs; so even if their glycemic index is high, their overall impact will be reduced because there are so few of them. The glycemic load is a measure of that *overall* impact. To find the glycemic load, multiply the glycemic *index* by the number of *net carbohydrates in a standard serving* (find the glycemic index for various foods at http://www.glycemicindex.com)

Consider the difference between carrots and pasta. Carrots have a glycemic index of 47, higher than that of whole-wheat spaghetti, which is only 32. If this was the only information you based your decision on, you'd think carrots were much worse, from a blood-sugar point of view. But while there are only 6 net (or effective) grams of carbs in a carrot, there are a whopping 48 grams of net carbs in the pasta! Let's calculate the glycemic load (index times net carbs): carrots would be 47 times 6, which is 282. But the calculations for the spaghetti would be 32 times 48, which is 1,536—more than 500% higher than carrots!

What's the Best Type of Protein Drink to Use?

Whey. It seems to be the best all-around source of protein, followed by soy that has been enriched with methionine (an amino acid that's very low in soy). Whey is absorbed the best and is the most available; it also increases levels of glutathione, perhaps the most powerful antioxidant in the body, which helps with immune function and has been shown to be helpful in weight loss.

What's the Difference between a Protein Drink and a Meal-Replacement Shake?

Protein powders are 100% (or almost 100%) pure protein. You can drink them by themselves or make a "meal-replacement" drink with them by adding a controlled amount of carbohydrates (berries are a good choice) and maybe some fat like nuts or nut butter (women can add flaxseed oil if they don't mind the taste). Designs for Health makes an excellent protein powder called Paleo Meal that is enriched with omega-3's and a number of other terrific ingredients (available on my website, http://www.jonny bowden.com).

Meal-replacement shakes have carbs, protein, and fat in different proportions depending on the philosophy of the company making them. Many are very high in carbs.

What's Wrong with Grains? Aren't They Supposed to Be Healthy?

Grains, grain products, starches, and sugars all share some common links: they turn into glucose (sugar) in your body very quickly, they promote addictive eating habits in a large percentage of people, and they trigger insulin release. All of these things result in weight gain and other health problems.[23] Grains also contain compounds called phytates and pyridoxine glucosides that block absorption of B vitamins, iron, zinc copper, and calcium and lead to possible mineral deficiencies that can slow metabolism. (For a full discussion of grains, see "The Problem with Grains" on page 213 and the discussion of wheat in chapter 4.) In addition, both gluten and certain protein fractions of gluten are a big problem for many people. It used to be thought that celiac disease—a sensitivity to gluten—was rare. We now know that it probably affects one in 33 people. That's a lot. There are an amazing number of toxins used in the processing of wheat and grains, and it is entirely possible that some of the problems that people have with wheat are actually caused by these toxins. (Other problems are certainly caused by the wheat itself.)[24] Clinically, an awful lot of problems seem to just magically "clear up" when you take grains, especially wheat, out of the diet. While whole grains are in theory better than refined grains, they're not nearly as common as you might think. The making of flour is itself a refining process. And the "wheat breads" in your grocery are no better than white bread. Couple this with the fact that grains usually have a very high-glycemic load, and you can see the potential problem. Obviously, not everyone will have a problem with grains, but cutting them out during the initial stages of a low-carb weight loss program is definitely a good idea.

Is Coffee Okay?

Probably. Those who argue against coffee are concerned with its possible effects on insulin and on the adrenal glands. Atkins didn't like it because he felt it caused unstable blood sugar. There is some research that suggests that caffeine increases insulin resistance[25] and that it raises insulin levels.[26] How much this matters as a practical consideration is debatable—the insulin insensitivity it produces in studies may be an insignificant amount as a practical matter and may be only temporary. There is also research showing that coffee actually *improves* insulin sensitivity[27] and contributes to *reducing* insulin,[28] as well as some research that says it has no effect on insulin at all.[29] And in one study, coffee was actually associated with a much *lower* risk of type 2 diabetes.[30]

While coffee is obviously a stimulant, drinking it is also a very pleasant experience for a lot of people, and that has to be factored into the mix. It's also high in antioxidants, such as chlorogenic acid, and by some accounts it's the biggest source of antioxidants in the American diet! Those who are very concerned about adrenal health (Dr. Diana Schwarzbein) recommend dumping it, but others say it's fine. From a weight-loss perspective, it's probably not going to hurt at all, and a fair amount of research shows that coffee drinking is associated with significantly less risk for diabetes, cardiovascular disease, and Parkinson's. According to Mark Houston, MD, new research has identified genes that are involved in the response to coffee/caffeine. Some people are "responders" and some are not, meaning the effect of coffee differs from person to person. If you respond with the jitters or disrupted sleep, it's probably a good idea to find another beverage (or drink less of it!).

Important note: it's not just the caffeine that's a problem (there's caffeine in green tea too, and that doesn't seem to hurt anyone): it's the enormous amount of toxins in the coffee plant. You can go a long way toward reducing any negative health impact of coffee by purchasing organically grown beans.

Are Diet Sodas Acceptable on My Low-Carb Diet?

You'd be *much* better off without them. If you can't give them up right away, put it on your goal list and at least start cutting back. Most of them use aspartame, which should definitely be eliminated (see next question); in addition, diet soda can stall weight loss in some people (up to 40% to 50%, by some estimations), possibly due to the citric acid they contain, possibly due to mechanisms not yet fully understood.

Many people do drink soda addictively (I had one client who routinely consumed sixteen cans a day), and the amounts consumed by people like this have never been tested for safety in long-term studies. Through a classical conditioning mechanism, like the one used to teach Pavlov's dogs to salivate at the sound of a bell, drinking diet soda may well trigger insulin production (as may the consumption of other artificial sweeteners). The sweetness without calories is also thought to deregulate our natural appetite mechanisms. And the chemicals, food colorings, flavorings, and other stuff in diet soda make it no picnic for the liver, either.

What about Aspartame?

Aspartame, the most common of the artificial sweeteners and the one used in most diet sodas, is a real problem. Even though it has been declared "safe," the FDA has received numerous reports of seizures and other problems that have been linked to it.[31] There's also good reason to believe that aspartame may be neurotoxic.[32] In a report to the Senate Labor and Human Resources Committee, Dr. Richard Wurtman, professor of neuroendocrine regulation at the Massachusetts Institute of Technology, stated that the most common side effects linked to aspartame include dizziness, visual impairment, disorientation, ear buzzing, a high level of SGOT (a liver enzyme), loss of equilibrium, severe muscle aches, episodes of high blood pressure, and other not-so-lovely stuff.[33] Other reports claim that in susceptible people, aspartame can produce symptoms ranging from sleep disturbances to headaches to fuzzy thinking to mood disturbances, and one recent article in the *Townsend Newsletter for Doctors and Patients* suggested that in susceptible people (called aspartame responders), the substance could be somewhat addictive. Kathleen Des Maisons, PhD, an expert in addictive nutrition, believes that the taste of any sweetener, for sugar-sensitive people, evokes a beta-endorphin response in the body that will create cravings.[34]

No integrative or holistic practitioner I interviewed had anything good to say about aspartame. The consensus of advice: stay away.

What about Artificial Sweeteners in General?

You basically have seven choices:

- Aspartame (Equal), is probably the most commonly used artificial sweetener these days, but it's also one that I *cannot* recommend (see previous question).
- Saccharin (Sweet'n Low) has been around for about a hundred years, and at one time it had a reputation as a cancer-causing agent because of studies in which rats got bladder tumors when they were fed incredibly high amounts (equivalent to what a human would get drinking eight hundred cans of diet soda a day). Recently, saccharine was declared safe, and probably is—in reasonable amounts. Next to sucralose and stevia, it's probably the best choice.
- Cyclamate (Sugar Twin, Sucaryl) also continues to have a cloud of smoke around it concerning cancer in rats, but it too has been added to food and beverages since the 1950s and is probably safe in small amounts.
- Acesulfame-K (Sunette) is in the same family as saccharin but isn't widely available in the States.
- Sucralose (Splenda) is the most promising of all. It is basically a slightly chemically altered version of sucrose (sugar) and is six hundred times sweeter. The chemical alteration prevents the digestive system from "recognizing" it and absorbing it, so it doesn't cause the rise in blood sugar and insulin associated with sucrose,

unless of course it turns out to cause an insulin rise through a conditioned response mechanism. The only possible problem with Splenda—and it is only theoretical—is that the chemical "alteration" involves adding chlorine molecules. Is that a good thing? Probably not, but only time will tell. As of this writing, there is a growing movement among "natural health" people to ban Splenda, due to enormous concerns about that chlorine molecule. The situation is evolving, so it's worth keeping an eye on.

- Erythritol is, in my opinion, one of the best "artificial" sweeteners currently available. It's a natural sugar alcohol, has virtually no glycemic impact, and tastes great. And you can use it in beverages. Erythritol is now available at supermarkets, sold under the brand name of Truvia. Personally, I'm a fan.

- Stevia is an herb sold as a food additive, which has basically no downside except a somewhat weird aftertaste that some people don't mind at all. You can get it at any health-food store. My personal favorite is the stevia sold by NuNaturals, a company that makes a number of stevia products, all of them high quality and reliable.

Note that not all of these sweeteners are suitable for cooking or baking, so be sure to check the label or check with the manufacturer.

Is Fructose Okay?

The short answer: Absolutely not. It's actually the most damaging part of sugar, and in the amounts we consume it, pretty close to metabolic poison. And that's whether it's coming from ordinary table sugar (50% glucose, 50% fructose), high-fructose corn syrup (55% fructose, 45% glucose), or agave nectar (up to 92% fructose).

Fructose doesn't raise blood sugar, so it used to be thought of as the perfect sweetener for diabetics. Bad idea. Even though it doesn't raise blood sugar, it induces insulin resistance in both animals[35] and humans.[36] Fructose is turned to fat in the liver, so it raises your triglycerides as well as contributing mightily to non-alcoholic fatty liver disease (NAFLD).

But fructose from reasonable amounts of fruits (and vegetables) is not as much of a problem, as there's less of it than in a concentrated sweetener, and it comes with a whole lot of other goodies such as fiber, antioxidants, and phytochemicals. When you consume fructose, make sure it comes in its natural container—fruit. Never use it as a sweetener, and don't make a habit of eating foods that are sweetened with it.

What about Protein Bars?

The problem is that many of these products are deceptively labeled. A lot of them will tell you they have only 2 or 3 grams of "usable" carbs, but don't be too quick to buy it. They are sweetened with sugar alcohols, which the manufacturers often decide not to count when telling you how many carbs the bar contains. The argument is that sugar alcohols don't have the same effect on blood sugar, which is true. But they're still carbs. Nutrition-labeling regulations don't require manufacturers to put the number of grams of sugar alcohols per serving *unless* they are making a claim related to sugar content, in which case it's mandatory. Since most of the low-carb bars don't claim to be sugar-free, they can get around this mandatory clause. Even Atkins does not count the glycerin (glycerol) that sweetens his Atkins Nutritional Bars as part of the carb gram count. The problem is that like all sugar alcohols, glycerin *is* a carbohydrate. The FDA's Office of Food Labeling states: "FDA nutrition labeling regulations require that when glycerin is used as a food ingredient, it must be included in the grams of total carbohydrate per serving declaration." So although sugar alcohols do behave differently in the body than sugar, you should still be aware of their presence.

The other concern about low-carb bars is calories. Just because they are low in carbs doesn't mean they're low in calories, so factor that in. In sugar-sensitive people, they can *easily* trigger cravings; these bars are, after all, very sweet, which is why they taste so good. And while most of them are better than candy bars, none is as good as real food.

So use them occasionally, but beware. Some low-carbers have found that these bars can stall weight loss, so if you're eating them a lot and you're stuck, they might be a good thing to let go of.

Can I Eat Dairy Products?

For many people, dairy—especially milk and cheese—will slow or stall weight loss. Many holistic practitioners recommend eliminating wheat, dairy, and sugar as the three biggest triggers of food reactions, subclinical allergies, and the like.

I don't believe homogenized, pasteurized milk is a good food. In addition to the pus cells (the FDA allows 1.5 million per cc of milk as "safe"), factory-farmed cows are treated with antibiotics, bovine growth hormone, and other drugs to fatten them and keep their milk production elevated to unnatural levels. The grain they eat, which is not their natural food, is irritating to their stomachs (one reason for the antibiotics) and contains a whole different set of toxins. (Raw organic milk, which may be available from local farmers, is a whole different story, but note that some states prohibit the sale of raw milk. For more information, see http://www.realmilk.com.) If you're not ready to eliminate milk, or if you want to consume it in small amounts, at the very least buy the organic kind. Excellent substitutes are the nut milks, like almond milk; or try goat's milk, which doesn't seem to present the same problems for most people. Many people who have a problem with milk are still able to tolerate fermented dairy foods like kefir and yogurt.

Cheese has stalled many a low-carber's weight loss. Although some plans allow it, if your weight loss isn't progressing, this might be one food to cut back on.

I'm Getting Bored with the Usual Low-Carb Fare. What Else Can I Eat?

Here are some terrific suggestions from low-carb chef and Internet guru Karen Barnaby.

- Thinly sliced radicchio, endive, and fennel with a fresh basil dressing, sprinkled with crisp bacon and goat cheese. Eat with roasted chicken.
- Raw, sautéed, or grilled mushrooms on romaine with blue cheese dressing. Eat with a steak.
- Fried peppers, mushrooms, and garlic. Serve on arugula, sprinkled with feta cheese, and eat with good Italian sausage.
- Thinly sliced cucumbers, radishes, and celery. Toss with lemon mayonnaise and serve on butter lettuce, along with a piece of salmon. Sprinkle with fresh dill.
- Cooked asparagus and Swiss chard. Serve a piece of halibut, cod, or sole on top and drown it in Hollandaise sauce.
- Sautéed spinach or julienned daikon seasoned with soy sauce and a few drops of sesame oil. Serve with grilled tuna on top and mayonnaise mixed with wasabi as a sauce.
- Marinated cubes of feta, Brie, or Camembert in basil, garlic, and lots of olive oil. Eat with sliced cucumbers as a snack or sprinkle on a salad. Have it alongside a hamburger. Use as an omelet filling with one fourth of a tomato, chopped.
- Make a cabbage slaw and jazz it up with mint, cilantro, green onions, and a bit of lime juice. Put canned tuna or salmon and hard-boiled eggs on top.

Here are some other ideas:

- Make omelets with fillings like bacon and Swiss cheese, mushroom and avocado, goat cheese and mushrooms, spinach and feta, or bacon and avocado.
- Add chopped nuts or sunflower seeds to cottage cheese.
- Make a "wrap" out of sliced turkey with cream cheese inside.
- Make a "wrap" out of sliced roast beef with cheddar, scallions, and a drop of sour cream (if dairy is on your program).
- Try deviled eggs.
- Use low-carb tortillas and make your own breakfast burritos.
- Keep varying the toppings on your salads. Try warm meats or shrimp, crab, or lobster. Try different cheeses, if that's on your program. Mix and match.
- Make a low-carb burger by putting a hamburger patty between two lettuce leaves (or red cabbage leaves). Add mayo and mustard if you like.
- Pan-fry some chicken and add feta cheese and olives.
- Eat a hot dog minus the bun and use mayo and mustard as dipping sauces.
- Steam some veggies and add butter, lemon, a handful of nuts, and maybe some soy sauce.
- Fill celery sticks with peanut butter, cream cheese, or tuna salad.
- Try beef jerky, turkey jerky, or veggie jerky.
- Mix sugar-free, all-natural peanut butter with whey protein powder and roll in cocoa powder.
- Combine whey protein powder with sour cream and Splenda; kneading this mixture renders a pretty interesting taffy. You must eat it within a couple of days, but it is great.

And here's one of my favorite ideas: "muffins" made with eggs and your choice of sausage, hamburger, shredded zucchini, mushrooms, onions, broccoli, cheeses, etc. Just pour the mixture into muffin tins, bake, and freeze for easy breakfasts on the go!

Plateaus

What Could Be Causing My Plateau?

The underlying premise of this book, and my philosophy of weight loss in general, is that *everybody's different* (the theory of biochemical individuality).

So you will not be surprised to find that I wholeheartedly believe there are *at least* a dozen or more reasons for the dreaded plateaus that you will inevitably reach in your weight-loss efforts. The Drs. Eades have called plateaus "the purgatory of dieting" for good reason. They drive everyone crazy (plateaus, not the Eadeses, who are very lovely people). Nevertheless, you need to learn to *expect* them and to deal with them. There is virtually no one who has successfully lost weight who has not experienced them. And the very first (and maybe most important) rule of dealing with them is this: don't panic, and don't give up.

Here are the top thirteen reasons plateaus occur:

1. **You are losing fat but building muscle.** If you are exercising, especially for the first time, you may be putting on muscle while you are losing fat. This change for the better will not show up on the scale, though it would definitely show up in a body-composition analysis. You will likely notice a small but definite change in your shape or the measurement of your waist, even though the scale isn't really moving. Don't worry—eventually, the scale will reflect the loss of body fat.

2. **Water retention masks fat loss.** You may be losing fat while holding on to water. This happens more often than you might imagine. Make sure you are drinking plenty of water. Not drinking enough water is one of the top reasons for plateaus and stalls.

3. **You are experiencing a period of adjustment.** Remember that when it comes to weight, your body operates something like the feedback loop of a thermostat. Your body needs periods of adjustment to catch up with the different amount and type of fuel it's getting, just like the thermostat needs to "catch up" with changes in the temperature of the air in your apartment. If you're resetting your "set point," it happens not all at once, but in stages. Being stuck at a certain weight for a few weeks may just be your body's way of reprogramming itself. Eventually, the scale will move again.

4. **Your carbohydrate level is too high.** The plans discussed in this book are contingent on careful monitoring of carbohydrates. Your carbohydrate intake may simply be too high for what *your* body needs to lose weight. You could easily be taking in more carbs than you're aware of, as many foods and drinks have what are known as "hidden carbs." There is a great hidden-carb counter listed in the Resources. If you suspect this may be the problem, check it out.

5. **Your carbohydrate level is too low!** This is one of the great paradoxes of low-carb dieting, because it is completely

counterintuitive. Nonetheless, I've seen it in action many times. More than one person wrote to me of weight loss stalled at a carb intake of 20 grams per day, which they were able to get going again by simply moving their carb intake *up* to about 40 or 50 grams. One possible explanation for this comes from the work of Dr. Diana Schwarzbein, who would argue that too low an intake of carbs creates higher levels of adrenaline and cortisol (which ultimately work against weight loss). While this scenario may not be true for everyone, upping your carbs is certainly worth a try.

6. **You are undereating.** Remember that the body responds to too few calories by simply becoming more efficient at extracting every single ounce of energy from its limited food supply. Too few calories literally slow down the metabolic rate.

7. **You are overeating.** At some point, every low-carber has to look at calories. Low-carb diets don't usually stress calorie-counting, because you're much less likely to overeat on healthy proteins and good fats than you are on junk carbohydrates. Nonetheless, calories still count to some degree. You may be eating too many of them.

8. **You aren't eating enough protein.** If you don't eat enough protein, you're more likely to break down your body's own protein for fuel. That means muscle loss, which in turn means a lowering of your metabolic rate. Make sure you're eating at least the minimum recommended amount of protein for your plan.

9. **You are not exercising.** Though weight loss is 80% diet, exercise definitely helps things along. The many things it does for both your health *and* your weight loss (and weight maintenance!) efforts are too lengthy to go into here. Just trust me. Do it.

10. **Medications are preventing optimum weight loss.** Many medications can interfere with weight loss. Steroid medications like prednisone are among the worst offenders, but there are plenty of others. Check this out with your doctor.

11. **You are experiencing food intolerances.** The usual suspects are foods that are generally reduced or eliminated on low-carb programs; if you're consuming them, try your own version of a modified elimination diet: remove the suspect food for a week or two and see what happens. The "sensitive seven" are wheat, milk, sugar, peanuts, soy, eggs, and corn.[37] (Refer to chapter 4 for a full discussion of the ways in which wheat, particularly, has a unique ability to keep you fat!) You may want to expand the wheat category to include all grains and the milk category to include cheese. Other well-known stallers that you might want to cut out for a while

include artificial sweeteners, especially aspartame (Equal); citric acid, found in diet sodas; glycerin, found in many low-carb meal-replacement bars, including those by Atkins; and alcohol.

12. **You have nutritional deficiencies.** A deficiency in some nutrient or nutrients may very well be interfering with how smoothly the energy-making cycles in your body run. This could easily account for you not burning fat at an optimal level. At the very least, take a high-potency multivitamin and mineral, although this is only the first line of defense—you probably need a lot more. Just as an example, in a paper in *Medical Hypotheses*, Dr. L.H. Leung noted that for reasons not completely understood, he had had a lot of success with weight-loss patients by simply adding pantothenic acid to their program.[38] (Nutritionist Barbara Marquette, MS, who teaches nutritional therapeutics in the University of Bridgeport's master's program in nutrition, has seen the identical effect.) This could be because of pantothenic acid's direct effect on the adrenal glands. However, this is only one example; there are easily a dozen other vitamin or mineral deficiencies that could prevent optimal fat loss.

13. **You're trying to do a low-fat version of low-carb.** Many people are so mired in the low-fat theology that even when they try a low-carb approach they're still constantly trying to keep fat intake low. Don't. Fat keeps you full and satiated and has many other healthful properties. And remember that saturated fat in particular "behaves" quite differently in a very-low-carb diet than it does when it's accompanied by high-carb intake.

How Do I Break a Plateau?

You can try a lot of things. You could up your carbs if the amount you've been eating is very low, or you could try lowering them (see the list of reasons for plateaus in previous question). Try cutting out treats and going back exclusively to unprocessed meat and dark green vegetables for a few days. Cut out the low-carb bars. Drink a lot more water. Or try one of the following techniques, which have been known to knock people off plateaus:

Try a vegetable-and-fruit fast. Eat nothing but vegetables and some fruit for about 3 days. This is very alkalinizing, in addition to being low in calories and very high in nutrients. Eat all you want, and feel free to add some good fat like flaxseed oil (for women), olive oil, or butter.

Try a vegetable-juice fast. This is a favorite of Dr. Allan Spreen, the "Nutrition Physician," and it's one of my favorites as well. Go a day or two on nothing but freshly squeezed vegetable juices. I'm not talking V8 here;

I'm talking the kind you make at home with a juicer. You can also drink hot water with lemon juice and, of course, all the fresh water you like.

Try raw foods for a few days. Be aware that not all people can tolerate this, and if your digestion isn't great, this may not be the best intervention for you.

Add digestive enzymes. Dr. John Hernandez, medical director of the Center for Health and Integrative Medicine in San Antonio, Texas, has found this to be one of the most useful weapons he has in his weight-loss arsenal.

Try the all-meat diet for a few days (no more than three). Eat nothing but meat and drink plenty of water. (The Dukan Diet uses this technique for one day a week during maintenance, and it suggests going back to the all-meat stage of the program for a few days if you ever get stuck on a plateau.) If you do this, don't try to make the meat too lean; a diet very high in lean meat without any fat can induce a condition known as "rabbit starvation." Doing this for a day or three poses very little risk for the vast majority of people, but you'll still feel better if your meat has some fat in it.

Do the Fat Fast. This is an Atkins technique, but it should be reserved for *only* the most metabolically resistant people who have been absolutely unable to move the scale any other way. It's based on the Kekwick and Pawan study in which researchers placed patients on a 1,000-calorie diet that was 90% fat and got better fat loss than on any other plan.[39] In the Atkins version, you eat only 1,000 calories, with 75% to 90% of it coming from fat. Atkins recommends five small meals of about 200 calories each. Sample 200-calorie choices include 1 ounce of macadamia nuts, 2 ounces of cream cheese or Brie, or 2 deviled eggs with 2 teaspoons of mayo. Atkins emphasizes that this is actually *dangerous* for anyone who is not metabolically resistant—the rate of weight loss is too rapid to be safe. Atkins used it only with people who could not lose weight any other way, to encourage them and to show them that weight loss was possible—but even then, he used it for only 4 or 5 days.

Exercise

What about Exercise?

Exercise is probably the most important predictor of whether you will keep weight off. Unfortunately, it doesn't really account for a great deal of the weight you will lose (maybe a few pounds a month), but if you don't do it, the odds of keeping the weight off tumble. Some lucky people are able to lose weight just by adding a lot of exercise to their daily routine without changing their diets much, but these are very rare people who usually don't have an awful lot of weight to lose.

That being said, there are many, many excellent reasons to begin an exercise program if you are not exercising already. The health benefits alone are legion, and exercise is one of the things that helps change your biochemistry to that of a leaner person. Exercise has an insulin-like effect on lowering blood sugar, it increases serotonin, and—except when very high-intensity—it decreases stress hormones.

Low-carb exercise gurus, such as Charles Poliquin, Robb Wolf, and Drs. Jade and Keoni Teta, recommend full-body circuit training for beginners (plus cardio interval training for all levels) as the ideal programs for low-carbers. I agree. These programs will maintain or even build a little muscle; yet they are not so overwhelmingly intense that you won't have the energy for them. You can supplement with cardio as you see fit: probably the more, the better. And don't worry about the fat-burning zone (see the following question). Just go as long and as hard as you can without exhausting yourself; or mix short, intense workouts with longer, slower ones.

Whatever you do, do *not* neglect weight training. Walking by itself is just not going to cut it as an exercise program for weight loss. Without using and challenging your muscles, you will lose them, slowly but surely, and that will slow down your metabolism. Weight training is the best way to boost a sluggish metabolism. The more muscle you have, the more calories you burn.

Do I Need to Exercise in the Fat-Burning Zone?

The need to exercise in the so-called fat-burning zone is a complete myth. You should exercise for as hard and as long as you safely and reasonably can, and go for the maximum amount of calories you can burn. It makes no real difference whether those calories come from fat or from sugar, any more than it matters if you pay for something with a check or with cash.

The average person uses about 70% fat and 30% sugar as "fuel" while they're sitting, sleeping, or relaxing. As they become more active, the percentages shift—the harder they exercise, the lower the proportion of fuel from fat and the higher the proportion of fuel from sugar. This is where the misunderstanding comes from. While the *percentages* of fuel do indeed change, so does the amount of calories burned. So, sure, at low levels of exercise, I'm burning about 70% of my calories from fat, but I'm burning only a couple of calories a minute! When I exercise harder, I may be burning only 40% fat, but I'm burning a lot more calories. Would you rather have 90% of all of my money or 10% of Donald Trump's?

I Have No Stamina for Exercise When I'm on a Low-Carb Diet. What Gives?

Lyle McDonald, one of the foremost experts on the ketogenic diet and author of a textbook in the field, works with many athletes, particularly bodybuilders. He believes that with very high-intensity exercise, the ketogenic diet can present a problem as far as energy goes. He therefore recommends that on exercise days you consume more carbohydrates than usual, then go back to your usual amount at the next meal. It's important to realize that he's talking only about super-high-intensity exercise. For more "regular" folks, a ketogenic—or any reduced-carb—diet will supply more than enough energy for circuit training, conventional weight training, and/or moderate aerobics. If it doesn't, it may be that you're not eating enough fat.

> *I've recently started both low-impact circuit training and a low-carb diet, and I haven't had any problems. As long as I don't overdo my workout, I have more energy than ever before.*
>
> *—Janice K.*

If, however, you still find that getting through your workouts is nearly impossible, try eating a small amount (5 to 25 grams) of carbohydrate about 30 minutes before your workout and see if that helps. If it does, you'll know that you are one of those people who need more carbs to work out effectively.

I'm a Runner and I Like to Run Races at My Local Runner's Club. I Thought "Carb Loading" Was a Must for Athletes. Can a Low-Carb Diet Work for Me?

Remember that the fuel you most want to use during endurance exercise is fat, not sugar. "Carb loading" simply ensures that your glycogen stores are full, which translates into using sugar for fuel. The better you are at fat-burning, the longer you'll be able to go. For what it's worth, Stu Mittleman, an exercise physiologist, nutritionist, ultramarathoner, and one of the greatest endurance athletes of all time, generally eats a diet of about 40% carbs, 30% protein, and 30% fat, but when he is in training for an event, he ups the *fat* to about 50%—not the carbs.

CHAPTER 11

Tricks of the Trade: The Top 50+ Tips for Making Low-Carb Work for You

I've put together more than fifty of the most useful tips for making low-carb eating a part of your life. The tips are organized into three categories—food and drink, motivation, and general. Occasionally, a tip in the "general" category may seem like it has nothing to do with low-carb eating, but believe me, if it's there, it has everything to do with making low-carb weight loss a success. Remember that no program that results in changing your body *and* your life can be based *just* around what foods to eat or not eat. We also need to know how to deal with the kinds of issues—boredom, anxiety, disappointment, failure, perseverance, and so on—that inevitably come up when we're talking about changing lifelong habits. By the way, before we get started, let me tell you the first and most important tip of all.

Don't Try to Do All the Tips

In low-carb dieting, as with many other things in life, you can easily and quickly get intellectually fatigued from information overload, a pitfall that causes many people to just throw up their hands and give up. Don't do this. Use the tips that make sense to you and that you can incorporate easily into your life. Don't worry about the rest. You can always go back and revisit them.

Now, let's get started!

Food and Drink

Drink Water

No kidding. This tip has been all over this book in various forms, including in the FAQ chapter, but it's so important that I'm going to stick it everywhere you might possibly see it. *Water can—and does—affect fat loss.* If you're on a ketogenic diet (Atkins induction phase, Protein Power phase 1, etc.), it's essential to flush out the ketones and waste products from the fat you're losing. Even if you're not on a ketogenic diet, it's essential to prevent constipation and to optimize kidney and liver function (remember that the liver is the main fat-processing factory in the body, and if it's not working properly, neither is fat metabolism). Eight glasses a day is the *minimum* and is not enough for most overweight people.

P.S.: If you need more motivation, water is number one in the antiaging arsenal of Dr. Nicholas Perricone, formerly of Yale University and the chairman of the International Conference on Aging and Aging Skin. Perricone says, "If I could teach my patients and students three things that would keep them forever young, they would be: one, drink water; two, drink water; and three, drink more water."

Watch Out for Protein Bars

Be careful with these. I definitely don't recommend them during the first 2 weeks, when you're adjusting to this new way of eating. For one thing, the market has been saturated with this new class of candy—I mean, snack food—and predictably, the bars vary in quality from complete junk to not so bad. Some of the best are Paleo Bar (available on my website, http://www.jonnybowden.com), Sears Labs' Omega-3 Zone (don't confuse them with the Zone bars found in every grocery store), and the Atkins bars, available everywhere. By the time you read this, there will undoubtedly be more. You can trust anything you find at http://www.rockwellnutrition.com, or on my own website, http://www.jonnybowden.com.

All protein bars are not created equal, and the term *energy bar* is a complete marketing scam. "Energy," in the parlance of nutrition, simply means "calories," but manufacturers want you to think that eating one of their bars will make you feel like running a marathon. Not so. In fact, most "energy" bars are loaded with carbs. Almost all have hydrogenated fats (trans-fats). Protein bars specifically have more protein and often fewer carbs, but you still have to read labels. Some are as high as 330 calories, not exactly snack food. In addition, they have sweeteners like sorbitol or mannitol, which are sugar alcohols that still need to be counted if you're counting carbs. Mannitol, especially, may give you gas. And even dear Dr. Atkins doesn't count the glycerine (also known as glycerol) when he tells you there's only 2 or 3 grams of effective carbs in his bars. That's controversial: glycerol—an odorless, colorless, sweet-tasting liquid—is used as a sweetener and is classified as a carbohydrate, but Atkins claims that because it does not impact blood sugar in the same way sugar does, it shouldn't be counted as part of the net (effective) carb content in his bars. Maybe; maybe not. Many low-carbers do find that it slows down their weight loss; others don't. In any case, stick with real food and hold off on the bars for a few weeks until you get your bearings in this new way of eating.

Consider Salmon for Breakfast . . . or Lunch or Dinner

I told you that not all tips would be applicable to all readers, but if you can make this one work, you'll reap a lot of results. Unfortunately, farmed salmon—which is what you'll get most often in restaurants—has all the problems other farm animals have. The fish are raised in pens, fed grain, and given antibiotics. As a result of the grain diet and the lack of exercise, their omega-3 fat content is not nearly as good as that of their wild brethren. However, with wild fish there is always the slight risk of mercury. So what to do? There are such huge benefits to eating salmon that I recommend it anyway. If you can get Alaskan wild salmon, that's great. Consider, however, some amazingly healthful varieties of canned salmon, which also taste delicious. The red sockeye kind is the best. You can get my *absolute* favorite, the hard-to-find gourmet Vital Choice salmon (which is also the choice of many other well-known nutrition and health gurus), through a link on my website, http://www.jonnybowden.com. They even have a special "Dr. Jonny Introductory Package" of salmon fillets, the best canned tuna on the planet, and three different kinds of organic berries.

Eat Breakfast Every Day

When you skip breakfast, among the many other negative things that happen is that insulin release is greater at the next meal than it would otherwise have been. Blood sugar is destabilized. You're more likely to be subject to cravings. In all likelihood, you're running on empty and masking it with coffee. If you're one of those people who has no appetite in the morning, it's probably because you've just conditioned yourself to this unnatural way of eating. A good place to start with the rehabilitation of your appetite is with a protein shake. Even people who are not hungry in the morning can get one of these babies down, especially if it's delicious and made with good extras like berries or a tablespoon of peanut butter. Eventually, you should transition to a real-food breakfast (at least for most days), and make sure it contains protein and some good fats.

If you need some additional motivation: at least seven studies have found a correlation between being overweight and skipping breakfast.[1]

Memorize This: Water Retention Can Mask Fat Loss!

This is one of those paradoxical situations that doesn't make sense on the surface—the less water you drink, the more water you retain. Why? Because when not enough water is coming into the body, a hormone called vasopressin acts on the kidneys to tell them to reabsorb the existing water in the body rather than urinating it; another hormone, aldosterone, tells the body to conserve sodium, leading to more water retention. Other factors—such as medications, hormones, menstrual cycles, and birth control pills—can also affect water retention. So sometimes your body is actually dropping fat, but because you're holding on to water, you might not notice it on the scale. Once again, the best advice is to keep drinking water.

Shop for Color

I read the women's magazines all the time to stay up-to-date on the kind of nutrition information being disseminated (I read the men's magazines too—but only, of course, for the articles.) One of the very best tips I ever read was this one: shop for color. If you don't want to memorize a whole bunch of antioxidants and proanthocyanidins and phytochemicals, the easiest way to ensure you're getting the best nutritional bang for your money is to look at what the contents of your cart look like on the checkout counter. Does it resemble one of those great postcard pictures of a European outdoor market? It should be overflowing in greens, reds, oranges, and even blues. All those colorings in fruits and vegetables are there because they are natural antioxidants that will serve a similar purpose in your body. If everything you buy is the color of cardboard, you're doing something wrong.

Shop the Outside Aisles

Want to magically reduce the number of calories you're eating from sugar, processed foods, and junk carbohydrates? Here's a simple trick: step away from the inner aisles of the supermarket. All the good stuff is on the outside. Spend your time in the periphery of the supermarket. (It also seems to be the secret to a good singles pickup; after all, no one ever turned to a stranger to ask, "How do you tell if this cereal box is fresh?")

Carry Protein-Rich Snack Food with You

Forget the vending machines, the airport kiosks, and the 7-Eleven stores. Start thinking of snack food in terms of real food, and start thinking of real food in terms of *protein* (and fat)—just what your hunting and gathering ancestors would most likely have been munching on while taking a break from stalking wild game. Think nuts, cheese (string cheese is a great choice), hard-boiled eggs, jerky, or some leftover chicken in a plastic bag. You can occasionally add a piece of fruit to the mix if your particular plan permits it, but what you *can't* do is grab a bag of chips or pretzels or a chocolate chip cookie—not if you want to get or stay slim!

STARBUCKS GOES "LOW-CARB"

In an example of low-carb going mainstream without much fanfare, Starbucks—which previously offered only extremely high-calorie, high-carb products, now offers a number of food items suitable for low-carbers, including nuts, cheese, and fruit.

My personal favorite is the high-protein snack plate to go, which is just about the best "mini-meal" I've seen in a large chain store. It beats just about any snack I've seen around, and I sometimes "re-create" it using my own ingredients when I want a high-protein meal of less than 300 calories.

The Starbucks "High Protein" meal-to-go consists of a whole egg, some grapes, some cheese, and a mini whole-grain bagel and peanut butter. Total calories: 260, with 13 grams of protein, 4 grams of fiber, and 9 grams of fat.

Now that's a healthful "fast-food" option!

Buy Some Cookbooks

If I had a mere nickel for every client who asked me "What can I eat?" or who complained of being bored with the same old choices, I would be one very rich nutritionist! The answer to the question became abundantly clear to me while researching this book. There are dozens—I mean dozens—of amazing cookbooks and recipes out there for virtually every level of ability and interest in cooking, from complete novice (me) to gourmet chef. (I've listed some cookbooks in Resources, and there are more coming out every month. I myself have written five with my coauthor, chef Jeannette Bessinger, and although they are not low-carb cookbooks per se, you'll find a lot of delicious recipes in there that keep sugar and junk ingredients to an absolute minimum.) In addition, virtually all websites with a low-carb bent have recipe sections, some of them incredibly diverse and interesting. There's a *lot* more to low-carb eating than just chicken and vegetables.

Don't Do Anything Else While You're Eating

You're trying to bring mindfulness and consciousness to the table when it comes to eating so that you can reduce some of the automatic eating that takes place when you're thinking about other things. A good way to do that is to make eating time *eating time*, not reading-the-paper time or watching-television time. The more you can do this, the better, and the less likely you are to consume food while you barely notice you're consuming it!

Eat Slowly and Savor Every Bite

Here's another tip you can file under "Grandmother knew best." The fact is that chewing your food slowly and thoroughly, putting your fork down between bites, and actually *enjoying* what you're eating can help you lose weight. Here's why. The brain doesn't really get the message "Hey, he's full!" from the stomach until about 20 minutes after you've eaten enough. That's how long it takes for the hormone CCK to do its job and signal "Enough!" to the brain. So fast eaters frequently overeat before their brain gets the signal that they're not really hungry anymore. You can go a long way toward enhancing natural appetite control by taking advantage of your body's excellent communication network, but you need to give it enough time to work! Also, eating slowly and actually *experiencing* your food works against the kind of unconscious, mindless eating that caused you to put on weight in the first place.

Eat the Bulk of Your Food Earlier in the Day

Nutritionist Adelle Davis used to say, "Eat breakfast like a king, lunch like a prince, and dinner like a pauper." She was right. One important study showed that when people were fed a 2,000-calorie meal for breakfast (and nothing else during the day), they lost weight, but when they were fed the exact same meal at night, they gained.[2] Spread your food out during the day to control your blood-sugar and insulin levels, but try not to eat too much in the evening.

Add Yogurt or Kefir to Your Daily Program

Cultured milk products restore healthful bacteria to your body and are usually well tolerated even by people who have problems with dairy. You need to eat the *plain yogurt* with the *real live cultures* (not the junk food with the tons of fruit on the bottom). Even better, use kefir. Here's the deal with the carb content: it's not as high as the package says. In fact, for ½ cup of yogurt, kefir, or buttermilk, you need to count only 2 grams of effective carbohydrate!

How can this be? It's because of the way the government measures carbs. They measure everything in the food—water, ash, protein, fat—and then assume that what's left is carbohydrate. This works fine for almost everything, including milk, but it doesn't work for *fermented* milk products. As Dr. Jack Goldberg of GO-Diet fame points out, when you ferment milk, you inoculate it with lactic-acid bacteria, which then "eats up" almost all of the milk sugar (lactose) and converts it into lactic acid, the stuff that curds the milk and gives the product its unique taste. So the milk *sugar* that the government thinks is left in the product is really just about gone—it's been "converted" in the fermenting process by the lactic acid bacteria. The "real" amount of carbohydrate left in ½ cup of plain yogurt or kefir is only 2 grams—this has been measured by Goldberg in his own lab. I recommend that you get the full-fat variety of kefir or yogurt and enjoy it almost daily.

Repeat After Me: Fruit Juice Is Not—and Never Was—a Health Food

One of the many triumphs of marketing by the giant food conglomerates was convincing America that fruit juice is good for you. There are ads that proclaim proudly that some stupid sugar-laden soft drink is actually 10% real fruit juice. Fruit juice is *not* fruit (and for carb addicts, even fruit itself has to be watched, at least in the beginning). Fruit juice is, plain and simple, junk food. It's loaded with sugar, it has none of the fiber of real fruit, it has a high glycemic load, and it contributes absolutely nothing of value to your diet except for a few measly vitamins that you can easily get elsewhere.

Eat Protein at Every Meal

Every single meal should have protein in it. Ideally, so should every snack (but see "Choose Your Battles" on page 328). Protein has less of an effect on insulin than carbs do, is more satisfying,[3] and requires more energy (calories) to break down and assimilate. The body recognizes protein (and fat) as something that you have a need for; therefore, the appetite-control mechanisms that send messages from your gut to your brain signaling that you've had enough food work well with protein (something they do not do with carbohydrates, as we saw in chapters 3 and 4). A greater ratio of protein to carbohydrate at a meal stabilizes blood sugar and reduces insulin response.[4] And research suggests that *leucine*, an amino acid found in protein, specifically helps you to maintain muscle mass while losing body fat during weight loss.[5]

WebMD Recommends Steak?

In what has to be considered the ultimate "turnaround," the ultra-conservative WebMD recently published an article called "Bad Foods that Are Good for Weight Loss."* Eggs and steak were at the top of the list.

Just remember that while both foods are indeed great for weight loss, commercial meat may not be so great for your health. Get the weight-loss benefits of protein by choosing grass-fed meat and cage-free eggs!

*http://www.webmd.com/diet/slideshow-bad-foods-that-are-good-for-weight-loss

---

"All-Natural" Doesn't Mean All-Good

Another triumph of the marketers was convincing us that "natural" on a food label actually *means* something. The term *all-natural* is a wholly unregulated, utterly meaningless term. Anyone can use it on anything. What's all-natural about frozen dinners, "energy" bars, or even cut-up chicken parts in the meat section of your supermarket? You mean they were "naturally" fed a diet they normally wouldn't eat, fed "natural" antibiotics, and then all by themselves just "naturally" morphed into chicken parts in little yellow "all-natural" Styrofoam containers? Forget the term *natural.* Toxic mushrooms are all-natural, and so is crude oil, but we don't eat those. Look for *real food,* preferably without a bar code. Think about what you could have hunted, fished for, gathered, plucked, or grown if you were with your original ancestors on the savanna. *That's* natural food. Eat it.

Replace Grains with Greens

There are lots of reasons why grains may not be the most healthful food in the world for most people. Grains contain little vitamin C and no vitamin A, and two of the major B-vitamin deficiency diseases are almost exclusively associated with excessive grain consumption.[6] Fiber—with very few exceptions—is present in paltry amounts in most processed grain products like cereals and breads and, in any case, can be gotten from vegetables and other sources. Though some people do okay with grains, if you've got a weight problem, you are probably not one of them. Get your carbohydrates from vegetables, at least most of the time. C. Leigh Broadhurst, PhD, author of *Diabetes: Prevention and Cure,* once told me that if she could have her overweight and diabetic clients make only a single change, the one that would have the most impact on their lives would be to remove wheat from their diets. Think about it. (And while you're thinking about it, go back and read chapter 4!)

Bring Your Own (Food, That Is)

One problem for a lot of my clients is that they don't know how to stay on their eating plan once they're out and about, running around, or stuck at the office. That's probably because the whole world is set up for quick-and-easy junk food, and chicken breasts don't fit in a vending machine. Don't be a victim of circumstance. Take control of your own life. Start thinking about packing your own lunches, or at the very least your own snacks. Bodybuilders have been doing it for decades. You can, too.

Use Green Drinks

Green drinks is the general category name for juices from barley, wheatgrass, or any combination of whole green foods. Green drinks pack an incredible nutritional wallop and usually have amazing phytonutrient and vitamin profiles. They are very alkalizing (and are thus a terrific balance to a higher-meat diet), they're usually made from organic sources, they're very low in calories, and most have no more than 3 to 4 grams of (low-glycemic) carbohydrate, an insignificant amount unless you are on the strictest of induction-stage diets (and even then, you can work them in). You can find them in most health-food and whole-food supermarkets, and you should definitely consider making them part of your program. My personal favorite is Barlean's Organic Greens.

Consider Eggs Rocky-Style

That's right. Raw eggs. I put two in a glass just about every day and drink 'em down. When I tell my clients this "tip," most look at me like I just stepped off a spaceship, but here's the deal: *there is no more perfect food on earth, and there is no more healthful way to eat it.* Dr. Joe Mercola says, "Raw whole eggs are a phenomenally inexpensive and incredible source of high-quality nutrients that many of us are deficient in, especially high-quality protein and fat." He also believes that the reason eggs are often allergenic is that they are cooked: heating the egg protein changes its chemical shape, which can lead to allergies. When consumed raw, the incidence of egg allergy virtually disappears. One great way to consume them—if you don't want to drink them straight—is in a protein shake. It'll add a creamy, delicious texture to the drink and beef up the protein and nutrient count.

What about salmonella? Well, first of all, understand this: the risk of getting an egg contaminated with salmonella is 1 in 30,000.[7] Second, nearly all of those contaminated eggs come from sick hens; if you get organic, free-range (and preferably omega-3-enriched) eggs, the risk virtually disappears. Third, even if you get it—and you probably won't—salmonella is a relatively benign, self-limiting illness in healthy people.[8] Ninety-four percent of those who get it don't even see a doctor.[9] And before you dismiss the idea of a raw egg or two as just too weird, remember how an egg cream was made at virtually every soda fountain in the world back in the "old days": chocolate syrup, seltzer, milk, and a raw egg!

Use Cabbage Leaves for "Bread"

You could use lettuce leaves, but red cabbage is stronger. You can make a "sandwich" (or a grain-free "wrap") of virtually any meat you like—deli turkey, real turkey, chicken, even a hamburger—by wrapping it in a big, hard leaf of cabbage or an outer leaf of lettuce. Try chicken with a few avocado slices or beef with tomato. Consider using this tip in conjunction with "Bring Your Own"!

Get a Coffee Grinder and Use It for Flaxseeds

This is just an all-around great health tip in general, but it can be especially useful to low-carbers for the following reason: flaxseeds (as opposed to flaxseed oil) are a significant source of fiber, which is not only protective against diseases like colon cancer but is also demonstrably related to weight loss. Fiber blunts blood-sugar response and adds to a feeling of fullness. At least a dozen clinical studies demonstrate the effect of fiber on weight loss. In addition, flaxseeds are one of the best sources of the omega-3 fat ALA (alpha-linolenic acid), which has documented heart-protective effects as well as being anti-inflammatory. Inflammatory chemicals (cytokines) are produced, among other places, in the fat cells, so the more fat cells you have, the higher your level of inflammation is likely to be. All in all, freshly ground flaxseeds are a terrific addition to your program. I use Barlean's FortiFlax on everything, from oatmeal to veggies, and even throw a spoonful or two in my protein drinks.

Sardines: The Health Food in a Can

You simply cannot beat sardines as a quick, easy, inexpensive source of first-class protein and omega-3 fats. I learned the usefulness of sardines as a fast and easy pick-me-up when I was traveling in Florida with the famous New York nutritionist Oz Garcia and giving seminars. We had a brutal schedule and almost no time between events to grab anything to eat. Whenever Oz felt his blood sugar dropping or his energy flagging, he would stop and run into the nearest convenience store or bodega and grab . . . *a can of sardines!* I learned firsthand how energizing and satisfying this food can be, right out of the can! If your particular low-carb program permits it, eat sardines with some low-carb, low-sugar crackers like Wasa bread. If you're in somewhat more relaxed circumstances than we were, sardines over any kind of green salad makes the perfect low-carb meal. The best kind (if you can find them) are packed in sardine oil. Do not buy the kind in soybean or cottonseed oils, as these are way too high in omega-6s.

When Eating Out, Send Back the Bread

Don't even let the waiter put it down. If it sits there, two things can happen to it—you can eat it, or you can *not* eat it. If you send it back, you eliminate the first possibility.

Eat Almonds—but Portion Them Out

Nuts are a great addition to the low-carb lifestyle—but they can also slow weight loss because they are so easy to overeat and are so high in calories. If you're going to eat them during the weight-loss phase of your program, divide them into appropriate portions. Fifteen almonds is a portion. If you buy those big convenience bags, don't take the whole bag with you to "snack" on—portion out your serving, put it in a little bag, and put the rest away.

Craving Sugar? Try Sautéed Almonds

Here's a neat treat that'll satisfy a craving for dessert: sauté some raw almonds in butter, or bake them and melt a little butter on top. Use a bit of sea salt if you like. Remember to watch the portion size (see previous tip).

Try This Super Craving Buster

Mix together 1 tablespoon each of sesame tahini and organic soy miso, and use the mixture as a spread on celery, lettuce, or even low-carb crackers like Wasa. It'll satisfy cravings and help reduce mineral deficiencies.

Crave-Bust with This Amino Acid

A tablespoon of powdered glutamine (an amino acid) sweetened with xylitol and dissolved in a tablespoon or two of heavy cream or half-and-half will disarm even the most demanding sugar craving.

Do Damage Control with Pasta

You don't have to give up pasta forever, especially once you're at your goal weight. But lower the glycemic load significantly by cooking it al dente. The less time you boil it, the more the long chains of starch molecules in the pasta remain closely packed, making it difficult for enzymes to break them down and thus lowering the impact the pasta has on your blood sugar. Better yet, get one of the new lower-carb, higher-fiber pastas and cook *that* al dente.

> *Giving up sugar was almost as hard as quitting smoking, but after about three months I found I didn't crave it anymore, and I felt 100% better.*
> *—Patricia M.*

Here's a Way to Become a Vegetable Lover Instantly

Even the most ardent antivegetable person is won over by a plate of roasted vegetables. Take a bunch of veggies—all kinds of peppers and root vegetables like carrots, parsnips, beets, and onions respond well to this method— cut them up, and arrange them in a roasting pan. Drizzle with olive oil and put 'em in the oven for 30 or 40 minutes. The roasting brings out sweetness and flavor you never knew existed.

Read Labels and Be a Sugar Detective

Manufacturers are required to list ingredients in order of amount; the first ingredient makes up the largest proportion of the product, and the last ingredient is present in the lowest proportion. Most manufacturers don't like saying that sugar is the main ingredient, even if it's true. So they label their products with small amounts of a ton of different forms of sugar—sucrose, glucose, corn syrup, corn sweetener, dextrose, fructose, lactose, maltodextrin, invert sugar, concentrated fruit juice, sorbitol, xylitol, mannitol, barley malt, malt extract, and the absolute worst of all, high-fructose corn syrup. By putting in small amounts of a mix of these, they can legally disguise the fact that the main ingredient in the packaged food you are holding is . . . sugar! If you want to know how many teaspoons of added sugar is in a food you are eating, just divide the number of grams of sugar on the label by 4. You'll be amazed to find that some cereals have 7 teaspoons of sugar per serving, and those serving sizes are tiny!

Watch Those "Legal" Desserts

Just because something is low-carb does not mean it is no-calorie and definitely does not mean you can eat unlimited amounts of it. Don't make the same mistake the low-fat dieters did when they consumed massive amounts of junk food, thinking it was perfectly okay because it was low-fat. There are plenty of delicious low-carb desserts, and it's nice to be able to have them once in a while, but if they trigger eating binges, then step away from the dessert! It's also not a good thing if they start to replace real food regularly (same problem with low-carb bars).

If You Need Dessert, Ask for Cheese and Berries or Berries and Cream

This is the dessert I see most of my "low-carbing colleagues" order when we go out. If you like, you can bring along some stevia or Truvia (which comes in single-size serving packages) and sweeten the berries just for good measure. Xylitol works equally well, but it's hard to find in a single-serving packet. Even better is to gradually come to appreciate the natural flavor and sweetness of the berries without any sweetener added.

Motivation

Keep a Journal

Virtually all of the successful low-carbers I interviewed for this book routinely kept food diaries, and journaling is one of four key behaviors consistently cited as a winning strategy by people who were successful in losing weight (at least 30 pounds, kept off for at least a year) in the National Weight Control Registry. It's also probably the one technique that every specialist, no matter where they stand on the "dieting" spectrum, recommends.

In my own "Unleash Your Thin" program, (available on my website, www.jonnybowden.com), the journal is an absolutely essential part. Here's why. You can't change something unless you know what it is you're changing—keeping records of what you're eating allows you to see what's working and what's not; it allows you to track changes in your eating behavior against changes in your weight (and energy, mood, and sleep); and it causes you to be aware of what you're eating, which keeps you rigorously honest.

In addition, for those who are so inclined, the journal can also be a terrific tool for self-discovery, and has been for many great artists throughout time. (Julia Cameron's *The Artist's Way* is based on this concept and has been a perennial bestseller since it was first published in 1992.) You can add recollections of the day's events as well as notations about your feelings, your moods, your resentments, your anxieties, and your joys. But don't feel you *have* to—all you really need to do to make this work from a weight-loss perspective is to keep a record of what you eat and drink—every single day. You don't have to do it forever, but the more you do it, the more successful you are likely to be.

Visit a Support Community Online

One of the best things about the Internet—besides instant messaging—is the way it has allowed people with similar interests to form long-distance communities of support and information sharing. We have a support board just for "Unleash Your Thin," and I've seen dozens of excellent community support boards scattered throughout the low-carb community. Take a look. You'll find bulletin boards with posts from people just like you (no matter what level you're at, your particular interest or concern, how much weight you have to lose, your age, or how sophisticated or unsophisticated you are about this stuff). If you don't like the first one you go to, just pick another; eventually, you'll find one where you feel at home.

Many of the low-carb sites also have links to the diet journals, called diet blogs, of people just like you who have been successful at losing weight.

Expect Stalls and Plateaus

There is no one on the planet who has lost weight who hasn't experienced these. They're a natural part of weight loss. Think of them as your body's way of "catching up" with the changes you're introducing to your lifestyle, kind of like a "reset" of the thermostat. They can occur for a million different reasons (see "Plateaus," page 295), but the important point is that they *do* and *will* occur, and you will be better off if you're prepared so that you don't get thrown when they happen.

Find a Diet Buddy

This works for both exercise and dieting. It may even be the secret behind the success of personal training. If you have a commitment that involves another person, you are far more likely to actually *do* it. A diet buddy is like your committed listener. By stating your goals—saying out loud to another person what you're going to eat, do, or accomplish today (or this week, or whenever)—you are giving your word a much greater reality than it might have if all you did was make a vague promise to yourself. And with the omnipresence of the Internet, there is no longer any reason not to take advantage of this secret dieting weapon. You can find a diet buddy anywhere, and you can set up the ground rules to include "check-ins" as frequently as you both need. I've seen this tip work time and time again with both exercise *and* diet, and I recommend it highly.

Don't Let Yourself Get Too Tired, Angry, Hungry, Lonely, or Bored

Emotional eating is a huge factor in weight gain, as most people reading this book know. In many ways, it is virtually impossible to separate the emotional component from the physiological components. All of these states of being—anger, sleep deprivation, hunger, loneliness, and boredom, not to mention anxiety, fear, nervousness, and stress—have been known to trigger overeating, nervous eating, comfort eating, or binge eating. The best cure in this case is a healthy dose of prevention.

Give Yourself a Nonfood Treat

Remember that changing your lifestyle is about breaking some old habits and replacing them with more empowering ones. One of the mental habits most in need of overhaul is telling yourself that food is your only reward and comfort. That doesn't mean there won't be a place in your life for comfort food or recreational eating, but you need to increase your repertoire of things that make you feel good.

Start looking for things that make you feel good besides food, and start finding time to do them! Give them to yourself as a reward, either for reaching a weight-loss goal or just for the hell of it. (I had one client who cut out a picture of the Armani suit he was going to buy when his waist got down to a 34 and put it on his refrigerator.) It might be a trip to a day spa, a manicure, some time on the golf course, reading a beach novel, or going to a museum. Better yet, take a tip from Julia Cameron's *The Artist's Way* and make a "play date" with yourself: just you, doing whatever you want, no agenda, no greater purpose than to have fun. It doesn't have to be an all-day deal. It would be really great if you could come up with a number of *little* things you could do that don't take a lot of time and that can be incorporated into your daily life—take a bath or spend some time meditating or even listening to one absolutely great song from the disco era ("To Be Real" brightens almost every day). When you feel the need to compulsively dig into the cookie jar, start to train yourself to substitute one of these nonfood treats. You'll be conditioning a new repertoire of behaviors that has nothing to do with food.

Focus on the Weight You Have Lost and Kept Off—and Remember "the Bowden Equation"

Focus on the weight you've lost rather than the weight you still have to lose. Focus on your successes rather than your "failures." And while you're at it, stop thinking of what hasn't happened yet as a "failure." Much better to reconceptualize those unmet goals as "challenges." I can't tell you the number of times I have seen a weight-loss effort bite the dust because the person continued to focus on how far she had to go rather than how far she'd come. Many studies have shown that weight-loss expectations tend to be greatly out of sync with what can realistically be attained. For example, most obesity programs consider the loss of 10% of original body weight a success, but when clients who are entering the program are asked what *they* think would be a successful outcome, they typically say that anything less than 25% would be a failure. This does not mean you should set your sights low—not at all. (Take a look at some of the before-and-after pics of real-life low-carb dieter—you can find tons of them on Google. They're amazing!) You can do this, too. But if you're expecting to lose 7 pounds a week consistently, you are going to be very, very disappointed, and if you are disappointed, you are going to feel like you failed—and if you feel like you're failing, you're much more likely to give up.

Remember my famous "Bowden Equation": *disappointment* equals the difference between *expectation* and *reality*. If you focus on the weight you have lost so far—even if it's a pound or two—you will be way better off in the long run and much more likely to keep going. Even better, focus on nonscale-related benefits, such as how you feel, lack of bloat, increased energy and well-being, lack of headaches, no more brain fog, or, best of all, lost inches and a changing shape. Remember that you lose weight exactly the same way you put it on—one pound at a time.

If You Get Stuck, Do Something Different

While stalls and plateaus are to be expected, they can be very frustrating. You may need to do something counterintuitive to start weight loss back up again. Some people have found that, strangely enough, adding *more* carbs gets things going again. Or try the Fat Fast outlined in Atkins or an "all-meat" day outlined in the Dukan Diet. Alternatively, go the other route and try a fruit-and-vegetable fast for a few days. None of these techniques will hurt—the fruit-and-vegetable one will probably do a lot of good—and any one of them may push you off a stall.

Take the Word "Cheating" Out of Your Vocabulary

Cheating implies lying or dishonesty. It's much more empowering to think about the low-carb lifestyle in terms of being "strict" or "not so strict." You may have some days when you are "not so strict." More than one very successful low-carber told me he would occasionally have days when he just had to have pizza, so he did. Then he'd get back on the "strict" track at the next meal. Usually, he didn't lose much momentum, and over time, the occasional lapse became meaningless. These people still lost a ton of weight over time by being strict more often than they were "not so strict."

Look in the Mirror and Talk to Yourself

Here's a tip from Dr. Jack Goldberg, who is clearly of the tough-love school of weight loss. He says that you shouldn't be angry with yourself if you lapse from your diet. Just look at yourself in the mirror and say the following to your image, in a loud voice so you can really hear yourself: "*Are you serious about losing weight? Then I don't want this to happen again. You are not a child. Grow up and take responsibility for yourself. There was no reason to eat that unhealthful junk.*"

Alternatively, you could use a more gentle, accepting approach and say to yourself something like this: "I'm human, and I love and accept myself, even if I don't always live up to my own high standards. I stand for having a good life in a healthy body. What I did (or ate) isn't in line with that, but now I'm willing to let it go and move on."

Whichever approach you take, remember that each new meal is an opportunity for a new decision, and you don't have to wait until "tomorrow" to start again!

General Tips

Read a Book

Actually, that's good advice for life in general, but it's essential for low-carbing. I've had dozens of people tell me they were "on Atkins," yet they had absolutely no idea what Atkins really said and had heard only diluted information third hand from their hairdresser. Obviously you're not averse to the act of reading, or you wouldn't have bought this book, so in a sense I'm preaching to the choir. But let *this* book whet your appetite for more info. Although you can clearly do the basic low-carb approach outlined in chapter 9 and get great results, one (or more) of the structured programs discussed in this book may have spoken to you in some way or piqued your interest. Consider my discussions of the diet programs in chapter 9 like CliffsNotes. Find a plan that appeals to you and invest in the book itself—it will give you far more detail, you'll know how to do the program correctly, and you'll probably learn a lot in the bargain. Even if you don't wind up sticking with that exact program, it'll give you a great jumping-off point.

Take Your Measurements

You want to know where you're starting from so that you can monitor your progress. Keeping your head in the sand accomplishes nothing. Many people lose inches before they lose pounds (or they lose both, which is even better). If you measure your waist, at the very least you'll be able to track changes that may be happening independently of the scale, and that can be a big motivator during those times when your actual weight doesn't move (and there *will* be those times—see "Plateaus," page 295). Measuring your chest, waist, hip, upper thigh(s), and upper arm(s) is best. Don't look for a significant change in measurement every week, but check in every now and again to see how far you've come. You won't be able to do that if you don't measure first!

Use the Scale

Yup. This suggestion meets with a lot of protest, so let's first deal with the objections. Many people, especially those who have suffered eating disorders in the past, have experienced the tyranny of the scale and have been obsessive about using it, driving themselves crazy in the bargain. For these people, throwing the scale out—and relying on how they feel and how they look—has been nothing short of a psychic liberation. I get that.

But here's the thing: there's a way to use the scale as an ally, as a means to an end, as a tool for empowerment. First of all, you have to get that the readout is just a number and not make it "mean" anything other than what it is. That number is not a statement about your self-worth, who you are, or anything else—*it's just the number of pounds you weigh at the moment.*

Second, you have to realize that, imperfect as it may be, the scale is your reality check. I've seen clients assume that they *must* have lost weight because they jogged that day or, conversely, that they gained all kinds of tonnage because they over-ate at the family barbecue. Don't kid yourself. Check in with the scale. Sure, you may gain some muscle while you're losing fat, and that won't be reflected on the scale, but eventually fat loss *will* be reflected in that digital readout! Using the scale also keeps you accountable and honest: if you see your weight go up the morning after you did some midnight pigging out, it's a good lesson in associating cause and effect. And don't think for a minute that you won't feel great when you finally see the scale move toward your goal, even if it is a pound at a time.

Speaking of the Scale, Use It the Right Way

Don't compare your weight on different scales at different times of day (like how much you weighed at the doctor's office versus how much you weighed at the gym). Scales are like clocks: no two agree perfectly; but if you keep checking the same one, it will accurately tell you how much time is passing. I recommend daily weigh-ins. There are two rules to using the scale correctly. One, always do it in the morning, wearing no clothes, before eating. Let that number be your reference. Two, average the results of the week. There are simply too many variables that can be responsible for a half-pound to pound variation, day to day, and it can make you crazy to see these minor variations (especially when they're in the wrong direction). Use the totals for the week to compute where you're going. (With all that said, some people may find daily weigh-ins emotionally just too tough. If that's you, at the very least do a weekly weigh-in, which will help you stay on track and prevent you from obsessing too much about the numbers.) Incidentally, I have seen clients of mine completely transform their weight loss results simply by making everyday weigh-ins a part of their program.

Eat Before You Shop for Food

Ever go shopping when you're hungry? Then you know why people buy things like chocolate-covered artichokes. *Anything* sounds good when you're starving. When you're hungry is *not* the time to hit the supermarket. You won't make any kind of rational decision about food. Much better: go after you've eaten, when your choices won't be dictated by a growling stomach and a craving brain.

Get a Calorie/Carb Counter

This is just part of the overall mandate for conscious eating. *You need to know what's going into your body.* It will keep you honest. If you're counting carbs, a carb counter is a must. It's nice to know the calorie, protein, and fat content as well. A good carb counter will provide information on net carbs, calories, protein, fat, fiber, and glycemic load rating (where applicable). Both Atkins and Protein Power have very good pocket carb guides, and new "carb counters" come out all the time. (I personally like *The Ultimate Guide to Accurate Carb Counting* by Gary Scheiner, MS.)

Get Enough Sleep

There is no way to overstate the effect sleep can have on your weight-loss efforts. Sleep, and lack of it, affects the body in several ways. One, lack of sleep is a stressor. Stress raises cortisol, which in turn sends a message to the body to store fat around the middle. (Chronically high levels of cortisol also produce a counter response from the body in the form of insulin release.) Two, the absence of deep, restful, restorative sleep prevents the body from building up a reserve of serotonin. Low serotonin states are associated with cravings and overeating (not to mention good old garden-variety depression). Three, without deep, restful sleep, your pituitary will not produce any significant amount of growth hormone, which assists in the building of muscle and the loss of fat. Fourth, lack of sleep causes people to be hungry and to overeat during the day.

Some experts feel so strongly about the role of a full night of uninterrupted sleep in successful weight loss that they will even prescribe medications (typically trazadone, brand name Desyrel) to regulate sleep patterns. They feel that you are much better off taking a fairly innocuous medication than you would be with not getting enough sleep. Sleep is so important I devoted an entire section to it in my book, *The Most Effective Ways to Live Longer*. Here's the bottom line: Lack of sleep will make you fat, and it will make you unhealthy—in more ways than you imagine. Pay attention to it. The old saying "I'll sleep when I'm dead" is for idiots.

Volunteer

Nothing contributes to your own life more than contributing to the lives of others. Too many of us have made weight our sole focus for too long. Try putting the focus on others. Choose an activity in which your weight is of no significance, like putting in some volunteer time in a hospital or an animal shelter, moderating an Internet group, mentoring a kid, or even helping out a friend or family member with a yard sale. Get out of the house and get out of your head. It'll help keep things in perspective.

Buy or Rent an Exercise Video (Then Use It!)

One great thing about living in a city is that there's always at least one video rental place, and virtually all of them carry exercise videos. There's a million of them, for every possible taste and style, from *Dancing to the Oldies* to entries from Kathy Smith, Jillian Michaels, and Denise Austin. Look around and you'll find everything from hardcore boot-camp stuff to the gentlest stretching. Try them on for size. If you're a beginner, just do one for a few minutes and watch yourself progress until you can do the whole thing. The best part of videos is that you don't have to be intimidated by anyone else in the class. And if you're not intimidated—and why in the world should you be, anyway?—there's always an exercise class at the local gym, YMCA/YWCA, or studio. Try one.

Clean Out Your Kitchen Cabinets and/or Your Refrigerator

Man, I can't tell you how many clients I've had who have lost weight just by doing this one thing! I call it *bulletproofing your environment*. In fact, whenever I go up a few pounds and need to lose it, this trick has been my salvation. For many people, the attitude about food—at least in the beginning, before they've really adopted this new Way of Life—is this: *if it's there, I'm gonna eat it*. Since a lot of our sabotage happens at night, when defenses are down (with television snacking or even midnight refrigerator raids), the best defense is a good offense. If it ain't there, you can't eat it. So get it out of there. That's not to say you couldn't get dressed, get in the car, go to the 24-hour convenience store, and buy some junk, but most of us won't go that far, even for a carb or sugar fix. We *will*, however, go as far as the freezer. So dump the junk from your house and give yourself an advantage. If you live with other people and this isn't really practical, try sectioning off parts of the fridge for your stuff and theirs, then think of the sections as truly separate. Pretend you're living with roommates who will get mad if you eat their food.

Stop Watching Television (Okay, Okay, Then Cut Back)

I know it seems like heresy to suggest this, but study after study has linked increased television watching with expanding waistlines,[10] not to mention the development of childhood obesity.[11] No one is quite sure exactly why, but it's true nonetheless. Speculation has ranged from the obvious—more TV watching means less activity and more snacking—to the slightly more subtle (the number of overt cues to eat that come with the commercials). Even the esoteric has been postulated, like the idea that certain brain states induced by staring aimlessly at the tube might be linked to a general slow-down of the metabolism.[12] Whatever. The bottom line is this: you watch more TV, you tend to be fatter. Try picking a few absolute favorites and then sticking with them. Watch them, enjoy them, then shut the TV off. And try turning it off when no one is watching it.

"Listening to Your Body": Not Always a Good Idea

Face it: our bodies lie. They're especially deceitful if we've been on the standard American diet for a long time. If we were back in the caveman days, eating only the food that was available to us by hunting, fishing, or gathering, our bodies would tell us exactly what we needed. Our sweet tooth, for example, was originally a great survival mechanism. It caused us to seek out sweet-tasting plants, which were generally safe to eat, and fruits, which we needed because we humans do not make our own vitamin C. Now that same sweet tooth causes us to roam the aisles of the 24-hour supermarket looking for cookies and ice cream. Our foolproof appetite regulators—such as *cholecystokinin*, the hormone that is released in the small intestine when our stomachs are full and we've had enough food—responds to protein and fat. It doesn't recognize carbohydrate very well, which is why it is so easy to overeat carbs.

So "listening to your body" may not always be such a great idea, as you can't count on it to tell the truth, especially when you begin this new way of eating. Our bodies often tell us what we *want*, which is a conditioned response, and confuse us by making us believe that it's what we *need*. They're not necessarily the same thing. We need to reeducate our bodies to tell us the truth, and we do that the same way we teach our kids to be honest—by training them. Once our bodies have been reconditioned to respond to real food, we can begin trusting them to give us reliable signals.

Finally . . .

If You Fall Off the Wagon

Don't let it be a big deal. Acknowledge that it happened, and just get back on, beginning with the very next meal.

CHAPTER 12

What We've Learned about Controlled-Carbohydrate Eating: Putting Together Your Program

S o, let's talk about putting together the perfect low-carb diet. The first step is to memorize the following: *there is no perfect diet.*

There's also no perfect dress size—the one that's perfect is the one that fits. If there's one nugget of truth that we can hang our collective philosophical hats on, it's the wisdom of the Romans: *De gustibus non disputandum est,* which means "Of taste, there is no disputing." Translated to the area of weight loss and diet, it means quite simply this: *everybody's different.* Each individual has his or her own emotional, psychological, and physical blueprint, as unique and special as fingerprints. No two people respond exactly the same way to anything—not to life, not to medicine, not to food, not to diet.

In interviewing dozens of people who have been low-carbing successfully for years, I was struck by the number of people who have done their own versions of programs discussed in this book, or who have come up with their own solutions, spins, and variations to make low-carbing work for them. Rick, for example, lost 50 pounds in 5 months by using the basic Atkins program, but he deviated from Atkins orthodoxy by drinking a glass of red wine per day right from the beginning and never bothering to check for ketosis. Laurie lost 144 pounds and went from a size 26 to a size 8 not by following any specific plan but by eating "only low-carb food, exercising every day, and, for the last 25 pounds, lowering the fat in my diet." Ari, who lost 50 pounds, did the Protein Power plan but monitored calories with an online diet tracker, making sure "not to go over 2,500 a day." Leigh—40 pounds, 10 inches down and still counting—is a strict lacto-ovo vegetarian and lost her weight on a pretty unusual low-carb diet without meat. She attributes her success to completely cutting out sugar in all forms. Carl, an award-winning amateur figure skater from Alaska, has dropped 116 pounds by lowering his carbs to 50–80 grams a day—higher on days he has to train hard—and carefully monitoring calories, which he keeps to about 1,500 to 1,800 a day. And Annie, a low-carber from England, lost 50 pounds on the Atkins program but found that she had to *increase* her carbs to continue losing weight. When she reached her goal weight, she switched to the Schwarzbein Principle.

Many people begin with a strict version of one of the programs discussed in this book and then "graduate" to a more customized variation of their own making. That is a terrific way to go for many people. The original structure serves a purpose, like training wheels on a bike. For some others, a program "off the rack" is going to fit them just fine and they can follow the recommendations of the plan precisely and get great results. Some of us are lucky enough to be able to buy clothes off the rack with no alterations. For most, custom tailoring will be necessary.

One-size-fits-all diets are finished. In the not-so-distant future, we will probably be able to determine, through a kind of functional genetics, which patients are most likely to respond to which medicines and nutrients and, possibly through some kind of metabolic/genetic/hormonal typing or through some kind of test not yet invented, who does better on what kinds of foods. But for now, we have only the low-tech way, a kind of informed version of trial and error: If it works, great. If not, move on to something else.

Low-Carb Is Not a Religion

Don't treat a low-carb lifestyle as a religion; it's much better to think of it as a *strategy*. Like any strategy, you use it to achieve a goal, and you use it until it stops working. Your goal may be to lose 10 pounds or 100, and to maintain that goal weight forever. Or your goal may be to live a healthier, richer life free of many of the risks from heart disease and diabetes that come with the standard American diet. In either case, or in *both* cases, you might find that you do much better on a more restricted plan, at least in the beginning. If that's the strategy that works for you, great. If you have less weight to lose and are less metabolically resistant, you may find that you get great results with a plan that is a little less restricted from the beginning, more like the second, ongoing weight-loss phase of some of the 3-phase plans (like Atkins, Protein Power, or Fat Flush). These plans allow anywhere between 40 and 90 grams of carbs per day. If you are already near your goal weight, don't have any serious problems with sugar metabolism, and simply want to improve your health and maintain your weight, the Zone, or the 3rd phase of one of the 3-phase plans, might be the perfect place for you. Find what works for you and do it. If it stops working, reassess.

Reassessment 101

Most people will lose weight on a low-carb program, whether it be on the restricted induction phase, the more lenient ongoing weight-loss phase, or a more general 50-gram-a-day starting plan. If you aren't losing any weight, or if your weight loss has stalled for more than a few weeks, it's time to go back to the drawing board.

You may be stalled because you need to reduce carbs further (say, to 20 to 30 grams). In some cases, it may even be because your carbs are a bit too *low*—remember, everybody's different! Equally likely is the possibility that your calories are too high, in which case you will need to begin measuring portions and keeping an eye on the amount of food you're taking in. You may have some nutrient or mineral deficiencies that could be slowing metabolic processes; consider at the very least supplementing with a high-quality multivitamin, essential fatty acids, and magnesium.

You may have sensitivities to some of the foods you are eating—a good game plan would then be to cut out all the usual suspects (especially wheat, dairy, and sugar) and see if the scale begins to move. Maybe you're sensitive to some of the sugar alcohols found in those low-carb protein bars—they've been known to stall weight loss in some people. So has the citric acid in diet sodas. The point is to be willing to experiment, fine-tune, and tweak your program. And in the words of Winston Churchill, "*Never give up!*"

Choose Your Battles

When you first begin low-carbing, don't allow yourself to be overwhelmed by too much information. It's especially easy to get caught up in the small battles among low-carb diet theorists about things like coffee, artificial sweeteners, diet sodas, sugar alcohols, protein bars, cheese, wine, and other minor areas of disagreement. Don't get sucked in. I've had clients who simply can't imagine giving up coffee; I tell them not to give it up. Same with diet sodas, wine, or even raspberry mocha–flavored coffee creamers! The important thing to remember is that you are trying to make changes on a *continuum*. The name of the game is *direction*, not *perfection*. If all that's standing between you and a more healthful low-carb diet is a couple of diet colas, keep the colas for now—maybe you'll give them up later (or maybe you won't). Learn to choose your battles. You don't have to do everything all at once.

Invest Time in the Kitchen

In 1970, we spent $6 billion on fast food. In the year 2000, we spent $110 *billion*—virtually 150% of the entire California budget deficit. (As of 2011, that figure had risen to an eye-popping $168 billion!) Fully 90% of the money spent on food in this country is spent on *processed* food. The typical American eats three fast-food burgers and four orders of fries *per week*. "We are," says Dr. Joe Mercola, "exchanging our health for convenience."

It's time to stop. Spend a little time in the kitchen. Prepare your own food. Make your own snacks. Cook your own breakfast. Begin to look at food as a *prescription drug*. As one Zone dieter on the Internet said, "Treating food in this new way is definitely a challenge and a learning experience—but it certainly beats my old way of eating that left me fat, tired, and depressed."

Junk Is Junk, High-Carb or Low-Carb

Americans' taste for simple solutions and a food industry more than willing to accommodate them could easily result in the following scenario: a vast, overweight population of "low-carbers" with swelling waistlines and skyrocketing health problems. A typical specimen of this committed "low-carber" strolls through Disneyland, one hand grasping a vat-size cup of sugar-free soda, the other holding any of a zillion "carbohydrate-free" snack foods yet to be invented—hot dogs on low-carb buns, low-carb *cotton candy*, low-carb candy bars, low carb-*popcorn*. You get the picture. And it's not pretty.

Cutting carbs is not enough. We have to cut the *junk*. We have to learn, unfortunately, that in most cases the food industry is not our friend. If "carb-free" becomes just another slogan like "low-fat" did and we become a nation addicted to carb-free, high-calorie, chemically enhanced junk food, we will have traded one idiotic notion for another, and our health will be in the same bad shape it was before.

This brings us to the question on the table: how *should* we proceed? What general principles can we extract from the collective wisdom of the diet authors discussed in this book and from the principles of controlled-carbohydrate eating that all subscribe to in one fashion or another? How can you put together a program that works for *your* life, that will allow *you* to lose weight, and that will promote and optimize *your* health for years to come?

Glad you asked.

Ten Simple Principles for a Successful Low-Carb Life

Principle #1: Begin with a 2-Week "Boot Camp" Period

Many of the diets discussed in this book make use of an initial restricted eating period of at least 2 weeks—what Atkins called the *induction phase*. This idea is common to many of the plans, and I recommend it highly and use it with my own clients all the time. During this time you do the following:

- Eat as much meat, poultry, and fish as you like.
- Eat unlimited vegetables.
- Eat as much of the healthful fats—butter, avocados, olive oil, coconut oil, fish oil—as you like. And, yes, "healthful fat" can include saturated

fat. But it doesn't include trans-fats or food that's been fried in reheated vegetable oil (i.e., almost all fast-food fare).

- Eliminate all *potatoes, rice, pasta, breads, cereals, and other starches and grains.*
- Eliminate sugar.
- Eliminate dairy.
- Eliminate alcohol.

Optional: the strictest version of this 2-week program also temporarily eliminates fruit. (On an "induction-lite" program, I allow my clients one or two small daily portions of berries, grapefruit, or an apple.)

You can have a cup or two of coffee, preferably organic; and if you like, you can sweeten your coffee with xylitol, stevia, or erythritol and lighten it with 2 tablespoons of cream. You need to drink *at least* 8 glasses of water a day, plus an additional 8 ounces for every 25 pounds of extra weight you are carrying. Hot water with lemon juice is fine, as are teas (green, black, oolong, white, and yerba matte). I personally do not object to caffeinated teas, though you are welcome to use herbals.

> *I always wondered why I felt tired after eating pasta and wide awake after eating meat. Now I know.*
> —Bill W.

If you prefer more specific guidelines for amounts, keep your protein portions to 3 to 4 ounces per meal and oils and butter to 4 tablespoons a day. Vegetables are essentially unlimited. You can eat 2 eggs a day with no problem, and you should use the whole egg, preferably from free-range chickens.

Principle #2: In the Beginning, Don't Be Concerned with Calories

First you want to make sure you're eating the right foods. There's plenty of time later to start fiddling with portion sizes. At this point in the game, I'm not concerned with calories; centering the diet on protein, fat, and fiber will generally cause you to be full before you've overeaten. For some lucky people, that's all that's necessary—calories will self-regulate. For most people, it will be necessary to deal with calories *if* weight doesn't come off (see principle #9).

Principle #3: Find Your Own Personal Level of Carb Restriction

Though to the nutritional establishment low-carb is low-carb, the truth is that low-carbing exists on a *continuum*. As you have seen, that can mean anything from the restrictive induction phase of Atkins (20 grams or less of carbs a day) to the much more lenient Zone (in the neighborhood of 150 grams a day for a man on a reduced-calorie program). That's a big range. Where you will fall on this continuum at any given time depends on a number of things:

- how metabolically resistant you are
- how much weight you have to lose
- how you feel, physically and mentally, at various levels of carb restriction
- whether your current strategy is working for you

I suggest you *begin* at about 50 grams of carbohydrate a day for the first week; use that as a baseline from which to determine whether the amount needs to be lower (or if you can tolerate more). If you're not into counting grams, simply eliminate all of the "forbidden foods" on the induction list (grains, starches, dairy, sugars, and fruits), and you will easily be where you should be to get good results without counting carbs.

> The whole concept of mindful eating—not doing twenty things while I was stuffing things into my face unconsciously— was really helpful to me. It just meant learning to put some time aside to actually enjoy and experience my food.
> —Melissa McN.

Principle #4: After the First 2 Weeks, Begin Adding Carbs Back Little by Little

After the initial "whoosh" of loss during the 2-week induction phase, your weight loss should stabilize, and you will probably wind up losing around 2 pounds a week. Some people find that they need to stay on an induction-phase eating plan to accomplish this, but most others can begin adding back *small* portions of foods on the "forbidden" list at this time. Virtually all of the plans agree on this principle and differ only on which foods should be added back and in what amounts. This is the place where you customize and individualize. I suggest that you constantly monitor how you feel, how you look, and what you weigh and, based on these factors, determine what can go back into your diet, as well as how much and how soon.

Principle #5: Add Back Foods According to the "Ladder of Desirability"

My suggestion is that you begin with low-glycemic fruits like berries. Some people will be able to add small amounts of cheese. Many will be able to add small amounts of nuts. (Remember that nuts and cheese, while perfectly okay for low-carb eating plans, are very dense in calories and very easy to overeat. When you get "stuck" at a plateau, it is often these foods that need to go first.) Grains should be the last on your "regular" diet to be added back in, if at all, and then only truly whole grains. The sprouted variety is best. Processed grains you can say good-bye to forever. Recreational foods include the ones we all know are not great for us but without which life would be just too boring—I include pizza, ice cream, and cheesecake on my list; you may have your own favorites. Obviously, they should be eaten infrequently!

Find the level of carbohydrate intake that suits you and allows you to keep losing consistently at a moderate rate (1 to 2 pounds a week, 3 at the most if you're very overweight), and stay at that level. Remember to expect plateaus and stalls (see page 295).

Principle #6: When You Add Back Foods, Add Them One at a Time and Watch for Reactions

One of the delightful unexpected "side effects" experienced by many low-carb dieters is that symptoms they've had for years—symptoms that are unrelated to weight—begin to clear up: notably headaches, allergic symptoms, inflammation, and assorted aches and pains. This is often because the low-carb diet, by its nature, eliminates many of the foods that are triggers for unrecognized food sensitivities as well as those that contribute to inflammation and pain (namely, grains—see chapter 4—and many of the omega-6 refined vegetable oils). When you begin to add back your carbs, don't do it haphazardly. Watch what you're adding, do it one food group at a time, and monitor yourself for any reactions. If you start to feel worse, the food you added back is not right for you. Dump it.

Principle #7: The Hard Work Begins with Maintenance

Difficult as it may seem, getting to a goal weight is not the really hard part. *Staying* there is. And, believe it or not, developing a strategy for maintenance can actually begin while you are still in the losing phase.

When I work with dieters on a weight-loss program, they inevitably ask me if they will have to "eat this way forever." Dieters who ask this question are invariably gritting their teeth and simply toughing it out, waiting to get to the goal so that they can relax and eat what they want. This is almost always a prescription for a disastrous result. You need to look at the weight-loss period as a kind of driver's ed for weight maintenance. The strategy you adopt for *losing* is like the strategy of an athlete training for an event; it's tougher and more rigorous than the "off-season" (maintenance). But every athlete also knows that getting to the top is only the first part of the journey; *staying there* is where the real action is.

So the answer to the question "Will I have to eat this way *forever?*" is "No."

But you *will* have to eat differently. To think that you can go back to eating the way you did when you got fat and get a completely different result is one definition of insanity. You will probably not have to be as restrictive and structured and disciplined as you have to be during the weight-loss phase, but you *will* have to be forever vigilant about preventing regain, which leads to principle #8.

Principle #8: Use the 4-Pound Rule

There will be times in life when recreational eating has an irresistible pull—weddings, birthdays, holidays, and just the plain old urge to get a couple of pizzas and beers once in a while. These situations do not have to be the end of the world; in fact, to never allow yourself these little pleasures would be a big mistake. The trick is to not allow these occasional "planned lapses" to generate a slide into chaos that culminates in a complete departure from the eating plan that allows you to keep your weight where you want it and maintain optimal health. So check in with the scale frequently. Choose a set number of pounds—let's use 4 as an example. If and when you see your weight climb 4 pounds above goal, immediately go back to your 2-week induction phase, and use that restrictive plan until you get back down to goal or even a couple of pounds under. Then you can go back to maintenance eating.

Principle #9: Don't Ignore Calories

Because some of the best-known low-carb plans do not make a big deal about calories (Atkins, Protein Power, Schwarzbein, Zone, Fat Flush, Paleo Solution, Unleash Your Thin), many people wrongly interpret this to mean that calories are irrelevant. No responsible low-carb author has ever said this. The lack of emphasis on calories per se has been because most of us believe that the regulation of hormones (namely insulin and glucagon) takes precedence over calorie-counting, which is an inefficient and unproductive (not to mention old-fashioned) way to lose weight.

This does *not* mean that calories don't count at all—they do. But the way calories behave in the human body is far more complicated than originally thought and way more individual than any formula could convey. (An interesting side note: When Dr. Jack Goldberg and Dr. Karen O'Mara first did a clinical test of their low-carb GO-Diet in a Chicago hospital, the person who lost the most weight on the diet consumed 1,200 calories a day—but the runner-up consumed 2,600!) Just as your level of carbohydrate restriction has to be determined by trial and error, so does your calorie intake.

> *The prejudice against fat people in the country is unbelievable. People always assume I have no self-control and they look at me like I'm somehow morally bankrupt.*
> *—Emma T.*

Many low-carbers have been stalled because, although they are eating all the right foods, they are just eating too darn many of them! This is where monitoring calories can come in handy. Though the point cannot be made strongly enough that each individual has to determine the appropriate number for his or her body, *in general*, women will lose on 1,200 to 1,400 calories per day and men on 1,500 to 1,800.

There will probably come a point at which it will be productive for you to know how many calories you are actually consuming so that you can make adjustments if necessary.

Principle #10: Low-Carb Doesn't Mean No-Carb

There is not a single low-carb diet writer who ever recommended a *no-carb* diet. You wouldn't know it from all the people who chatter on about their "all-protein" diet, but such a diet does not exist anywhere in the responsible literature. Low-carb diets restrict carbohydrates, sometimes to very low amounts (especially in induction phases), but *never* to zero, and even the induction phases are not meant to last indefinitely. You can always have vegetables. You *should* always have vegetables. And even at the strictest induction levels, you can eat a fair amount of them for your 20 to 30 grams of effective carb content (much, much more when you move up to ongoing weight loss and finally to maintenance phases).

Make Low-Carb Part of a System of Self-Care

If you think of low-carbing as nothing more than a way to get skinny, you are missing out on one of the great benefits of this lifestyle. Low-carbing does not have to be merely a weight-loss strategy. It can, and should, be the cornerstone of an entire system of self-care that enhances your health and your life in dozens of ways. Keeping carbs low is only the first step, and not even the most important. You can use the tools in this book to change your entire relationship to food and, by extension, to the whole notion of how you care for yourself. Some of the terrific benefits noted by low-carbers have to do with other changes in their diet and lifestyle that have accompanied their switch to low-carbohydrate foods.

> *It was almost like a religious experience for me when I finally gave up all the "white stuff"—potatoes, rice, pasta, bread. For the first time in 20 years I didn't feel bloated all the time.*
>
> *—Brian C.*

Here are ten important ways in which you can make low-carbing work for you forever.

1. Eliminate trans-fats. Because trans-fats are found in most of the foods that are eliminated on low-carb diets, low-carbers automatically reduce their intake of this dangerous, health-robbing fat, which is found in baked goods, cookies, cakes, snack foods, and especially foods deep-fried in vegetable oils. Avoid anything that includes *partially hydrogenated oil* on the label. Fats are vitally important for the integrity of the cells and as precursors to important hormones in the body, but if the good stuff isn't around, the body will make those structures out of the reject materials. Don't feed your body damaged goods. Give it the good stuff. Dump the trans-fats.

2. Consume more omega-3s and way fewer omega-6s. Omega-3s are found in fish and flax. Omega-6s are found mainly in (highly processed) vegetable oils on your grocer's shelf. Omega-6s are pro-inflammatory; omega-3s are anti-inflammatory. You need both, but they need to be in balance. Many nutritionists believe that one of the greatest health problems of our time is the imbalance between these two classes of fats in the diet. Our Paleo ancestors consumed omega-6s and omega-3s in a very healthy 1:1 ratio. We

currently consume something like a 20:1 ratio in favor of the pro-inflammatory omega-6s. Those polyunsaturated, highly processed vegetable oils contribute to a wide range of health problems. By reducing your consumption of vegetable oils and increasing your consumption of fish and flax (with food, supplements, or both), you help to restore the ideal ratio of fatty acids and go a long way toward improving your overall health.

3. Eliminate sugar. The destructive effects of sugar on human health have been addressed by nearly every one of the low-carb–diet authors and have been discussed in some depth in chapter 3. For those who want to delve deeper into the subject, there are several excellent books about sugar. There is absolutely no—I repeat, *no*—need for refined sugar in the human diet. You may not be able to completely eliminate sugar from your diet, but you can sure try. The greater your success, the greater the benefit to your overall health and well-being.

4. Eliminate processed foods. In the ideal diet—low-carb or otherwise—you would eat only what you could hunt, fish, gather, pluck, grow, or possibly milk. While that may not be practical or possible in today's world, it's the bull's-eye to aim for. The more you can make foods with bar codes a smaller part of your diet, the better off you'll be. With food processing, the rule should be *none is best and less is better*. The closer a food is to the way nature created it, the better it is for your health. Eliminating processed foods also goes a long way toward eliminating a big source of exogenous toxins like chemicals, preservatives, deodorizers, colorings, flavorings, and especially trans-fatty acids.

5. Build your meals around protein, fat, and vegetables. As you can see from the Jonny Bowden Healthy Low-Carb Life Pyramid on page 338, these three food groups should form the basis of your diet. The exact proportions of the three will vary from person to person. There have been hunter–gatherer societies that existed on almost all protein and fat (like the Inuit) and others that existed primarily on plant foods, but there have been no hunter–gatherer societies that thrived on TV dinners. Your individual metabolism and preferences will determine how much of a contribution each of these three categories—protein, fat, and vegetables—makes to your overall diet, but whatever the mix, these should be the three major sources for most of your calories.

6. Drink plenty of water. Water has been discussed in many places in this book, but drinking it still earns a place on the top-ten

list of health habits to cultivate in order to make low-carb living synonymous with great health. Get in the daily habit of washing out metabolic waste products as well as the toxins in the fat cells you'll be emptying. Refresh, replenish, and restore your body's fluids on a constant basis with water. Just do it.

7. Get plenty of sleep. All together now, one more time: *stress makes you fat.* And one of life's biggest stressors is lack of sleep. Important hormones (like human growth hormone) and neurotransmitters (like serotonin) simply don't get made in sufficient quantities if you're not sleeping soundly and deeply for at least 7 to 8 hours a night. Sleep is a weight-loss drug. It has no bad side effects. And it's free!

8. Exercise every day. Not only will this increase your metabolic rate and burn calories, but doing it regularly—at least 5 days a week— is the single best predictor of whether you will be successful in keeping weight off. Exercise will change your mood, keep you lean, and very likely extend your life. Do you really need a better reason to get out and move?

9. Get 25 to 50 grams of fiber every single day. Getting the right amount of fiber will help you lose weight, help stabilize your blood sugar, lower the glycemic load of food, keep hunger at bay, and in all likelihood help protect against certain cancers. You get fiber in vegetables, nuts, and fiber supplements. And don't buy into the nonsense about needing foods like bread for fiber. Bread's a fiber lightweight. Much better to get it from vegetables, fruits, beans, and foods like avocados, which are surprisingly high in fiber!

10. Expand joy in your life. In the words of Robert Crayhon, "Pleasure is a nutrient." Never forget that sadness is not a Prozac deficiency. Some natural serotonin boosters are playing with kids, petting a dog, making love, being in the sunshine, and doing things for others. Find the things in your life that raise your spirits, lift your soul, and make you happy—then *do* them. Often!

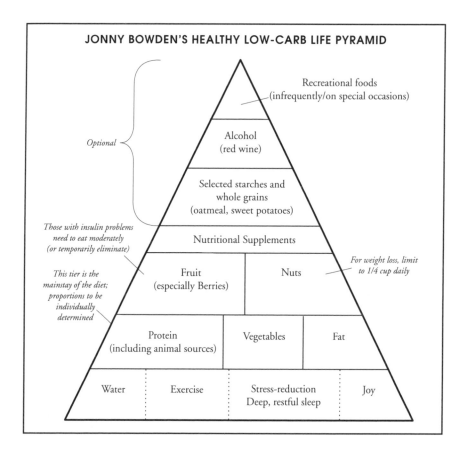

JONNY BOWDEN'S HEALTHY LOW-CARB LIFE PYRAMID

Recreational foods
(infrequently/on special occasions)

Optional

Alcohol
(red wine)

Selected starches and
whole grains
(oatmeal, sweet potatoes)

*Those with insulin problems
need to eat moderately
(or temporarily eliminate)*

Nutritional Supplements

*This tier is the
mainstay of the diet;
proportions to be
individually
determined*

Fruit
(especially Berries)

Nuts

*For weight loss, limit
to 1/4 cup daily*

Protein
(including animal sources)

Vegetables

Fat

Water · Exercise · Stress-reduction
Deep, restful sleep · Joy

You Can Lose Weight: Believing Is Seeing

Until 1954, it was generally believed that human beings could not run a mile in fewer than 4 minutes. The world agreed that there was an innate physiological limitation that prevented anyone from breaking this barrier. But the world forgot to tell Roger Bannister, a neurologist who, on May 6, 1954, ran a mile in 3 minutes, 59.4 seconds, the first sub-4-minute mile.

But that's not the interesting part of the story.

The interesting part of the story is that the *next* guy after Bannister to break the 4-minute-mile barrier—John Landy—did it 46 days later. For decades it had never been done, and then it was done *twice* in fewer than 2 months. By the end of 1957, sixteen runners had surpassed the record. The number who've done it as of the writing of this book is in the hundreds.

What happened? Certainly, the aerobic capacity of human beings didn't suddenly expand in 1954. What happened was that the shared belief that it was not possible to run that fast evaporated. As soon as people *saw* that it was possible, they *believed* it could be done. Those sixteen runners who broke the sub-4-minute barrier were never stopped by a physiological barrier—they were stopped by their *belief* in a physiological barrier. When they saw that it could be done, they believed it was possible.

And then they did it.

This book is about giving you the best information available today about weight loss and diet. But in the long run, successful weight loss has never been just about information. Information is the first step. Information puts you on a level playing field. But the real action is what you *do* with that information—how you let it empower you, how you apply it to your life.

Weight loss is about taking control of your life.

If you can *see* it for yourself, as Bannister did, you can *believe* in it. And if you can *believe* in it, you can *do* it. Weight loss is just the medium in which you can practice mastery—of your environment, your mind, and your body.

Master these things and you master your life. The only limits that are there for you are those you believe in.

Enjoy the journey.

CHAPTER 13

Research Relating to Low-Carb Diets: An Updated Summary for Your Doctor (or for You)

I n my experience, doctors who disagree with the low-carb approach fall into one of two categories.

The first category consists of well-intentioned and sincere physicians who honestly don't know about the copious research on low-carb diets. They worry about the "dangers" of such diets, especially when it comes to heart disease. Doctors who fall into this category may be surprisingly open to seeing the amount of positive research that has been done on low-carbing, and the papers included in this chapter should go a long way toward reassuring them that low-carb eating is a perfectly safe (and very effective) strategy that will benefit you in a variety of ways. Your doctor may want to use this research as a starting point for his or her own investigations, and should be very reassured by the studies presented in this chapter.

The second category of doctors is simply convinced that low-carb diets will kill you, and they are not particularly interested in hearing any facts that might cause them to have to reconsider their positions. They are true believers—and behave more like zealots than scientists. You won't have any luck convincing this group of anything; their minds are already made up.

But this chapter is not just for your doctor. It's also so that you can be reassured that there is a ton of research on the low-carb approach to weight loss, diabetes, and metabolic syndrome. You'll also find review papers on saturated fat and protein, two studies that specifically looked at the effect of protein on calcium and bones, and one paper on low-carb diets and polycystic ovary syndrome. This is far from a complete picture of the positive research that has been done on low-carb and ketogenic diets, but it is a good representative sampling.

The National Cholesterol Education Program Diet versus a Diet Lower in Carbohydrates and Higher in Protein and Monounsaturated Fat

Reference: Y. W. Aude, et al., "The National Cholesterol Education Program Diet versus a Diet Lower in Carbohydrates and Higher in Protein and Monounsaturated Fat," *Archives of Internal Medicine*, 164, no 19.(October 2004):2141–2146.

In this study, researchers tested a conventional low-fat diet recommended by the National Cholesterol Education Program against a "modified low-carb" diet with higher protein and higher monounsaturated fat. Weight loss was greater in the higher protein, higher monounsaturated fat, low carb group. There were no differences between the groups in cholesterol or triglycerides, but within the modified low-carb diet group there were significant favorable changes.

The Effects of Low-Carbohydrate versus Conventional Weight Loss Diets in Severely Obese Adults: One-Year Follow-up

Reference: L. Stern, N. Iqbal, P. Seshadri, et al., "The Effects of Low-Carbohydrate versus Conventional Weight Loss Diets in Severely Obese Adults: One-Year Follow-up of a Randomized Trial," *Annals of Internal Medicine*, 140, no. 10 (May 2004): 778–785.

In this study, obese adults were assigned to either a low-carb diet or a low-fat conventional diet. After one year, both groups had similar weight loss, but triglycerides decreased significantly more in the low-carb group and HDL cholesterol (the so-called "good" cholesterol) decreased less. And for those with diabetes, the low-carb dieters had a greater improvement in long-term blood sugar control than the low-fat dieters.

A Low-Carbohydrate, Ketogenic Diet versus a Low-Fat Diet to Treat Obesity and Hyperlipidemia: A Randomized, Controlled Trial

Reference: W. S. Yancy Jr., M. K. Olsen, J. R. Guyton, R. P. Bakst, E. C. Westman, Center for Health Services Research in Primary Care, Department of Veterans Affairs Medical Center, and Duke University Medical Center, Durham, North Carolina, "A Low-Carbohydrate, Ketogenic Diet versus a Low-Fat Diet to Treat Obesity and Hyperlipidemia: A Randomized, Controlled Trial," *Annals of Internal Medicine*, 140, no. 10 (May 18, 2004): 769–777.

This study tested a low-fat diet against a low-carb diet for 6 months on overweight volunteers. The low-carb group lost more weight and more fat mass than the high-carb group. The low-carb group also had a significantly greater increase in HDL (so-called "good") cholesterol than the low-fat group, as well as a significant decrease in triglycerides.

A Randomized Trial Comparing a Very Low Carbohydrate Diet and a Calorie-Restricted Low-Fat Diet on Body Weight and Cardiovascular Risk Factors in Healthy Women

Reference: B. J. Brehm, R. J. Seeley, S. R. Daniels, D. A. D'Alessio, "A Randomized Trial Comparing a Very Low Carbohydrate Diet and a Calorie-Restricted Low-Fat Diet on Body Weight and Cardiovascular Risk Factors in Healthy Women," *The Journal of Clinical Endocrinology & Metabolism*, 88, no. 4 (April 2003): 1617–1623.

In this study, healthy obese females were put on either a very low carbohydrate diet (with no restrictions on calories), or a calorie restricted diet (with <30% fat). Both groups wound up eating about the same number of calories. **The very low carb group lost more weight.** There were no increased risk factors for cardiovascular disease in either group.

Effects of a Low-Carbohydrate Diet on Weight Loss and Cardiovascular Risk Factor in Overweight Adolescents

Reference: S. B. Sondike, N. Copperman, M. S. Jacobson, "Effects of a Low-Carbohydrate Diet on Weight Loss and Cardiovascular Risk Factor in Overweight Adolescents," *The Journal of Pediatrics*, 142, no. 3 (March 2003): 253–258.

In this landmark study, overweight adolescents were put on either a low-carb diet or a low-fat diet (<30% fat). The low-carb diet group was Atkins Induction (<20g carbs per day) for two weeks, then <40g per day for 10 weeks. They were told to eat low carb foods whenever hungry. **The low-carb group lost twice as much weight.** In neither group were there any adverse effects on blood lipids.

Premenopausal Women Following a Low-Carbohydrate/High-Protein Diet Experience Greater Weight Loss and Less Hunger Compared to a High-Carbohydrate/Low-Fat Diet

Reference: S. M. Nickols-Richardson, J. J. Volpe, M. D. Coleman, "Premenopausal Women Following a Low-Carbohydrate/High-Protein Diet Experience Greater Weight Loss and Less Hunger Compared to a High-Carbohydrate/Low-Fat Diet," Abstract presented at FASEB Meeting on Experimental Biology: Translating the Genome, April 17–21, 2004, Washington, DC.

In this study, premenopausal women were instructed to follow either an Atkins-type diet or a high-carbohydrate/low-fat diet for six weeks. **The women on the low-carb diet lost significantly more weight than the women on the high-carb diet. Only in the low-carb group did hunger scores decrease significantly.** The authors report that "a low carbohydrate diet appears to be superior to a higher carbohydrate diet as it results in **greater percentage change in body weight with lower scores in hunger.**"

A Low-Carbohydrate as Compared with a Low-Fat Diet in Severe Obesity

Reference: F. F. Samaha, N. Iqbal, P. Seshadri, K. L. Chicano, D. A. Daily, J. McGrory, T. Williams, M. Williams, E. J. Gracely, L. Stern, "A Low-Carbohydrate as Compared with a Low-Fat Diet in Severe Obesity," *The New England Journal of Medicine*, 348 (May 2003): 2074–2081.

In this study, severely obese subjects were assigned to either a low carb diet or a low calorie/ fat-restricted diet. **Those on the low-carb diet lost more weight and had greater decreases in triglycerides. Insulin sensitivity**, measured only in subjects without diabetes, **also improved more among subjects on the low-carbohydrate diet.**

Comparison of Energy-Restricted Very Low-Carbohydrate and Low-Fat Diets on Weight Loss and Body Composition in Overweight Men and Women

Reference: J. S. Volek, M. J. Sharman, A. L. Gómez, D. A. Judelson, M. R. Rubin, G. Watson, B. Sokmen, R. Silvestre, D. N. French, and W. J. Kraemer, "Comparison of Energy-Restricted Very Low-Carbohydrate and Low-Fat Diets on Weight Loss and Body Composition in Overweight Men and Women," *Nutrition & Metabolism*, 1, no. 13 (London: 2004).

In a population of overweight men and premenopausal women, two diets were compared. One was a very low-carb ketogenic diet (i.e. the first stage of Atkins); the other was a standard low-fat diet. The low-carb diet had almost three hundred more calories than the low-fat diet (1855 calories per day on low-carb vs. 1562 calories per day on low-fat. The majority of men and women experienced greater overall weight loss and greater body fat loss on the very low-carb diet than on the low-fat one. The researchers concluded, "This study shows a clear benefit of a very low-carb ketogenic diet over low-fat diet for short-term body weight and fat loss, especially in men."

Weight-loss with Low or High Carbohydrate Diet?

Reference: A. Golay, C. Eigenheer, Y. Morel, P. Kujawski, T. Lehmann, N. de Tonnac, "Weight-Loss with Low or High Carbohydrate Diet?" *International Journal of Obesity and Related Metabolic Disorders*, 20, no. 12 (December 1996):1067–1072.

This was a study that seemed to show no significant difference in weight loss between a "low carb" and a "high carb" diet, and is sometimes quoted as "evidence" that low-carb has no particular advantage over the standard diet. But the "low carb" diet was 25% carbs (which is much higher than many other studies and higher than many low-carb diets recommend) while the "high carb" diet was more like the Zone (45% carbs), so can in no sense be considered a true "high carb" diet. That said, even though both programs produced the same amount of weight loss, the lower carb group had more improvement in fasting blood insulin and triglyceride levels.

Very Low Carbohydrate Diet Improves Cholesterol and Triglyceride Levels

Reference: J. S. Volek, M. J. Sharman, and A. L. Gómez, et al., "An Isoenergetic Very Low Carbohydrate Diet Improves Serum HDL Cholesterol and Triacylglycerol Concentrations, the Total Cholesterol to HDL Cholesterol Ratio and Postprandial Lipemic Responses Compared with a Low Fat Diet in Normal Weight, Normolipidemic Women," *The Journal of Nutrition*, 133, no. 9, (September 2003): 2756–2761.

Researchers compared the effects of a very low carbohydrate diet with a low fat diet on cholesterol and other cardiac risk factors. Compared with the low fat diet, the low carb diet did raise cholesterol; but it raised good cholesterol (HDL) twice as much as it raised bad cholesterol (LDL) **resulting in a much improved cholesterol** *ratio*. **The low carb diet also reduced triglycerides.** The authors conclude that the **low carb diet produced "favorable effects on cardiovascular disease risk status."**

Clinical Use of a Carbohydrate-Restricted Diet to Treat the Dyslipidemia of the Metabolic Syndrome

Reference: Joseph T. Hickey, Lisa Hickey, William S. Yancy Jr., et. al., "Clinical Use of a Carbohydrate-Restricted Diet to Treat the Dyslipidemia of the Metabolic Syndrome," *Metabolic Syndrome and Related Disorders*, 1, no. 3 (September 2003): 227–232.

An analysis of patients attending a preventive medicine clinic found that carbohydrate restriction led to a **13% reduction in total cholesterol, 16% reduction in LDL cholesterol, 38% reduction in triglycerides, and a 13% increase in HDL cholesterol**. Carbohydrate-restriction also led to an **82% reduction in the dangerous LDL-pattern B molecules** while simultaneously producing a **30% increase in the large (very good) HDL molecules**. The researchers concluded that a **carbohydrate-restricted diet should be considered as a treatment for the metabolic syndrome**.

Carbohydrate Restriction Has a More Favorable Impact on the Metabolic Syndrome than a Low Fat Diet

Reference: J. S. Volek, S. D. Phinney, C. E. Forsythe, et al., "Carbohydrate Restriction has a More Favorable Impact on the Metabolic Syndrome than a Low Fat Diet," *Lipids*, 44, no. 4 (April 2009): 297–309.

The researchers compared two diets of equal calories (1500) in subjects with risk factors for heart disease and metabolic syndrome. One group ate a low-carb diet and one group ate a low-fat diet. Those following the low-carb diet had consistently reduced blood sugar, improved insulin sensitivity, greater weight loss, lower triglycerides and greater HDL cholesterol.

Very Low-Carbohydrate and Low-Fat Diets Affect Fasting Lipids and Postprandial Lipemia Differently in Overweight Men

Reference: M. J. Sharman, A. L. Gomez, W. J. Kraemer, J. S. Volek, "Very Low-Carbohydrate and Low-Fat Diets Affect Fasting Lipids and Postprandial

Lipemia Differently in Overweight Men," *Journal of Nutrition*, 134, no. 4 (April 2004): 880–885.

In a population of overweight men, researchers compared the effects of a very low-carb diet and a low-fat diet. The low-carb dieters lost more weight. While both diets had the same effect on total cholesterol and on fasting insulin, triglycerides and fasting blood sugar were reduced more by the low-carb diet. Only those on the low-carb diet had an improvement in LDL particle size, meaning the big, harmless particles increased while the small dense athrogenic particles decreased.

Low Carbohydrate Diet. Its Effects on Selected Body Parameters of Obese Patients

Reference: F. A. Alnasir, B. E. Fateha, "Low Carbohydrate Diet. Its Effects on Selected Body Parameters of Obese Patients," *Saudi Medical Journal*, 24, no. 9 (September 2003): 949–952.

In this study, 13 obese patients were put on a low-carb diet. After six weeks there was a significant reduction in both body weight and waist circumference. Furthermore, both blood cholesterol and fasting blood sugar were reduced. The researchers concluded that a "low carbohydrate diet could help in reducing body weight without any significant harmful effect."

Note: this was one of the very few studies where they did not get improvements in triglycerides with a low carbohydrate diet.

Beneficial Effect of Low Carbohydrate in Low Calorie Diets on Visceral Fat Reduction in Type 2 Diabetic Patients with Obesity

Reference: Y. Miyashita, N. Koide, M. Ohtsuka, et al., "Beneficial Effect of Low Carbohydrate in Low Calorie Diets on Visceral Fat Reduction in Type 2 Diabetic Patients with Obesity," *Diabetes Research and Clinical Practice*, 65, no. 3 (September 2004): 235–241.

Two low calorie diets were tested in a group of type II diabetics: Low carb, and High carb. Both diets had the same number of calories (1000 per day).

Both groups lost weight and improved blood sugar. But the low carb group had greater decreases in visceral fat, greater improvements in fasting insulin and greater increases in HDL ("good") cholesterol.

A Low-Carbohydrate, Ketogenic Diet for Type 2 Diabetes Mellitus

Reference: W. S. Yancy, M. E. Foy, E. C. Westman, "A Low-Carbohydrate, Ketogenic Diet for Type 2 Diabetes Mellitus," *Journal of General Internal Medicine*, 19, no. 1S (2004): 110.

Patients with Type ll Diabetes were put on a low-carb ketogenic diet (<20 gram carbohydrate per day) after which they increased carbohydrates by a small amount each week as needed (essentially the Atkins diet). They were also instructed to take a multivitamin and consume 6-8 glasses of fluids daily.

After 16 weeks, the 19 men and women completing the study had significant improvements in glycemic control (HbA1c decreased 15%) and triglyceride levels, a significant weight loss of 7%, and improvements in fasting serum glucose. Diabetes medications were discontinued or reduced in 68% of the participants.

A Pilot Trial of a Low-Carbohydrate, Ketogenic Diet

Reference: W. S. Yancy Jr., M. C. Vernon, E. C. Westman, "A Pilot Trial of a Low-Carbohydrate, Ketogenic Diet in Patients with Type 2 Diabetes," *Metabolic Syndrome and Related Disorders*, 1, no. 3 (September 2003): 239–243.

In this small pilot study, 21 overweight diabetic patients were put on a very low carb ketogenic diet (initially <20 g carbohydrates a day). Diabetes medications were discontinued in 7 participants and reduced in 10 others. Mean body weight decreased 6.6% and triglycerides decreased 42%. There were improvements in several measures relating to metabolic syndrome (blood pressure, waist circumference, blood sugar control).

Randomized Trial on Protein vs Carbohydrate in Ad Libitum Fat Reduced Diet for the Treatment of Obesity

Reference: A. R. Skov, S. Toubro, B. Ronn, L. Holm, A. Astrup, "Randomized Trial on Protein vs Carbohydrate in Ad Libitum Fat Reduced Diet for the Treatment of Obesity," *International Journal of Obesity and Related Metabolic Disorders*, 23, no. 5 (May 1999): 528–536.

The purpose of this study was to see what happens when you replace carbohydrates in the diet with protein. Two groups of obese men were tested. In half the men, they replaced the carbs in their high carb diet with protein. Weight loss and fat loss was greater in the high protein group. More people lost weight in the high protein group. Those in the high protein group (but not the high carb group) lowered their triglycerides.

Meat, Fish and Egg Intake and Risk of Breast Cancer

Reference: M. D. Holmes, G. A. Colditz, D. J. Hunter, et al., "Meat, Fish and Egg Intake and Risk of Breast Cancer," *International Journal of Cancer*, 104, no. 2 (March 2003): 221–227.

Researchers examined the results of the Nurses' Health Study, which followed almost 90,000 women for 18 years, to see if there was any significant increase breast cancer risk for those eating meat or fish. The answer was no.

They found no increase that eating animal protein, red meat or fish during mid-life and later was associated with any increased risk of breast cancer.

Effect on Dietary Protein Supplements on Calcium

Reference: B. Dawson-Hughes, S. S. Harris, H. Rasmussen, et al., "Effect of Dietary Protein Supplements on Calcium Excretion in Healthy Older Men and Women," *Journal of Clinical Endocrinology and Metabolism*, 89, no. 3 (2004): 1169–1173.

This study was done to test the impact of additional protein in the diet on bone health. In this study of older men and women, researchers found that higher protein intakes did not impact calcium excretion and that higher protein intakes have a *favorable* effect on bones.

Low Protein Intake: The Impact on Calcium and Bone *Homeostasis in Humans*

Reference: J. E. Kerstetter, K. O. O'Brien, K. L. Insogna, "Low Protein Intake: The Impact on Calcium and Bone Homeostasis in Humans," *The Journal of Nutrition*, 133, no. 3 (March 2003): 855S–861S.

There's frequently more calcium excreted in the urine of people on higher protein diets, leading many to believe that high protein diets cause bone loss. The authors suggest the opposite. They found that a low protein diet produced *reduced* calcium absorption, meaning people eating the lowest protein diets absorbed the *least* amount of calcium. The authors review several studies showing *reduced* bone density and *increased* bone loss in people on low protein diets. They state that there are no definitive nutrition intervention studies that show a detrimental effect of a high protein diet on the skeleton.

High-Protein Weight Loss Diets and Purported Adverse Effects: Where Is the Evidence?

Reference: A. H. Manninen, "High-Protein Weight Loss Diets and Purported Adverse Effects: Where Is the Evidence?" *Sports Nutrition Review Journal*, 1, no. 1 (2004): 45–51.

This review article evaluated the literature regarding the effects of high-protein, low-carbohydrate weight loss diets on cardiac, renal, bone, and liver functions. This paper looked at over 40 studies on high-protein low carbohydrate weight loss diets. It concluded that there is no evidence protein is associated with heart problems. Some studies actually show the risk of heart disease is lower when protein replaces some carbs. Higher protein intake is actually associated with greater bone mineral density and lower risk of osteoporosis.

A Pilot Study of a Low-Carbohydrate, Ketogenic Diet for Obesity-Related Polycystic Ovary Syndrome

Reference: E. C. Westman, W. S. Yancy, J. Hepburn, et al., "A Pilot Study of a Low-Carbohydrate, Ketogenic Diet for Obesity-Related Polycystic Ovary Syndrome," *Journal of General Internal Medicine*, 19, no 1S (2004): 111.

Polycystic ovary syndrome (PCOS), an endocrine disorder characterized by central obesity and insulin resistance, is common in women of reproductive age.

Researchers studied the effects of a low carbohydrate ketogenic diet on PCOS.

Women between the ages of 18-45 with PCOS were counseled to follow Atkins Induction (less than 20 grams of carbohydrate per day) and proceed onto On-Going Weight Loss (increasing carbohydrates as tolerated).

They were also instructed to take a multivitamin and consume 6-8 glasses of water a day. After 24 weeks, the five women who completed the study (45% retention) lost a significant amount of weight (average loss of 27 pounds) and decreased their free testosterone. Although not significant, there were improvements in insulin, glucose, testosterone, HbA1c, perceived body hair, and triglycerides.

A Low-Glycemic Index Diet in the Treatment of Pediatric Obesity

Reference: L. E. Spieth, J. D. Harnish, C. M. Lenders, L. B. Raezer, M. A. Pereira, S. J. Hangen, D. S. Ludwig, "A Low-Glycemic Index Diet in the Treatment of Pediatric Obesity," *Archives of Pediatrics & Adolescent Medicine*, 154, no. 9 (September 2000): 947–951.

Term to Know: GI- glycemic index

The purpose of this study was to examine the effects of a low-glycemic index (GI) diet compared with a standard reduced-fat diet in the management of childhood obesity. Obese children were put on either a conventional low-fat diet or a low-glycemic diet. The kids on the low-glycemic diet lost more weight.

Glycemic Load and Chronic Disease

Reference: J. C. Brand-Miller, "Glycemic Load and Chronic Disease," *Nutrition Reviews*, 61, no. 5, pt. 2 (May 2003): S49–55.

This paper discusses the implications of a low-glycemic diet on chronic disease. Noting that diets with a high glycemic load are associated with increased risk of type ll diabetes and cardiovascular disease, it reviews evidence that low glycemic diets may protect against obesity, colon cancer and breast cancer and suggests that high glycemic diets affect health differently in insulin resistant people.

Abnormal Glucose Tolerance and the Risk of Cancer Death in the United States

Reference: S. H. Saydah, C. M. Loria, M. S. Eberhardt, et al., "Abnormal Glucose Tolerance and the Risk of Cancer Death in the United States," *American Journal of Epidemiology*, 157, no. 12 (2003): 1092–1100.

Abnormal glucose tolerance is a well-established risk factor for cardiovascular disease. This study suggests that impaired glucose tolerance is also an independent predictor for cancer mortality.

High Dietary Fructose Induces a Hepatic Stress

Reference: G. L. Kelley, G. Allan, S. Azhar, "High Dietary Fructose Induces a Hepatic Stress Response Resulting in Cholesterol and Lipid Dysregulation," *Endocrinology*, 145, no. 2 (2004): 548–555.

This study demonstrates that high fructose diets cause liver stress, inflammation and elevated triglycerides.

Increasing Refined Sugars in the American Diet Can Be Linked to US Epidemic of Type 2 Diabetes

Reference: L. S. Gross, LiLi, E. S. Ford, et al., "Increased Consumption of Refined Carbohydrates and the Epidemic of Type 2 Diabetes in the United States: An Ecological Assessment," *American Journal of Clinical Nutrition*, 79, no. 5 (May 2004): 774–779.

Researchers examined the relationship of refined sugar in the diet and Type ll Diabetes. They found a strong *positive* correlation between Type ll Diabetes and the consumption of refined sugar, particular high-fructose corn syrup.

They found a *negative* correlation between Type ll Diabetes and fiber consumption (less fiber in the diet correlated to higher incidence of Diabetes).

Consumption of High-Fructose Corn Syrup in Beverages May Play a Role in the Epidemic of Obesity

Reference: G. A. Bray, S. J. Nielsen, B. M. Popkin, "Consumption of High-Fructose Corn Syrup in Beverages May Play a Role in the Epidemic of Obesity," *American Journal of Clinical Nutrition*, 79, no. 4 (April 2004): 537–543.

The most conservative estimate of the consumption of high-fructose corn syrup indicates an average of 132 calories of HFCS per day for all Americans. An analysis of food consumption patterns in the US found a clear association between the consumption of high-fructose corn syrup and weight gain and obesity.

Saturated Fats: What Dietary Intake?

Reference: J. B. German, C. J. Dillard, "Saturated Fats: What Dietary Intake?", *American Journal of Clinical Nutrition*, 80, no. 3 (September 2004): 550–559.

This excellent review paper looked at various saturated fatty acids and pointed out that many of them have significant health benefits. The paper argued that we should not be so quick to try to reduce intake of saturated fat to zero.

A Review of Low-Carbohydrate Ketogenic Diets

Reference: E. C. Westman, J. Mavropoulos, W. S. Yancy, et al., "A Review of Low-Carbohydrate Ketogenic Diets," *Current Atherosclerosis Reports*, 5, no. 6 (November 2003): 476–483.

This review article summarizes the published research on low-carbohydrate ketogenic diet. The authors concluded that individuals tend to lose more weight on carbohydrate restricted diets than on conventional, higher carbohydrate diets. The authors also conclude that these diets have shown favorable effects on risk factors associated with heart disease.

Resources and Support for a Low-Carb Lifestyle

http://www.jonnybowden.com

Sign up for my free video course, "7 Nutritional Lies That Are Making You Sick and Fat" and get my free newsletter at www.jonnybowden.com. Follow me on Twitter @jonnybowden.

The following blogs are highly recommended:

The blog of Michael R. Eades, MD:
http://www.proteinpower.com/drmike

Jimmy Moore's "Living La Vida Low-Carb":
http://www.livinlavidalowcarb.com

Stephan Guyenet's "Whole Health Source":
http://wholehealthsource.blogspot.com

Mark Sisson's "Mark's Daily Apple": http://www.marksdailyapple.com

Denise Minger's "Raw Food SOS": http://www.rawfoodsos.com

Dr. Wiliam Davis's "Track Your Plaque":
http://www.trackyourplaque.com/blog

Robb Wolf's blog: http://www.robbwolf.com

Dr. Robert K. Su's "Carbohydrates Can Kill":
http://www.carbohydratescankill.com/blog

Jackie Eberstein's "Controlled Carbohydrate Nutrition":
http://www.controlcarb.com

These videos are highly recommended:

Sugar: The Bitter Truth by Robert H. Lustig, MD (UCSF professor of
pediatrics in the Division of Endocrinology). Available on YouTube.

The Battle of the Diets: Is Anyone Winning (At Losing?) by
Christopher Gardner, Stanford School of Medicine. Available on
YouTube.

Overcoming the Addiction to Sugars and Flours: Living Smart,
episode 313, an interview with addictive nutrition specialist Joan
Ifkland, PhD. Available on YouTube.

Exercise

In addition to training countless Olympians, bodybuilders, and sports
teams, Charles Poliquin, M.Sc, knows so much about nutrition that he frequently lectures at medical and naturopathic schools. If you're really serious about getting in shape on a carb-controlled diet, you should visit his
website: http://www.charlespoliquin.com.

Two new exercise gurus that I've become a huge fan of since the original edition of this book are Drs. Jade and Keoni Teta. These guys—like
Poliquin—are superb trainers who really know their nutrition. You can find
them at http://www.metaboliceffect.com.

JJ Virgin is well known as a "celebrity nutritionist," but she's also one of
America's top trainers. Check out her programs at http://www.jjvirgin.com.

Helpful Tools

Calculate your BMI (body mass index): BMI is the accepted way
of calculating whether you are overweight or obese; 25–29.9 is
considered overweight and over 30 is obese. Go to
http://www.nhlbisupport.com/bmi.

Glycemic Index and Load: The definitive site for glycemic values
can be found by Google-ing "glycemic index" or "glycemic load,"
and that's the site that will come up. Remember, the load is far
more important than the index. For a useful list of foods divided
into categories of "high," "medium," and "low," go to
http://www.mendosa.com/common_foods.htm.

Nutritional Data: You can find the nutritional facts on just about any food you can think of at this site: http://www.nutritiondata.com, which also features a great tool that lets you search the database for foods with the most amount of any particular vitamin, essential fat, or mineral.

Another way to look for nutrition facts is the good old USDA database: http://www.nal.usda.gov/fnic/foodcomp/search.

Health and General-Interest Sites of Value to Low-Carbers

The Weston A. Price Foundation, a nonprofit educational organization, is a clearinghouse of information on healthful lifestyles, ecology, sound nutrition, alternative medicine, humane farming, and organic gardening: http://www.westonaprice.org.

The International Network of Cholesterol Skeptics (THINCS) is a group of international researchers, MDs, and PhDs who question the theory that animal fat and high cholesterol are dangerous to your heart and vessels. Its president and spokesperson is the iconoclast researcher Uffe Ravnskov, MD, PhD, author of The Cholesterol Myths (see "Recommended Reading"). The site is copiously researched and referenced: http://www.thincs.org.

Second Opinions: Barry Groves, an Englishman with a PhD in nutritional science, runs this site, which was called, by the London Sunday Times Magazine (October 2002), one of only five reliable and informative websites for dietary information. Groves devotes his site to "exposing dietary and medical misinformation" about such things as low-calorie diets, fats, cholesterol, heart disease, and other "dietary and medical bits and bobs." The (long) article titled "The Cholesterol Myth," copiously referenced, is a highlight. Highly recommended: http://www.second-opinions.co.uk.

Vitamins and Supplements

Here are the top four things *not* to bargain shop for:

- Parachutes
- Tattoos
- Scuba equipment
- Vitamins

All vitamin and supplements are not created equal. Two ingredients lists may look similar, but that does not mean they're of the same quality: both Mercedes and Hyundais have engines, but they are hardly the same animal. Fish oils may become rancid or may contain the same pollutants fish do unless they are scrupulously tested—minerals like magnesium and calcium come in a half dozen different forms (magnesium oxide, magnesium glycinate, etc.), some cheap, some expensive. A supplement may officially contain carnitine, but it may be present in a meaningless amount. The vitamins I recommend are the ones that are generally marketed to health professionals, and they are many cuts above what is found in the average health-food store.

All the companies I carry in the online store on my website are of this quality—I hope you will check them out at http://www.jonnybowden.com.

Another wonderful place to buy the highest quality supplements online is at http://www.rockwellnutrition.com.

Recommended Reading

The Great Cholesterol Myth (Jonny Bowden, PhD, CNS and Stephen Sinatra, MD). This book goes into great detail about why we have been completely misled about cholesterol and why the real culprit in the modern diet is not fat at all, but sugar.

The Cholesterol Con: The Truth About What Really Causes Heart Disease and How to Avoid (Dr. Malcolm Kendrick). An utterly spellbinding account, heavily referenced, of the shakiness of the evidence that animal fat and cholesterol are the true causes of heart disease.

The Cholesterol Myths (Uffe Ravnskov, MD, PhD). A detailed, systematic expose in which Ravnskov, a brilliant Swedish scientist and researcher, takes on the cholesterol establishment and literally debunks every major premise of the anti–saturated fat and cholesterol dogma.

Why We Get Fat (Gary Taubes). This is the user-friendly version of Taubes's masterpiece, *Good Calories, Bad Calories.* Highly recommended. And if you have the patience, try *Good Calories, Bad Calories* as well!

Wheat Belly (William Davis, MD). This is one of the most insightful and interesting books on the hazards of high-carb diets and, specifically, wheat. Spoiler alert: it's *not* just about gluten.

Dangerous Grains: Why Gluten Cereal Grains May Be Hazardous to Your Health (James Braly, MD and Ron Hoggan, MA). This is an excellent and thought-provoking book about gluten sensitivity by a renowned food-allergy expert and a respected patient advocate. The authors discuss the impact of grains on a range of conditions, including autoimmune disease, chronic pain, osteoporosis, digestive problems, and brain disorders.

The Gluten Connection: How Gluten Sensitivity May Be Sabotaging Your Health (Shari Lieberman, PhD, CNS). An absolutely indispensible book by one of the great nutritionists of our time, delineating how undetected sensitivity to grains can undermine our health.

The Art and Science of Low-Carbohydrate Living (Jeff Volek, RD, PhD and Stephen Phinney, MD). Though this superb book was written for professionals, it's not too dense or difficult for the reader who wants more depth and detail than is usually available in consumer books. Written by two of the premier researchers in the field of low-carb diets.

The Hungry Gene: The Science of Fat and the Future of Thin (Ellen Ruppel Shell). Science journalism at its best. An account of obesity research through the years, it makes a case that obesity is not a matter of weak will or gluttony but of vulnerable genes preyed upon by a hostile environment. It also exposes the unholy alliance between schools and Coke, Pepsi, Pizza Hut, and McDonald's.

Waistland: The (R)evolutionary Science behind Our Weight and Fitness Crisis (Deirdre Barrett, PhD). A Harvard psychologist takes a novel and fascinating look at exactly what makes us fat and what we can do about it.

What Your Doctor May Not Tell You About Hypertension (Mark Houston, MD, Barry Fox, PhD, and Nadine Taylor, MS, RD). Hypertension overlaps with heart disease, diabetes, and obesity in many ways, and this book should be on the shelf of anyone interested in a more modern and enlightened approach to its treatment.

Beat Sugar Addiction Now!: The Cutting Edge-Program That Cures Your Type of Sugar Addiction and Puts You on the Road to Feeling Great—and Losing Weight! (Jacob Teitelbaum, MD and Chrystle

Fiedler). The best-selling author of *From Fatigued to Fantastic* uncovers four different types of sugar addiction and gives a step-by-step plan for resolving their underlying causes.

Sugars and Flours: How They Make Us Crazy, Sick and Fat, and What to Do About It (Joan Ifland). Ifland is a specialist in addictive nutrition and is the chair of the Refined Food Addiction Research Foundation. She knows what she's talking about!

Atkins Diabetes Revolution (Mary C. Vernon, MD, CMD, and Jacqueline A. Eberstein, RN). This book was essentially written by two highly respected medical associates of Dr. Robert Atkins, and if there is any justice in the world, it will become the bible for diabetes treatment. Dr. Mary Vernon and Jacqueline Eberstein, a nurse, built on Dr. Atkins's copious notes and treatment protocols, added their own spin, and came up with nothing less than a blueprint for the way diabetes should be treated. An absolute must-read.

Syndrome X (Jack Challem, Burton Berkson, MD, and Melissa Diane Smith). Though there have been a number of books written about metabolic syndrome, or Syndrome X (a precursor to diabetes that centers on insulin resistance), this is one of the best.

The False Fat Diet (Elson Haas, MD) This is an excellent book on the connection between food sensitivities and food allergies to weight gain.

Livin' La Vida Low-Carb: My Journey from Flabby Fat to Sensationally Skinny (Jimmy Moore). An inspiring story by a man who went from 410 pounds to 180 pounds on a low-carb program and became one of the country's leading crusaders for the low-carb point of view.

Cookbooks

1,001 Low-Carb Recipes: Hundreds of Delicious Recipes from dinner to Dessert That Let You Live Your Low-Carb Lifestyle and Never Look Back (Dana Carpender). The updated and expanded recipe guide from the queen of low-carb cooking.

500 Low-Carb Recipes: 500 Recipes, from Snacks to Dessert, That the Whole Family Will Love (Dana Carpender). From the proprietor of the popular site http://www.holdthetoast.com and the author of *How I Gave Up My Low-Fat Diet and Lost 40 Pounds,* Dana Carpender's sample fare includes Heroin Wings (so named because they are supposedly addictive!), Mockahlua Cheesecake, Meatza (pizza without the crust), and the secret to low-carb stuffing.

300 15-Minute Low-Carb Recipes: Hundreds of Delicious Meals That Let You Live Your Low-Carb Lifestyle and Never Look Back (Dana Carpender). Another solid title from Dana Carpender.

200 Low-Carb Slow Cooker Recipes: Healthy Dinners That Are Ready When you Are! (Dana Carpender). Carpender turns her talents to the slow-cooker.

The New Atkins for a New You Cookbook: 200 Simple and Delicious Low-Carb Recipes in 30 Minutes or Less (Colette Heimowitz). Atkins-friendly recipes for the New Atkins program, a more flexible and easier-to-maintain lifestyle. All the recipes have a prep time of 30 minutes or fewer and most use 10 or fewer ingredients.

The Primal Blueprint Cookbook (Mark Sisson and Jennifer Meier). The first cookbook from the author of *The Primal Blueprint,* this excellent cookbook has dishes based on meat, foul, seafood, and eggs, as well as desserts (baked coconut milk custard, anyone?) and "primal substitute" recipes for such comfort foods as jambalaya and enchiladas.

Primal Blueprint Quick & Easy Meals (Mark Sisson and Jennifer Meier). Delicious, primal-approved meals you can put together in under 30 minutes. By the author of *The Primal Blueprint.*

The Low-Carb Comfort Food Cookbook (Mike Eades, MD and Mary Dan Eades, MD with Ursula Solom). This revolutionary cookbook from the best-selling authors of *Protein Power* will satisfy all your comfort-food cravings without breaking the carbohydrate bank!

Everyday Paleo (Sarah Fragoso). Fragoso is an active mother of three who gives detailed instructions for using the Paleo lifestyle to improve the health and longevity of your family. Introduction by Robb Wolf of Paleo Solution fame.

The Low-Carb Baking and Dessert Cookbook (Ursula Solom). With a foreword by none other than Mary Dan Eades, MD, coauthor of

Protein Power, this book offers scores of recipes for breads, biscuits, pastries, cookies, pies, and the like that are not only low-carb but delicious.

The Paleo Diet Cookbook: More than 150 Recipes for Paleo Breakfasts, Lunches, Dinners, Snacks and Beverages (Loren Cordain). This cookbook, from the author of the original *Paleo Diet*, contains low-carb breakfasts, brunches, lunches, dinners, snacks, and beverages and features 2 weeks of meal plans and shopping tips.

The Low-Carb Cookbook: The Complete Guide to the Healthy Low-Carbohydrate Lifestyle— with over 250 Delicious Recipes (Fran McCullough). Written by a well-known cookbook editor and writer who lost more than 60 pounds herself the low-carb way, this book has been a favorite for a long time and has an introduction by Drs. Michael and Mary Dan Eades.

Nourishing Traditions: The Cookbook That Challenges Politically Correct Nutrition and the Diet Dictocrats (Sally Fallon with Mary Enig, PhD). While this is technically a cookbook, it is also a lot more. It contains wonderful recipes using whole natural foods (no fat-free substitutes here) and a running commentary that challenges conventional dietary wisdom. Be forewarned that this is not specifically a low-carb book, but it belongs on your bookshelf anyway.

JONNY BOWDEN COOKBOOKS

While not specifically low-carb, all my cookbooks have a common theme: low sugar, whole foods, no trans-fats, lowomega-6s, high omega-3s, fiber, and lots of nutrients. You will find lots of low-carb options in all of these, and for those whose personal carb allowance is a bit higher, there will be even more to choose from. Many of the recipes and meals in these books represent a middle ground between very strict low-carb and moderate-carb, making them suitable for a wider variety of occasions.

The Healthiest Meals on Earth (Jonny Bowden and Jeannette Bessinger).

The Healthiest 15-Minute Recipes on Earth (Jonny Bowden and Jeannette Bessinger).

The Most Effective Ways to Live Longer Cookbook (Jonny Bowden and Jeannette Bessinger).

Endnotes

Chapter 1: Low-Carb Redux: The Updated Truth about Low-Carbohydrate Diets

1. William S. Yancy, Jr., MD, MHS; Maren K. Olsen, PhD; et al., (2004). "A Low-Carbohydrate, Ketogenic Diet versus a Low-Fat Diet To Treat Obesity and Hyperlipidemia." *Annals of Internal Medicine* 140 (10): 769–777 (2004); Linda Stern, MD; Nayyar Iqbal, MD; Prakash Seshadri, MD, et al., "The Effects of Low-Carbohydrate versus Conventional Weight Loss Diets in Severely Obese Adults: One-Year Follow-up of a Randomized Trial." *Annals of Internal Medicine* 140 (10): 778–85. (2004).

2. "Moderately Reduced Carbohydrate Diet Keeps People Feeling Full Longer," *Science Daily*, http://www.sciencedaily.com/releases/2009/06/090611142405.htm (June 11, 2009).

3. Thomas L. Halton, Simin Liu, et al., "Low-Carbohydrate-Diet Score and Risk of Type 2 Diabetes in Women," *American Journal of Clinical Nutrition* 87, no. 2 (2008): 339–346.

4. Thomas L. Halton, Walter C. Willett, et al., "Low-Carbohydrate-Diet Score and the Risk of Coronary Heart Disease in Women," *New England Journal of Medicine* 355, no. 19 (2006): 1991–2002.

5. R. N. Smith, A. Braue, et al., "The Effect of a Low Glycemic Load Diet on Acne Vulgaris and the Fatty Acid Composition of Skin Surface Triglycerides," *Journal of Dermatological Science* 50, no. 1 (2008): 41–52.

6. C. C. Douglas, B. A. Gower, et al., "Role of Diet in the Treatment of Polycystic Ovary Syndrome," *Fertil Steril* 85, no. 3 (2006): 679–688.

7. P. Crawford, S. L. Paden, M. K. Park, "Clinical Inquiries: What Is the Dietary Treatment for Low HDL Cholesterol?" *Journal of Family Practice* 55, no. 12 (2006): 1076–1078.

8. C. J. Chiu, A. Taylor, et al., "Dietary Carbohydrate and the Progression of Age-Related Macular Degeneration: A Prospective Study from the Age-Related Eye Disease Study," *American Journal of Clinical Nutrition* 86, no. 4 (2007): 1210–1218; C. J. Chiu, L. D. Hubbard, et al., "Dietary Glycemic Index and Carbohydrate in Relation to Early Age-Related Macular Degeneration," *American Journal of Clinical Nutrition* 83, no. 4 (2006): 880–886.

9. R. J. Wood, M. L. Fernandez, et al., "Effects of a Carbohydrate-Restricted Diet with and without Supplemental Soluble Fiber on Plasma Low-Density Lipoprotein Cholesterol and Other Clinical Markers of Cardiovascular Risk," *Metabolism* 56, no. 1 (2007): 58–67.

10. "Comparison of the Atkins, Zone, Ornish, and LEARN Diets for Change in

Weight and Related Risk Factors among Overweight Premenopausal Women," *Journal of the American Medical Association*, http://jama.ama-assn.org/cgi/content/abstract/297/9/969 (March 7, 2007).

11. Personal communication, interview with Christopher Gardner.

12. C. B. Ebbeling, M. M. Leidig, et al., "Effects of a Low-Glycemic Load vs. Low-Fat Diet in Obese Young Adults: A Randomized Trial," *Journal of the American Medical Association* 297, no. 19 (2007): 2092–2102.

13. S. M. Nickols-Richardson, M. D. Coleman, et al., "Perceived Hunger is Lower and Weight Loss is Greater in Overweight Premenopausal Women Consuming a Low-Carbohydrate/High-Protein vs. High-Carbohydrate/Low-Fat Diet," *Journal of the American Dietetic Association* 105, no. 9 (2005): 1433–1437.

14. G. Boden, K. Sargrad, et al., "Effect of a Low-Carbohydrate Diet on Appetite, Blood Glucose Levels, and Insulin Resistance in Obese Patients With Type 2 Diabetes," *Annals of Internal Medicine* 142, no. 6 (March 15, 2005): 403–411.

15. David J. A. Jenkins, et al., "The Effect of a Plant-Based Low-Carbohydrate ("Eco-Atkins") Diet on Body Weight and Blood Lipid Concentrations in Hyperlipidemic Subjects, *Journal of the American Medical Association* http://archinte.jamanetwork.com/article.aspx?articleid=415074 (June 2009).

16. Anssi H. Manninen, "Metabolic Effects of the Very-Low-Carbohydrate Diets," http://www.ncbi.nlm.nih.gov/pmc/articles/PMC2129159 (December 31, 2004).

Chapter 2: The History and Origins of Low-Carb Diets

1. William Banting, *Letter on Corpulence* (self, 1864); full text available at http://www.lowcarb.ca/corpulence/corpulence_1.html.

2. Dr. Phil McGraw, *The Ultimate Weight Solution: The 7 Keys to Weight Loss Freedom* (New York: Free Press, 2003).

3. Vance Thompson, *Eat and Grow Thin* (New York: E.P. Dutton, 1914).

4. Alfred Pennington, *New England Journal of Medicine* 248 (1953): 959; *American Journal of Digestive Diseases* 21 (1954): 69.

5. Alfred Pennington, *Holiday Magazine*, June 1950. Quoted in Richard Mackarness, *Eat Fat and Grow Slim* (London: Harvill, 1958).

6. Vilhjalmur Stefansson, "Adventures in Diet," *Harper's Monthly Magazine* (November 1935, December 1935, January 1936).

7. Ibid.

8. Ibid.

9. Evelyn Stefansson, preface to *Eat Fat and Grow Slim*, by Richard Mackarness (London: Harvill, 1958).

10. Ibid.

11. Blake Donaldson, *Strong Medicine* (New York: Doubleday, 1960).

12. Alan Kekwick and Gaston L.S. Pawan, "Calorie Intake in Relation to Body Weight Changes in the Obese," *Lancet* 2 (1956): 155; "Metabolic Study in Human Obesity with Isocaloric Diets High in Fat, Protein or Carbohydrate," *Metabolism* 6, no. 5 (1957): 447–460; "The Effect of High Fat and High Carbohydrate Diets on Rates of Weight Loss in Mice," *Metabolism* 13, no. 1 (1964): 87–97.

13. Bonnie J. Brehm, et al., "A Randomized Trial Comparing a Very Low Carbohydrate Diet and a Calorie-Restricted Low Fat Diet on Body Weight and

Cardiovascular Risk Factors in Healthy Women," *Journal of Clinical Endocrinology and Metabolism* 88, no. 4 (2003): 1617–1623.

14. Richard Mackarness, *Eat Fat and Grow Slim* (London: Harvill, 1958).

15. Christian B. Allan and Wolfgang Lutz, *Life Without Bread* (Los Angeles: Keats, 2000).

16. Richard Mackarness, *Eat Fat and Grow Slim* (London: Harvill, 1958).

17. Anonymous, *Beyond Our Wildest Dreams: A History of Overeaters Anonymous as Seen by a Cofounder* (Rio Rancho, NM: Overeaters Anonymous, 1996).

18. Herman Taller, *Calories Don't Count* (New York: Simon & Schuster, 1961).

19. Ibid.

20. Ancel Keys, "Coronary Heart Disease in Seven Countries," *Circulation* 41, suppl. 1 (1970): 1–211.

21. Uffe Ravnskov, *The Cholesterol Myths* (Washington, DC: New Trends, 2000); Malcolm Kendrick, "Why the Cholesterol-Heart Disease Theory Is Wrong," http://www.thincs.org/Malcolm.choltheory.htm (July 31, 2012); Uffe Ravnskov, "Is Atherosclerosis Caused by High Cholesterol?" *QJM* 95, no. 6 (June 2002): 397–403.

22. Mary Enig, "The Oiling of America," http://www.westonaprice.org/know-your-fats/the-oiling-of-america; C.V. Felton, et al., "Dietary Polyunsaturated Fatty Acids and Composition of Human Aortic Plaques," *Lancet* 344 (1994): 1195–1196; P.A. Godley, et al., "Biomarkers of Essential Fatty Acid Consumption and Risk of Prostatic Carcinoma," *Cancer Epidemiology Biomarkers & Prevention* 5, no. 11 (November 1996): 889–895; M.S. Micozzi and T.E. Moon, *Investigating the Role of Macronutrients*, vol. 2, Nutrition and Cancer Prevention Series (New York: Marcel Dekker, 1992).

23. Laura Fraser, *Losing It: False Hopes and Fat Profits in the Diet Industry* (New York: Plume, 1998).

24. Irwin Stillman, *The Doctor's Quick Weight Loss Diet* (New York: Dell, 1967).

25. Marjorie R. Freedman, et al., "Popular Diets: A Scientific Review," *Obesity Research* 9 suppl. (2001): 5S–17S.

26. Ancel Keys, "Coronary Heart Disease in Seven Countries," *Circulation* 41, suppl. 1 (1970): 1–211.

27. George V. Mann, *Coronary Heart Disease: The Dietary Sense and Nonsense* (London: Janus, 1993).

28. Uffe Ravnskov, *The Cholesterol Myths* (Washington, DC: New Trends, 2000).

29. George V. Mann, et al., "Atherosclerosis in the Masai," *American Journal of Epidemiology* 95 (1972): 26–37.

30. John Yudkin, *Sweet and Dangerous* (New York: Wyden, 1972).

31. Ancel Keys, "Letter: Normal Plasma Cholesterol in a Man Who Eats 25 Eggs a Day," *The New England Journal of Medicine* 325 (1991): 584.

32. National Heart, Lung, and Blood Institute, National Cholesterol Education Program, http://www.nhlbi.nih.gov/about/ncep.

33. Apex Fitness Group, *Apex Fitness Systems Certification Manual*, 3rd ed. (Thousand Oaks, CA: Apex Fitness Group, 2001).

34. Dean Ornish, "Intensive Lifestyle Changes for Reversal of Coronary Heart Disease," *Journal of the American Medical Association* 280, no. 23 (December 16, 1998): 2001–2007.

35. Marjorie R. Freedman, et al., "Popular Diets: A Scientific Review," *Obesity Research* 9 (2001): 5S–17S, tables 6 and 7, http://www.nature.com/oby/journal/v9/n3s/full/oby2001113a.html.

36. Walter Willett, "R&D: Discover Dialogue," *Discover* 24, no. 3, online edition, http://www.discover.com (March 2003); "Too Many Carbs in Your Diet?" http://www.ABCnews.com (January 9, 2002); Walter Willett, *Eat, Drink, and Be Healthy* (New York: Fireside, 2001).

37. USDA Millennium Lecture Series Symposium on the Great Nutrition Debate, http://www.cnpp.usda.gov/publications/otherprojects/symposiumgreatnutritiondebatetranscript.txt (July 31, 2012).

Chapter 3: Why Low-Carb Diets Work

1. Woodson Merrell, "How I Became a Low-Carb Believer," *Time* (November 1, 1999).

2. Gary Taubes, "What If It's All Been a Big Fat Lie?" *New York Times Magazine*, (July 7, 2002).

3. Sharon H. Saydah, et al., "Abnormal Glucose Tolerance and the Risk of Cancer Death in the United States," *American Journal of Epidemiology* 157 (June 15, 2003): 1092–1100; B.A. Stoll, "Upper Abdominal Obesity, Insulin Resistance and Breast Cancer Risk," *International Journal of Obesity and Related Metabolic Disorders* 26, no. 6 (June 2002): 747–753.

4. Nancy Appleton, *Lick the Sugar Habit* (New York: Avery, 1996).

5. C. Leigh Broadhurst, *Diabetes: Prevention and Cure* (New York: Kensington, 1999); Christian B. Allan and Wolfgang Lutz, *Life Without Bread* (New York: McGraw-Hill, 2000).

6. Walter Willett, *Eat, Drink, and Be Healthy* (New York: Fireside, 2001).

7. C. Leigh Broadhurst, *Diabetes: Prevention and Cure* (New York: Kensington, 1999); W. M. Ringsdorf, et al., "Sucrose, neutrophilic phagocytosis and resistance to disease," *Dental Survey* 52, no. 12 (1976): 46–48; E. Kijak, et al., *Southern California State Dental Association Journal* 32, no. 8 (September 1964).

8. Ron Rosedale, "Insulin and Its Metabolic Effects," lecture given at Boulderfest Nutrition Conference, Boulder, CO, 1999.

9. J. Lemann, et al., "Evidence That Glucose Ingestion Inhibits Net Renal Tubular Reabsorption of Calcium and Magnesium in Man," *American Journal of Clinical Nutrition* 70 (1967): 236–245.

10. John Yudkin, et al., "Effects of High Dietary Sugar," *British Journal of Medicine* 281 (November 22, 1980): 1396.

11. Ron Rosedale, "Insulin and Its Metabolic Effects," lecture given at Boulderfest Nutrition Conference, Boulder, CO, 1999.

12. J. Michael Gaziano, "Fasting Triglycerides, High-Density Lipoprotein, and Risk of Myocardial Infarction," *Circulation* 96 (1997): 2520–2525.

13. Gerald Reaven, "An Interview with Gerald Reaven," interview by Louise Morrin, *The Canadian Association of Cardiac Rehabilitation Newsletter*, September 2000.

14. Calvin Ezrin, with Kristen L. Caron, *Your Fat Can Make You Thin* (Lincolnwood, IL: Contemporary Books, 2001).

15. Adam Marcus, "Low-Fat Mice Hold Clue to Obesity Treatment," *Reuters Magazine* (December 7, 2000).

16. Mitchell Lazar, et al., *Nature* (January 18, 2001); N. Seppa, "Protein May Tie Obesity to Diabetes," *Science News* 159 (January 20, 2001): 36.

17. Calvin Ezrin, with Kristen L. Caron, *Your Fat Can Make You Thin* (Lincolnwood, IL: Contemporary Books, 2001).

18. D.K. Layman, et al., "A Reduced Ratio of Dietary Carbohydrate to Protein Improves Body Composition and Blood Lipid Profiles During Weight Loss in Adult Women," *Journal of Nutrition* 133, no. 2 (February 2003): 411–417; D.K. Layman, et al., "Increased Dietary Protein Modifies Glucose and Insulin Homeostasis in Adult Women During Weight Loss," *Journal of Nutrition* 133, no. 2 (February 2003): 405–10.

19. D.K. Layman, et al., "The Role of Leucine in Weight Loss Diets and Glucose Homeostasis," *Journal of Nutrition* 133, no. 1 (January 2003): 261S–267S.

20. Y.O. Chang and C.C. Soong, "Effect of Feeding Diets Lacking Various Essential Amino Acids on Body Composition of Rats," *International Journal for Vitamin and Nutrition Research* 45, no. 2 (1975): 230–236.

21. D.K. Layman, et al., "A Reduced Ratio of Dietary Carbohydrate to Protein Improves Body Composition and Blood Lipid Profiles during Weight Loss in Adult Women," *Journal of Nutrition* 133, no. 2 (February 2003): 411–417.

22. C.S. Johnson, et al., "Postprandial Thermogenesis Is Increased 100% on a High-Protein, Low-Fat Diet versus a High-Carbohydrate, Low-Fat Diet in Healthy, Young Women," *Journal of the American College of Nutrition* 21, no. 1 (February 2002): 55–61.

23. American Association of Clinical Endocrinologists, "Findings and Recommendations on the Insulin Resistance Syndrome" (American Association of Clinical Endocrinologists, Washington, DC, August 25–26, 2002).

24. Ibid.

25. Ibid.

26. Ibid.

27. American Diabetes Association, "Diabetes Statistics," http://www.diabetes.org/diabetes-basics/diabetes-statistics (January 26, 2011).

28. American Association of Clinical Endocrinologists, "Findings and Recommendations on the Insulin Resistance Syndrome" (American Association of Clinical Endocrinologists, Washington, DC, August 25–26, 2002); John E. Gerich, "Contributions of Insulin-Resistance and Insulin-Secretory Defects to the Pathogenesis of Type 2 Diabetes Mellitus," *Mayo Clinic Proceedings* 78 (April 2003): 447–456.

29. E.S. Ford, et al., "Prevalence of the Metabolic Syndrome among US Adults" *Journal of the American Medical Association* 287 (2002): 356–359.

30. Dara Myers, "Diabetes Diet War," *U.S. News & World Report* (July 14, 2003): 48–49.

31. Richard Bernstein, *The Diabetes Solution* (New York: Little, Brown, 1997); C. Leigh Broadhurst, *Diabetes: Prevention and Cure* (New York: Kensington, 1999).

32. American Association of Clinical Endocrinologists, "Findings and Recommendations on the Insulin Resistance Syndrome" (American Association of Clinical Endocrinologists, Washington, DC, August 25–26, 2002).

33. Laure Morin-Papunen, "Insulin Resistance in Polycystic Ovary Syndrome," PhD diss. University of Oulu, Finland, 2000.

34. Mark Perloe "Treatment of Polycystic Ovary Syndrome with Insulin Lowering Medications," http://www.ivf.com/pcostreat.html.

35. Ron Rosedale, "Insulin and Its Metabolic Effects," lecture given at Boulderfest Nutrition Conference, Boulder, CO, 1999.

36. Vincenzo Marigliano, et al., "Normal Values in Extreme Old Age," *Annals of the New York Academy of Sciences* 673 (December 22, 1992): 23–28.

37. J. Salmeron, et al., "Dietary Fat Intake and Risk of Type 2 Diabetes in Women," *American Journal of Clinical Nutrition* 73, no. 6 (June 2001): 1019–1026.

38. B.V. Mann, "Metabolic Consequences of Dietary Trans-Fatty Acids," *Lancet* 343 (1994): 1268–1271.

39. Elson Haas, *The False Fat Diet* (New York: Ballantine, 2000).

40. US Department of Health and Human Services: National Digestive Diseases Information Clearinghouse (NDDIC) website, http://digestive.niddk.nih.gov/ddiseases/pubs/celiac/#common.

41. James Braly with Ron Hoggan, *Dangerous Grains* (New York: Avery, 2002).

42. Joseph Mercola with Alison Rose Levy, *The No-Grain Diet* (New York: Dutton, 2003).

43. S. Liu, et al., "A Prospective Study of Dietary Glycemic Load, Carbohydrate Intake, and Risk of Coronary Heart Disease in U.S. Women," *American Journal of Clinical Nutrition* 71, no. 6 (June 2000): 1455–1461.

44. Walter Willett, et al., "Glycemic Index, Glycemic Load, and Risk of Type 2 Diabetes," *American Journal of Clinical Nutrition* 76, no. 1 (July 2002): 274S–280S.

Chapter 4: The Major Culprits in a High-Carb Diet: Wheat and Fructose

1. American Diabetes Association, "Diabetes Statistics," http://www.diabetes.org/diabetes-basics/diabetes-statistics/ (January 26, 2011).

2. National Heart, Lung, and Blood Institute, "What Is Metabolic Syndrome?" http://www.nhlbi.nih.gov/health/health-topics/topics/ms (June 4, 2012).

3. ObesityinAmerica.org, "Obesity-Related Diseases," http://www.obesityinamerica.org/understandingObesity/diseases.cfm (June 4, 2012).

4. A. Galassi, et al., "Metabolic Syndrome and Risk of Cardiovascular Disease," *The American Journal of Medicine* http://www.ncbi.nlm.nih.gov/pubmed/17000207 (October 2006).

5. US Department of Health & Human Services, "Overweight and Obesity: Health Consequences," http://www.surgeongeneral.gov/library/calls/obesity/fact_consequences.html (June 6, 2012).

6. National Diabetes Information Clearinghouse, "Diabetes, Heart Disease, and Stroke," http://diabetes.niddk.nih.gov/dm/pubs/stroke/#connection (September 13, 2011).

7. Ibid.

8. Cleveland Clinic, "High Blood Pressure and Heart Attack," http://my.clevelandclinic.org/disorders/hypertension_high_blood_pressure/hic_high_blood_pressure_and_heart_attack.aspx (September 13, 2011).

9. Rik P. Bogers, et al., "Association of Overweight with Increased Risk of Coronary Heart Disease Partly Independent of Blood Pressure and Cholesterol Levels," *Archives of Internal Medicine* 167, no. 16, http://archinte.ama-assn.org/cgi/content/abstract/167/16/1720 (September 2007).

10. John N. Fain, "Release of Inflammatory Mediators by Human Adipose Tissue is Enhanced in Obesity and Primarily by the Nonfat Cells," *Mediators of*

Inflammation, http://www.hindawi.com/journals/mi/2010/513948 (June 6, 2012).

11. S. A. Silvera, et al., "Dietary Carbohydrates and Breast Cancer Risk: A Prospective Study of the Roles of Overall Glycemic Index and Glycemic Load. *International Journal of Cancer* 114, no. 4 (Apr 20, 2005): 653–658.

12. S. Sieri, et al., "Dietary Glycemic Load and Risk of Coronary Heart Disease in a Large Italian Cohort," *Archives of Internal Medicine* 170, no. 7, http://www.ncbi .nlm.nih.gov/pubmed/20386010 (April 12, 2010).

13. A. Esfahani, et al., "The Glycemic Index: Physiological Significance," *Journal of the American College of Nutrition* 28 suppl. http://www.ncbi.nlm.nih.gov/ pubmed/20234030(August 2009).

14. "Study of Obese Diabetics Explains Why Low-Carb Diets Produce Fast Results." *Science Daily.* http://www.sciencedaily.com/ releases/2005/03/050326095632.htm (March 26, 2005).

15. Ibid.

16. Kay M. Behall, et al., "Diets Containing High Amylose vs Amylopectin Starch: Effects on Metabolic Variables in Human Subjects" *American Journal of Clinical Nutrition* 49 (1989): 337–344.

17. Kaye Foster-Powell, Susanna H. A. Holt, Janette C. Brand-Miller, "International Table of Glycemic Index and Glycemic Load Values," *American Journal of Clinical Nutrition* 76, no. 1(2002): 5–56.

18. Davis, William, *Wheat Belly,* (New York: Rodale, 2011): 35.

19. Martin R. Cohen, et al., "Naloxone Reduces Food Intake in Humans," *Psychosomatic Medicine* 47, no. 2 (March/April 1985): 132–138.

20. A. Drewnowski, et al., "Naloxone, an Opiate Blocker, Reduces the Consumption of Sweet High-Fat Foods in Obese and Lean Female Binge Eaters," *American Journal of Clinical Nutrition* 61 (1995): 1206–1212.

21. Marian T. Hannan, et al., "Effect of Dietary Protein on Bone Loss in Elderly Men and Women: The Framingham Osteoporosis Study," *Journal of Bone and Mineral Research* 15, no. 12 (December 2000): 2504–2512.

22. Annebeth Rosenvinge Skov, et al., "Effect of Protein Intake on Bone Mineralization during Weight Loss: A 6-Month Trial," *Obesity Research* 10, no. 6 (2002): 432–438.

23. Anthony Sebastian, et al., "Estimation of the Net Acid Load of the Diet of Ancestral Pre-Agricultural Homo Sapiens and Their Hominid Ancestors," *American Journal of Clinical Nutrition* 76, no. 6, (December 2002): 1308–1316.

24. X. Ouyang, et al., "Fructose Consumption as a Risk Factor for Non-Alcoholic Fatty Liver Disease," *Journal of Hepatology,* http://www.ncbi.nlm.nih.gov/ pubmed/18395287 (June 2008); K. Nomura, T. Yamanouchi, "The Role of Fructose-Enriched Diets in Mechanisms of Nonalcoholic Fatty Liver Disease," *The Journal of Nutritional Biochemistry* 23, no. 3, http://www.ncbi.nlm.nih.gov/ pubmed/22129639 (March 2012); Manal F. Abdelmalek, et al., "Increased Fructose Consumption is Associated with Fibrosis Severity in Patients with NAFLD," *Hepatology* 51, no. 6, http://www.ncbi.nlm.nih.gov/pmc/articles/ PMC2922495 (June 2010).

25. Wendy Loo, "Fructose, Not Fats, the Main Cause of NAFLD Epidemic," *Medical Tribune, MIMS Malaysia* (accessed Mar 24, 2012).

26. Robbert Meerwaldt, et al., "The Clinical Relevance of Assessing Advanced

Glycation Endproducts Accumulation in Diabetes," *Cardiovascular Diabetology*, http://www.cardiab.com/content/7/1/29 (2008); Andries J. Smith, et al., "Advanced Glycation Endproducts in Chronic Heart Failure," *Annals of the New York Library of Science*, http://onlinelibrary.wiley.com/doi/10.1196/annals.1433.038/abstract?systemMessage=Wiley+Online+Library+will+be+disrupted+3+Dec+from+10-12+GMT+for+monthly+maintenance (April 2008); Jasper W. L. Hartog, et al., "Advanced Glycation End-Products (AGEs) and Heart Failure: Pathophysiology and Clinical Implications," *European Journal of Heart Failure* 9, no. 12, http://eurjhf.oxfordjournals.org/content/9/12/1146.full (2007).

27. Kimber L. Stanhope, et al., "Consumption of Fructose and High Fructose Corn Syrup Increase Postprandial Triglycerides, LDL-Cholesterol, and Apoliprotein-B in Young Men and Women," *The Journal of Clinical Endocrinology & Metabolism* http://jcem.endojournals.org/content/early/2011/08/11/jc.2011-1251 (August 17, 2011); "Fructose Consumption Increases Risk Factors for Heart Disease," *Science Daily*, http://www.sciencedaily.com/releases/2011/07/110728082558.htm (July 28, 2011); Kimber L. Stanhope and Peter J. Havel, "Endocrine and Metabolic Effects of Beverages Sweetened with Fructose, Glucose, Sucrose, or High-Fructose Corn Syrup," *The American Journal of Clinical Nutrition* 88, no. 6, http://www.ajcn.org/content/88/6/1733S.abstract (December 2008).

28. Gary Taubes, "Is Sugar Toxic?" *New York Times*, http://www.nytimes.com/2011/04/17/magazine/mag-17Sugar-t.html?pagewanted=all (April 13, 2011).

29. Luc Tappy, et al., "Metabolic Effects of Fructose and the Worldwide Increase in Obesity," *Physiological Reviews* 90, no.1 (January 2010): 23–46; M. Dirlewanger, et al., "Effects of Fructose on Hepatic Glucose Metabolism in Humans, *American Journal of Physiology - Endocrinology and Metabolism* 279 (2000): E907–E911.

30. S. S. Elliott, N. L. Keim, J. S. Stern, et al., "Fructose, Weight Gain, and the Insulin Resistance Syndrome." *The American Journal of Clinical Nutrition* 76, no. 5 (November 2002): 911–922; K. A. Lê, L. Tappy, "Metabolic Effects of Fructose," *Current Opinion in Clinical Nutrition & Metabolic Care* 9, no. 4 (2006): 469–475; Y. Rayssiguier, E. Gueux, W. Nowacki, et al., "High Fructose Consumption Combined with Low Dietary Magnesium Intake May Increase the Incidence of the Metabolic Syndrome by Inducing Inflammation," *Magnesium Research* 19, no. 4 (2006): 237–243.

31. A. C. Rutledge, K. Adeli, "Fructose and the Metabolic Syndrome: Pathophysiology and Molecular Mechanisms," *Nutrition Reviews* 65 no. 6 pt. 2, S13–S23; K. A. Lê, L. Tappy "Metabolic Effects of Fructose," *Current Opinion in Clinical Nutrition & Metabolic Care* 9, no. 4 (2006): 469–475.

32. "Fructose Metabolism by the Brain Increases Food Intake and Obesity," *Science Daily*, http://www.sciencedaily.com/releases/2009/03/090325091811.htm (March 25, 2009).

33. Ann Harding, "Diabetes Doubles Alzheimer's Risk," *CNN Health*, http://www.cnn.com/2011/09/19/health/diabetes-doubles-alzheimers/index.html (September 19, 2011); "Getting Diabetes Before 65 More than Doubles Risk for Alzheimer's Disease," *Science Daily*, http://www.sciencedaily.com/releases/2009/01/090127152835.htm (January 27, 2009).

Chapter 5: The Cholesterol Connection: Have We All Been Misled?

1. "Low-Carb Diet Reduces Inflammation and Blood Saturated Fat in Metabolic Syndrome," *Science Daily,* http://www.sciencedaily.com/releases/2007/12/071203091236.htm (December 3, 2007).

2. "Food Fried in Vegetable Oil May Contain Toxic Compound," *Bio-Medicine,* http://news.bio-medicine.org/biology-news-3/Food-fried-in-vegetable-oil-may-contain-toxic-compound-11958-1 (May 2005).

3. James H. Hays, Angela DiSabatino, et al., "Effect of a High Saturated Fat and No-Starch Diet on Serum Lipid Subfractions in Patients with Documented Atherosclerotic Cardiovascular Disease," *Mayo Clinic Proceedings* 78, no. 11 (November 2003): 1331–1336.

4. Jeff Volek and Cassandra Forsythe, "The Case for Not Restricting Saturated Fat on a Low Carbohydrate Diet," *Nutrition & Metabolism* 2 (2005): 21, http://www.pubmedcentral.nih.gov/articlerender.fcgi?artid=1208952.

5. Walter C. Willett and Alberto Ascherio, "Commentary: Trans-Fatty Acids: Are the Effects Only Marginal?" *American Journal of Public Health* 84 (1994): 722–724.

6. M. A. French, K. Sundram, and M. T. Clandinin, "Cholesterolaemic Effect of Palmitic Acid in Relation to Other Dietary Fatty Acids," *Asia Pacific Journal of Clinical Nutrition* 11 Suppl 7 (2002): S401–S407.

7. H. M. Krumholz, S. S. Seeman, et al., "Lack of Association between Cholesterol and Coronary Heart Disease Mortality and Morbidity and All-Cause Mortality in Persons Older than 70 Years," *Journal of the American Medical Association* 272, no. 17 (November 2, 1994), 1335–1340, http://jama.ama-assn.org/cgi/content/abstract/272/17/1335.

8. Chris Kresser, "Cholesterol Doesn't Cause Heart Disease" (June 10, 2008), http://chriskresser.com/cholesterol-doesnt-cause-heart-disease.

9. Michel de Lorgeril, et al., "Mediterranean Diet, Traditional Risk Factors, and the Rate of Cardiovascular Complications After Myocardial Infarction: Final Report of the Lyon Diet Heart Study," *Circulation* 99 (1999): 779–785, http://circ.ahajournals.org/cgi/content/full/99/6/779.

10. Antonio M. Gotto Jr., "Triglyceride: The Forgotten Risk Factor," *Circulation* 97, no. 11 (1998): 1027–1028.

11. J. Michael Gaziano, et al., "Fasting Triglycerides, High-Density Lipoprotein, and Risk of Myocardial Infarction," *Circulation* 96 (1997): 2520–2525.

12. J. Michael Gaziano, et al., "Fasting Triglycerides, High-Density Lipoprotein, and Risk of Myocardial Infarction," *Circulation* 96 (1997): 2520–2525.

13. Cleveland Clinic, Miller Family Heart & Vascular Institute, "Nutrition—Cholesterol Guidelines," http://my.clevelandclinic.org/heart/prevention/nutrition/atp3.aspx.

14. Stephen R. Daniels, Frank R. Greer, and the Committee on Nutrition, "Lipid Screening and Cardiovascular Health in Childhood," *Pediatrics* 122, no. 1 (July 2008): 198–208, http://aappolicy.aappublications.org/cgi/content/full/pediatrics;122/1/198 (note that the "122/1/198" at the end *is* part of the URL).

15. Walter Willett, "Got Fat? Exploding Nutrition Myths," *World Health News* (March 29, 2000), http://www.diabetesincontrol.com/results.php?storyarticle=243.

Chapter 6: The Biggest Myths about Low-Carb Diets

1. Anssi H. Manninen, "Metabolic Effects of the Very-Low-Carbohydrate Diets: Misunderstood 'Villains' of Human Metabolism," *Journal of the International Society of Sports Nutrition* 1, no. 2 (2004): 7–11, http://www.pubmedcentral.nih.gov/articlerender.fcgi?artid=2129159; Ekhard E. Ziegler and L. J. Filer (eds.), *Present Knowledge in Nutrition: Seventh Edition* (Washington, DC: ILSI Press, 1996), chapter 5: Carbohydrates (Szepesi).

2. Institute of Medicine (IOM) of the National Academies, *Dietary Reference Intakes: Energy, Carbohydrate, Fiber, Fat, Fatty Acids, Cholesterol, Protein, and Amino Acids* (Washington, DC: National Academies Press, 2002); http://books.nap.edu/openbook.php?record_id=10490&page=275.

3. "Metabolic Effects of the Very-Low-Carbohydrate Diets: Misunderstood "Villains" of Human Metabolism" Anssi H Manninen, J Int Soc Sports Nutr. 2004; 1(2): 7–11 Published online 2004 December 31. doi: 10.1186/1550–2783-1-2-7. Also available at: http://www.pubmedcentral.nih.gov/articlerender.fcgi?artid=2129159.

4. Donald Voet and Judith Voet, *Biochemistry* (New York: John Wiley and Sons, 1998).

5. Richard L. Veech, et al., "Ketone Bodies: Potential Therapeutic Uses," *IUBMB Life* 51 (2001): 241–247.

6. Matthew J. Sharman, et al., "A Ketogenic Diet Favorably Affects Serum Biomarkers for Cardiovascular Disease in Normal-Weight Men," *Journal of Nutrition* 132, no. 7 (July 2002): 1879–1885.

7. Eric C. Westman, et al., "Effect of 6-Month Adherence to a Very Low Carbohydrate Diet Program," *American Journal of Medicine* 133, no. 1 (2002): 30–36.

8. Bonnie J. Brehm, et al., "A Randomized Trial Comparing a Very Low Carbohydrate Diet and a Calorie-Restricted Low Fat Diet on Body Weight and Cardiovascular Risk Factors in Healthy Women," *Journal of Clinical Endocrinology and Metabolism* 88, no. 4 (2003): 1617–1623.

9. Marian T. Hannan, et al., "Effect of Dietary Protein on Bone Loss in Elderly Men and Women: The Framingham Osteoporosis Study," *Journal of Bone and Mineral Research* 15, no. 12 (December 2000): 2504–2512.

10. Jane E. Kerstetter, et al., "Dietary Protein, Calcium Metabolism, and Skeletal Homeostasis Revisited," *American Journal of Clinical Nutrition* 78, no. 3 (September 2003): 584S–592S; Jane E. Kerstetter, et al., "Dietary Protein Affects Intestinal Calcium Absorption," *American Journal of Clinical Nutrition* 68, no. 4 (1998): 859–865.

11. Annebeth Rosenvinge Skov, et al., "Effect of Protein Intake on Bone Mineralization During Weight Loss: A 6-Month Trial," *Obesity Research* 10 (2002): 432–438.

12. Robert P. Heaney, "Editorial: Protein and Calcium: Antagonists or Synergists?" *American Journal of Clinical Nutrition* 75, no. 4 (April 2002): 609–610.

13. Eric L. Knight, et al., "The Impact of Protein Intake on Renal Function Decline in Women with Normal Renal Function or Mild Renal Insufficiency," *Annals of Internal Medicine* 138 (2003): 460–467.

14. Thomas B. Wiegmann, et al., "Controlled Changes in Chronic Dietary Protein Intake Do Not Change Glomerular Filtration Rate," *American Journal of Kidney Diseases* 15, no. 2 (February 1990): 147–154.

15. Annebeth Rosenvinge Skov, et al., "Changes in Renal Function During Weight Loss Induced by High vs. Low-Protein Low-Fat Diets in Overweight Subjects," *International Journal of Obesity and Related Metabolic Disorders* 23, no. 11 (November 1999): 1170–1177.

16. Marjorie R. Freedman, et al., "Popular Diets: A Scientific Review," *Obesity Research* 9 suppl. (2001): 5S–17S.

17. Stephen B. Sondike, et al., "Effects of a Low-Carbohydrate Diet on Weight Loss and Cardiovascular Risk Factor in Overweight Adolescents," *Journal of Pediatrics* 142, no. 3 (March 2003): 253–258.

18. Gary D. Foster, et al., "A Randomized Trial of a Low-Carbohydrate Diet for Obesity," *New England Journal of Medicine* 348, no. 21 (May, 22 2003): 2082–2090; Frederick F. Samaha, et al., "A Low-Carbohydrate as Compared with a Low-Fat Diet in Severe Obesity," *New England Journal of Medicine* 348, no. 21 (May 22, 2003): 2074–2081.

19. Alain Golay, et al., "Weight-Loss with Low or High Carbohydrate Diet?" *International Journal of Obesity and Related Metabolic Disorders* 20, no. 12 (December 1996): 1067–1072.

20. Alain Golay, et al., "Similar Weight Loss with Low- or High-Carbohydrate Diets," *American Journal of Clinical Nutrition* 63, no. 2 (February 1996): 174–178.

21. Walter C. Willett, "Dietary Fat Plays a Major Role in Obesity: No," *Obesity Reviews* 3, no. 2 (May 2002): 59–68.

22. Walter C. Willett and Rudolph L. Leibel, "Dietary Fat Is Not a Major Determinant of Body Fat," *American Journal of Medicine* 113, suppl. 9B (30 December 30, 2002): 47S–59S.

23. Jackie L. Boucher, et al., "Weight Loss, Diets, and Supplements: Does Anything Work?" *Diabetes Spectrum* 14, no. 3 (August 2001): 169–75.

24. Ibid.

25. John S. Yudkin, "Diet and Coronary Thrombosis: Hypothesis and Fact," *Lancet* 2 (1957): 155–162.

26. Uffe Ravnskov, *The Cholesterol Myths* (Washington, DC: New Trends, 2000).

27. Malcolm Kendrick, "Why the Cholesterol-Heart Disease Theory Is Wrong," http://www.thincs.org/Malcolm.choltheory.htm (July 31, 2012).

28. Ancel Keys, "Letter: Normal Plasma Cholesterol in a Man Who Eats 25 Eggs a Day," *New England Journal of Medicine* 325, no. 8 (August 22, 1991): 584.

29. Eugene Braunwald, "Shattuck Lecture: Cardiovascular Medicine at the Turn of the Millennium: Triumphs, Concerns, and Opportunities," *New England Journal of Medicine* 337, no. 19 (November 6, 1997): 1360–1369.

30. Ian A. Prior, et al., "Cholesterol, Coconuts, and Diet on Polynesian Atolls: A Natural Experiment: The Pukapuka and Tokelau Island Studies," *American Journal of Clinical Nutrition* 34, no. 8 (August 1981): 1552–1561.

31. Alberto Ascherio and Walter C. Willett, "Health Effects of Trans Fatty Acids," *American Journal of Clinical Nutrition* 66, suppl. 4 (October 1997): 1006S–1010S.

32. Mary G. Enig, *Know Your Fats: The Complete Primer for Understanding the Nutrition of Fats, Oils and Cholesterol* (Brookhaven, PA: Bethesda Press, 2000).

33. Ibid.

34. Gary Taubes, "The Soft Science of Dietary Fat," *Science* 291 (March 30, 2001): 2536.

35. Darlene M. Dreon, et al., "A Very-Low-Fat Diet Is Not Associated with Improved Lipoprotein Profiles in Men with a Predominance of Large, Low-Density

Lipoproteins," *American Journal of Clinical Nutrition* 69, no. 3 (March 1999): 411–418.

36. J. Michael Gaziano, "Fasting Triglycerides, High-Density Lipoprotein, and Risk of Myocardial Infarction," *Circulation* 96 (1997): 2520–2525.

37. Dean Ornish, et al., "Intensive Lifestyle Changes for Reversal of Coronary Heart Disease," *Journal of the American Medical Association* 280, no. 23 (December 16, 1998): 2001–2007.

38. Alberto Ascherio and Walter C. Willett, "Health Effects of Trans Fatty Acids," *American Journal of Clinical Nutrition* 66, suppl. 4 (October 1997): 1006S–1010S.

39. Alberto Ascherio, et al., "Dietary Fat and Risk of Coronary Heart Disease in Men: Cohort Follow Up Study in the United States," *British Medical Journal* 313 (July 13, 1996): 84–90.

40. Alain Golay, et al., "Weight-Loss with Low or High Carbohydrate Diet?" *International Journal of Obesity and Related Metabolic Disorders* 20, no. 12 (December 1996): 1067–1072.

Chapter 7: But What about the China Study?

1. T. C. Campbell, B. Parpia, and J. Chen. "Diet, Lifestyle, and the Etiology of Coronary Artery Disease: The Cornell China Study." *American Journal of Cardiology* 82, no. 10B (November 26, 1998): 18T–21T.

2. Junshi C et al. *Diet, Life-style and Mortality in China*, p. 608; J. V. Pottala, et al., "Blood Eicosapentaenoic and Docosahexaenoic Acids Predict All-Cause Mortality in Patients with Stable Coronary Heart Disease: The Heart and Soul Study." *Circulation: Cardiovascular Quality and Outcomes* 3, no. 4 (July 2010): 406–412; A. Manerba, et al., "N-3 PUFAs and Cardiovascular Disease Prevention." *Future Cardiology* 6, no. 3 (May 2010): 343–350; Y. Wang, et al., "Fish Consumption, Blood Docosahexaenoic Acid and Chronic Diseases in Chinese Rural Populations." *Comparative Biochemistry and Physiology Part A: Molecular and Integrative Physiology* 136, no. 1 (September 2003): 127–140.

3. Braly, James, MD, and Ron Hoggan, MA, *Dangerous Grains*, (New York: Penguin Putnam, 2002): 124.

4. T. Colin Campbell, et al., *The China Study* (New York: BenBella, 2004), 7.

5. R. Hakkak, et al., "Dietary Whey Protein Protects against Azoxymethane-Induced Colon Tumors in Male Rats," *Cancer Epidemiology Biomarkers & Prevention* 10, no. 5 (May 2001): 555–558.

6. T. C. Campbell, et al., "Effect of Dietary Intake of Fish Oil and Fish Protein on the Development of L-azaserine-Induced Preneoplastic Lesions in the Rat Pancreas." *Journal of the National Cancer Institute* 75, no. 5 (November 1985).

7. Ibid.

8. "Geographic Study of Mortality, Biochemistry, and Diet in Rural China," http://www.ctsu.ox.ac.uk/~china/monograph (June 6, 2012).

9. Denise Minger, "Heart Disease and the China Study, Post #1.5," *Raw Food SOS*, http://rawfoodsos.com/2010/10/09/heart-disease-and-the-china-study-post-1-5 (June 6, 2012).

10. Denise Minger, "The China Study: Fact or Fallacy?" *Raw Food SOS*, http://rawfoodsos.com/2010/07/07/the-china-study-fact-or-fallac (June 6, 2012).

11. "Reply to T. C. Campbell," *The American Journal of Clinical Nutrition* 71, no. 3, http://www.ajcn.org/content/71/3/850.full (March 2000).

12. Susan Lang, "Eating Less Meat May Help Reduce Osteoporosis Risk, Studies Show," *Cornell Chronicle,* http://www.news.cornell.edu/chronicle/96/11.14.96/osteoporosis.html (June 6, 2012).

13. T. C. Campbell, et al., "Dietary Calcium and Bone Density among Middle-Aged and Elderly Women in China," *The American Journal of Clinical Nutrition* 58, no. 2 http://www.ajcn.org/content/58/2/219.full.pdf+html (August 1993).

14. Ibid.

15. Ronald G. Munger, et al., "Prospective Study of Dietary Protein Intake and Risk of Hip Fracture in Postmenopausal Women," *The American Journal of Clinical Nutrition* 69, no. 1, http://www.ajcn.org/content/69/1/147.full (January 1999).

16. Marian T. Hannan, et al., "Effect of Dietary Protein on Bone Loss in Elderly Men and Women," *Journal of Bone and Mineral Research* 15, no. 12, http://onlinelibrary.wiley.com/doi/10.1359/jbmr.2000.15.12.2504/full (December 2000).

17. Joanne H. E. Promislow, et al., "Protein Consumption and Bone Mineral Density in the Elderly: The Rancho Bernardo Study," *American Journal of Epidemiology* 155, no. 7 http://aje.oxfordjournals.org/content/155/7/636.full (2002).

18. Zamzam K. (Fariba) Roughead, et al., "Controlled High Meat Diets Do Not Affect Calcium Retention or Indices of Bone Status in Healthy Postmenopausal Women," *The Journal of Nutrition* 133, no. 4, http://jn.nutrition.org/content/133/4/1020.full (April 1, 2003).

19. Robert P. Heaney, "Protein Intake and Bone Health," *The American Journal of Clinical Information* 73, no. 1, http://www.ajcn.org/content/73/1/5.full?ijkey=4cb6e2c476005c7b83fa6ad532f803db8a3b65ec&keytype2=tf_ipsecsha (January 2001).

20. M. Delmi, et al., "Dietary Supplementation in Elderly Patients with Fractured Neck of the Femur," *Lancet* 355 (1990): 1013–1016; M. D. Bastow, J. Rawlings, S. P. Allison. "Benefits of Supplementary Tube Feeding After Fractured Neck of Femur." *British Medical Journal* 287 (1983): 1589–1592.

21. M. A. Schürch, et al., "Protein Supplements Increase Serum Insulin-like Growth Factor-I Levels and Attenuate Proximal Femur Bone Loss in Patients with Recent Hip Fracture. *Annals of Internal Medicine* 128 (1998): 801–809; J. P. Bonjour, et al., "Nutritional Aspects of Hip Fractures," *Bone* 18 (1996): 139S–44S.

22. Robert P. Heaney, "Protein Intake and Bone Health," *The American Journal of Clinical Nutrition* 73, no. 1 (2001): 5–6.

23. Robert P. Heaney, "Protein Intake and Bone Health," *The American Journal of Clinical Nutrition* 73, no. 1 (2001): 5–6.

24. Campbell, *The China Study* (New York: BenBella, 2004), 220.

25. National Agricultural Library, *The USDA National Nutrient Database,* http://ndb.nal.usda.gov (June 6, 2012).

26. W. X. Fan, et al., "Erythrocyte Fatty Acids, Plasma Lipids, and Cardiovascular Disease in Rural China," *The American Journal of Clinical Nutrition* 52, no. 6 (December 1990): 1027–1036.

27. Ibid.

Chapter 8: My Big Fat Diet: The Town That Lost 1,200 Pounds

1. Mary Bissell, *My Big Fat Diet* (documentary film), http://www.mybigfatdiet.net.

2. Cassandra E. Forsythe, Stephen D. Phinney, et al., "Comparison of Low Fat and Low Carbohydrate Diets on Circulating Fatty Acid Composition and Markers of Inflammation", *Lipids* 43, no. 1 (January 2008): 65–77.
3. "Low-Carb Diet Reduces Inflammation and Blood Saturated Fat in Metabolic Syndrome," *Science Daily,* http://www.sciencedaily.com/releases/2007/12/071203091236.htm (December 4, 2007).
4. Stuart G. Jarrett, Julie B. Milder, et al., "The Ketogenic Diet Increases Mitochondrial Glutathione Levels," *Journal of Neurochemistry* 106, no. 3, (August 2008): 1044–1051.

Chapter 9: Twenty-three Modern Low-Carb Diets and What They Can Do for You

1. Marjorie R. Freedman, et al., "Popular Diets: A Scientific Review," *Obesity Research* 9 suppl. (2001): 5S–17S.
2. Kathleen DesMaisons, personal communication with author, August 2003.
3. Beatrice A. Golomb, et al., "Insulin Sensitivity Markers: Predictors of Accidents and Suicides in Helsinki Heart Study Screenees," *Journal of Clinical Epidemiology* 55, no. 8 (August 2002): 767–773.
4. Calvin Ezrin, with Kristen L. Caron, *Your Fat Can Make You Thin* (Lincolnwood, IL: Contemporary Books, 2001).
5. David Leonardi, personal communication with author, August 2003; Richard K. Bernstein, *The Diabetes Solution* (New York: Little, Brown, 1997), 43.
6. Loren Cordain, "Cereal Grains: Humanity's Double-Edged Sword," *World Review of Nutrition and Dietetics* 84 (1999): 19–73.

Chapter 10: Frequently Asked Questions

1. "Health and Medicine," *U.S. News & World Report* (July 14, 2003).
2. Ibid.
3. Ibid.
4. Calvin Ezrin, with Kristen L. Caron, *Your Fat Can Make You Thin* (Lincolnwood, IL: Contemporary Books, 2001).
5. Ellen Ruppel Shell, *The Hungry Gene: The Science of Fat and the Future of Thin* (New York: Atlantic Monthly Press, 2002).
6. *Natural Medicines Comprehensive Database, Monograph: Bitter Orange* (Stockton, CA: Therapeutic Research, 2003).
7. M. Blumenthal, et al., *Herbal Medicine Expanded Commission E Monographs* (Atlanta: Integrative Medicine Communications, 2000).
8. Gioacchino Calapai, et al., "Antiobesity and Cardiovascular Toxic Effects of *Citrus aurantium* Extracts in the Rat: A Preliminary Report," *Fitoterapia* 70, no. 6 (December 1, 1999): 586–592.
9. *Natural Medicines Comprehensive Database, Patient Handout: Bitter Orange* (Stockton, CA: Therapeutic Research, 2003).
10. Joanne Carroll and Dorcas Koenigsberger, "The Ketogenic Diet: A Practical Guide for Caregivers," *Journal of the American Dietetic Association* 98, no. 3 (March 1998): 316–321.

11. Lyle McDonald, *The Ketogenic Diet*, (http://www.theketogenicdiet.com, 1998).

12. Jenkins, et al., "The Effect of a Plant-Based Low-Carbohydrate ("Eco-Atkins") Diet on Body Weight and Blood Lipid Concentrations in Hyperlipidemic Subjects," *Archives of Internal Medicine* 169, no. 11 (2009): 1046-1054.

13. Donald S. Robertson, *The Snowbird Diet* (New York: Warner Books, 1986).

14. Mary Enig, "Letter to Dr. Mercola," http://www.mercola.com (January 16, 2000).

15. S. Sadeghi, et al., "Dietary Lipids Modify the Cytokine Response to Bacterial Lipopolysaccharide in Mice," *Immunology* 96, no. 3 (March 1999): 404–410.

16. Mary Enig, *Indian Coconut Journal* (September 1995).

17. Ian A. Prior, et al., "Cholesterol, Coconuts, and Diet on Polynesian Atolls: A Natural Experiment," *American Journal of Clinical Nutrition* 34, no. 8 (August 1981): 1552–1561.

18. Mary Enig, "Coconut: In Support of Good Health in the 21st Century," http://coconutoil.com/coconut_oil_21st_century.

19. Mary Enig, *Know Your Fats: The Complete Primer for Understanding the Nutrition of Fats, Oils and Cholesterol* (Silver Spring, MD: Bethesda Press, 2000).

20. Kathleen DesMaisons, *The Sugar Addict's Total Recovery Program* (New York: Ballantine, 2000).

21. Kathleen DesMaisons, *Your Last Diet* (New York: Ballantine, 2001).

22. Jennie Brand-Miller, et al., *The New Glucose Revolution* (New York: Marlowe, 2002).

23. Joseph Mercola, *The No-Grain Diet* (New York: Dutton, 2003).

24. John Hernandez, "Weight Loss Protocols," lecture given at Boulderfest Nutrition Conference, Boulder, CO, 2000.

25. Gerben B. Keijzers, et al., "Caffeine Can Decrease Insulin Sensitivity in Humans," *Diabetes Care* 25, no. 2 (February 2002): 364–369; M. Sachs, et al., "Effect of Caffeine on Various Metabolic Parameters In Vivo," *Zeitschrift für Ernahrungswissenschaft* 23, 23, no. 3 (September 1984): 181–205.

26. Terry E. Grahm, et al., "Caffeine Ingestion Elevates Plasma Insulin Response in Humans During an Oral Glucose Tolerance Test," *Canadian Journal of Physiology and Pharmacology* 79, no. 7 (July 2001): 559–565.

27. S.P. Tofovic, et al., "Renal and Metabolic Effects of Caffeine in Obese (fa/fa(cp)) Diabetic, Hypertensive ZSF1 Rats," *Renal Failure* 23, no. 2 (March 2001): 159–173.

28. Koutarou Muroyama, et al., "Anti-Obesity Effects of a Mixture of Thiamin, Arginine, Caffeine and Citric Acid in Non-Insulin Dependent Diabetic KK Mice," *Journal of Nutritional Science and Vitaminology* 49, no. 1 (February 2003): 56–63.

29. A. Pizziol, et al., "Effects of Caffeine on Glucose Tolerance: A Placebo-Controlled Study," *European Journal of Clinical Nutrition* 52, no. 11 (November 1998): 846–849.

30. Rob M. van Dam, et al., "Coffee Consumption and Risk of Type 2 Diabetes Mellitus," *Lancet* 360 (November 9, 2002): 1477–1478.

31. L. Tllefson, et al., "An Analysis of FDA Passive Surveillance Reports of Seizures Associated with Consumption of Aspartame," *Journal of the American Dietetic Association* 92, no. 5 (May 1992): 598–601.

32. Russell L. Blaylock, *Excitotoxins: The Taste That Kills* (Albuquerque, NM: Health Press, 1996).

33. David Voreacos, "Experts Tell Panel of Continued Concern over Use of Aspartame," *Los Angeles Times*, November 4, 1987, p. 19.

34. Kathleen DesMaisons, *The Sugar Addict's Total Recovery Program* (New York: Ballantine, 2000).

35. Sharon S. Elliott, et al., "Fructose, Weight Gain, and the Insulin Resistance Syndrome," *American Journal of Clinical Nutrition* 76, no. 5 (November 2002): 911–922.

36. M. Dirlewanger, et al., "Effects of Fructose on Hepatic Glucose Metabolism in Humans," *American Journal of Physiology, Endocrinology and Metabolism* 279, no. 4 (October 2000): E907–E911.

37. Elson Haas, *The False Fat Diet* (New York: Ballantine Books, 2000).

38. L. H. Leung, "Pantothenic Acid as a Weight-Reducing Agent: Fasting Without Hunger, Weakness and Ketosis," *Medical Hypotheses* 44, no. 5 (May 1995): 403–405.

39. Alan Kekwick and Gaston L.S. Pawan, "Metabolic Study in Human Obesity with Isocaloric Diets High in Fat, Protein or Carbohydrate," *Metabolism* 6, no. 5 (1957): 447–460.

Chapter 11: Tricks of the Trade: The Top 50+ Tips for Making Low-Carb Work for You

1. C.D. Summerbell, et al., "Relationship Between Feeding Pattern and Body Mass Index in 220 Free-Living People in Four Age Groups," *European Journal of Clinical Nutrition* 50 (August 1996): 513–519; R. M. Ortega, et al., "Differences in the Breakfast Habits of Overweight/Obese and Normal Weight Schoolchildren," *International Journal for Vitamin and Nutrition Research* 68, no. 2 (1998): 125–132; R. M. Ortega, et al., "Associations Between Obesity, Breakfast-Time Food Habits, and Intake of Energy and Nutrients in a Group of Elderly Madrid Residents," *Journal of the American College of Nutrition* 15, no. 1 (February 1996): 65–72.

2. F. Halberg, "Chronobiology and Nutrition," *Contemporary Nutrition* 8, no. 9 (1983): 2 pages (unpaginated).

3. Donald K. Layman, et al., "A Reduced Ratio of Dietary Carbohydrate to Protein Improves Body Composition and Blood Lipid Profiles during Weight Loss in Adult Women," *Journal of Nutrition* 133, no. 2 (February 2003): 411–417.

4. Donald K. Layman, et al., "Increased Dietary Protein Modifies Glucose and Insulin Homeostasis in Adult Women During Weight Loss," *Journal of Nutrition* 133, no. 2 (February 2003): 405–410.

5. Donald K. Layman, "The Role of Leucine in Weight Loss Diets and Glucose Homeostasis," *Journal of Nutrition* 133, no. 1 (January 2003): 261S–267S.

6. Joseph Mercola, *The No-Grain Diet* (New York: Dutton, 2003).

7. B. K. Hope, et al., "An Overview of the *Salmonella enteritidis* Risk Assessment for Shell Eggs and Egg Products," *Risk Analysis* 22, no. 2 (April 2002): 203–218.

8. Joseph Mercola, "Raw Eggs for Your Health—Major Update," http://www.mercola.com/2002/nov/13/eggs.htm.

9. B. K. Hope, et al., "An Overview of the *Salmonella enteritidis* Risk Assessment for Shell Eggs and Egg Products," *Risk Analysis* 22, no. 2 (April 2002): 203–218.

10. Larry A. Tucker and Marilyn Bagwell, "Television Viewing and Obesity in Adult Females," *American Journal of Public Health* 81 (1991): 908–911.

11. W. H. Dietz, Jr., and S. L. Gortmaker, "Do We Fatten Our Children at the Television Set?" *Pediatrics* 75 (1985): 807–812.

12. Michael Murray, et al., *Encyclopedia of Natural Medicine*, 2nd ed. (Rocklin, CA: Prima Health, 1998): 681.

Index